Current Topics in Pathology

74

Editors

C.L. Berry E. Grundmann W.H. Kirsten

Dermatopathology

Contributors

S.M. Burge · A.C. Chu · B.M. Goudie · R.B. Goudie
A.S. Jack · T.J. Ryan · W. Sterry · D. Weedon · N.A. Wright

Editor

Colin Leonard Berry

With 94 Figures

Springer-Verlag
Berlin Heidelberg NewYork Tokyo 1985

C.L. BERRY, Professor Dr., Department of Morbid Anatomy. The London Hospital Medical College, GB-London E1 1BB

E. GRUNDMANN, Professor Dr., Gerhard-Domagk-Institut für Pathologie der Universität, Domagkstraße 17, D-4400 Münster/Westfalen

W.H. KIRSTEN, Professor Dr., Department of Pathology, The University of Chicago, 950 East 59th Street, Chicago, IL 60637, USA

Library of Congress Cataloging in Publication Data. Main entry under title: Dermatopathology. (Current topics in pathology; 74) Includes bibliographies and index. 1. Skin—Diseases. I. Burge, S.M. (Susan M.) II. Berry, Colin Leonard, 1937– . III. Series: Current topics in pathology; v. 74. [DNLM: 1. Skin Diseases—pathology. W1 CU821H v. 74 / WR 105 D435] RB1-E6 vol. 74 616.07 s 84–25472 [RL95] [616.5]
ISBN-13: 978-3-642-69576-6 e-ISBN-13: 978-3-642-69574-2
DOI: 10.1007/ 978-3-642-69574-2

Typesetting: Universitätsdruckerei H. Stürtz AG, D-8700 Würzburg
2122/3130-543210

List of Contributors

BURGE, Dr. SUSAN M.	Department of Dermatology, The Slade Hospital, Oxfordshire Health Authority, Headington, Oxford OX3 7JH, Great Britain
CHU, Dr. A.C.	Unit of Dermatology, Royal Postgraduate Medical School, Hammersmith Hospital Ducane Road, London, W12, Great Britain
GOUDIE, Dr. B.M.	Department of Pathology, Royal Infirmary University of Glasgow, Glasgow G4 OSF, Great Britain
GOUDIE, Prof. Dr. R.B.	Department of Pathology, Royal Infirmary University of Glasgow, Glasgow G4 OSF, Great Britain
JACK, Dr. A.S.	Department of Pathology, Royal Infirmary University of Glasgow, Glasgow G4 OSF, Great Britain
RYAN, Dr. T.J.	Department of Dermatology, The Slade Hospital, Oxfordshire Health Authority, Headington, Oxford OX3 7JH, Great Britain
STERRY, Priv.-Doz. Dr. med. W.	Abteilung Dermatologie und Venerologie, Klinikum der Christian-Albrechts-Universität Kiel, Schittenhelmstraße 7, D-2300 Kiel
WEEDON, Prof. Dr. D.	Department of Pathology, Princess Alexandra Hospital, The University of Queensland, Brisbane 4102, Australia
WRIGHT, Prof. Dr. N.A.	Department of Histopathology, Hammersmith Hospital, Royal Postgraduate Medical School, University of London, Ducane Road, London W12 OHS, Great Britain

Preface

In any histopathology department, cutaneous biopsies form the major part of the workload. In many instances these may be readily dealt with by experienced pathologists and their documentation represents an essential step in organising therapy. However, in a number of areas dramatic changes have occurred in dermatopathology. The rapidly changing incidence of pigmented lesions of the skin and the availability of diagnostic cell markers in the complex cutaneous lymphomas have meant that for many pathologists a review in these fields will be valuable. The distribution and pattern of skin pigmentation may allow us to make important assertions and draw important conclusions about the genetics of skin disease, but also about human variability. Cutaneous vasculitis is a difficult problem where clinicopathological consultation is vital in diagnosis and the review presented has been written with this very much in mind. In the same way, many diagnostic difficulties exist in assessing buttous lesions in the skin and for this reason a review was invited.

Finally, our understanding of certain skin diseases has been radically altered by knowledge of the dynamics of the changes seen, a field which has also been studied with advantage in other systems in pathology.

This volume is intended as an aide to those many pathologists and dermatologists who, often together, are responsible for the provision of clinical care in this demanding field.

London C.L. Berry

Contents

Indexed in ISR

Melanoma and Other Melanocytic Skin Lesions

D. WEEDON

Introduction

The literature on malignant melanoma and other melanocytic skin lesions has expanded greatly in recent years making it difficult for the average clinician and pathologist to keep abreast of the recent trends. The introduction of new statistical techniques such as multiple regression analyses and the Cox proportional hazards model has provided new insights into the important prognostic variables in melanoma. Furthermore, several new concepts such as the dysplastic naevus syndrome and minimal deviation melanoma have emerged in recent years which have profound significance on the interpretation of some melanocytic lesions. It therefore seems timely to review this subject, with an emphasis on those aspects which have been published in recent years, or which are neglected in standard textbooks of dermatopathology.

1. Lesions with Basal Hyperpigmentation

Increased melanin can be found in the basal layer in many different circumstances. These include racial pigmentation, chloasma of pregnancy, in a freckle, associated with heavy metal pigmentation, certain endocrine disturbances, Albright's syndrome, Peutz Jegher's syndrome, urticaria pigmentosa, acromelanosis and the various punctate and reticulate hyperpigmentation syndromes. These have recently been reviewed (FULK 1984), and it is not proposed to discuss this group further.

2. Lesions with Basal Melanocyte Proliferation

2.1 Lentigo Simplex

Simple lentigos are small, usually uniformly pigmented macules without predilection for sun-exposed areas. Multiple lentigines may be unilateral in distribution (THOMPSON & DIEHL 1980) or generalized, the latter form sometimes being a marker of underlying developmental defects. These syndromes which include the Leopard syndrome have recently been reviewed, and will not be considered further (FULK 1984). Atrial myxoma has also been reported in association with lentigines (PETERSON & SERRILL 1984).

On histological examination, a lentigo shows basal hyperpigmentation with an increased number of single melanocytes within the basal layer. There is usually epidermal hyperplasia with regular elongation of the rete ridges. There is often a sparse lymphohistiocytic infiltrate in the papillary dermis, including scattered melanophages. Some lesions form junctional nests and evolve into lentiginous naevi (ACKERMAN & RAGAZ 1984). These lesions are discussed in Section 2.5.

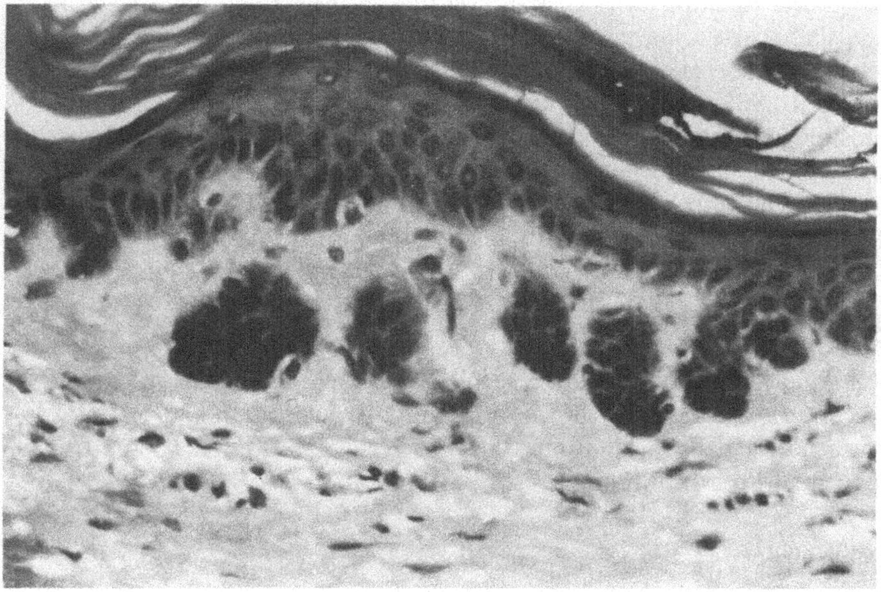

Fig. 1. Solar lentigo. There is bulbous expansion of the rete ridges

2.2 Solar Lentigo

Solar (senile) lentigos are light to dark brown macules, usually 5–15 mm in diameter which develop on the sun-damaged skin of elderly patients. They are often multiple. They may increase in size slowly over many years. Ackerman & Ragaz (1984) believe that patches of solar lentigo evolve into reticulated seborrhoeic keratoses.

On histological examination, there is elongation of the rete ridges, some of which are short and bulb-like, while others have finger-like rete ridges connecting with adjacent rete to form a reticular framework (Fig. 1). These latter lesions resemble so-called seborrhoeic keratoses of reticulate type. There is basal hyperpigmentation, usually some melanophages in the papillary dermis, and often solar elastosis. There is an increase in melanocytes, particularly at the bases of the clubbed and budding rete ridges (Montagna et al. 1980), although sometimes the increase is not noticed on casual examination of a slide. On electron microscopy, the melanosome complexes inside the keratinocytes are much larger than those found in non-involved skin (Montagna et al. 1980).

2.3 Becker's Melanosis

Becker's melanosis, also known as Becker's naevus is usually found in the region of the shoulder girdle of young men as unilateral, hyperpigmented, irregular areas. Hypertrichosis develops after the pigmentation. Recently, lesional tissue has been found to show an increased level of androgen receptors, suggesting that exquisite local androgen sensitivity may explain the clinical manifestations (PERSON & LONGCOPE 1984). There may be associated structural abnormalities (GLINICK et al. 1983).

On histological examination there may be slight acanthosis, with basal hyperpigmentation and some melanin incontinence. Melanocyte proliferation is mild and not always obvious. Hair follicles may be enlarged and there may be smooth muscle hyperplasia or hamartomas in the dermis.

2.4 Café au Lait Spots

In routine H and E sections, no increase in basal melanocytes can be recognized, although an increase has been shown by quantitative studies. In DOPA-stained epidermal sheets, giant melanosomes may be seen in café-au-lait spots from many patients with neurofibromatosis.

2.5 Lentiginous Naevus

This is a neglected entity which is usually grouped with lentigo simplex. It has also been called naevoid lentigo and naevus incipiens (STEWART et al. 1978). It appears to represent the progression of a lentigo into a junctional and then a compound naevus (ACKERMAN & RAGAZ 1984). They usually present clinically as deeply pigmented lesions on the trunk of adults between the ages of 20 and 40 years. Because of their deep pigmentation they often cause undue worry when found on medical practitioners and their relatives, and they are therefore removed. Their small size and regular margin contrast with that of malignant melanoma.

At the advancing edge there is a lentiginous proliferation of melanocytes, usually associated with some elongation of the rete. In the central area of the lesion there is junctional nest formation, and in some lesions intradermal nests are also present. There are usually melanin-containing macrophages in the dermis. They should not be confused with dysplastic naevi on histological examination. Similar lesions were reported recently by ENG (1983) as small junctional naevi.

2.6 Speckled Lentiginous Naevus

Speckled lentiginous naevus (STEWART et al. 1978) is the preferred term for a lesion composed of small dark hyperpigmented speckles, superimposed on a tan-brown macular background. They often have a zosteriform distribution (MATSUDO et al. 1973; SIMÕES 1981). They may be present at birth or appear in childhood.

On histological examination, the background pigmented area resembles lentigo simplex, while the speckled areas show the features of a lentiginous naevus with lentigo-like areas progressing to junctional and compound naevi (STEWART et al. 1978).

Similar cases have been reported under the term naevus spilus (ITO & HAMADA 1952; COHEN et al. 1970), but this name should be used in its original sense for a large light to dark brown plaque showing mild epidermal thickening and basal hyperpigmentation, without an increase in basal melanocytes or naevus-cell nest formation (STEWART et al. 1978).

The term zosteriform lentiginous naevus has also been used in a confusing way. It has been used synonymously with speckled lentiginous naevus (MATSUDO et al. 1973) and for lesions without a background macular pigmentation (PORT et al. 1978). These latter lesions are really clusters of lentiginous naevi, in a zosteriform distribution (RUTH et al. 1980). The term spotted grouped pigmented naevus has been used by the Japanese for lesions which are similar to the speckled lentiginous naevus and which have been present since birth. They have shown greater maturation on histological examination, with well-formed intradermal naevi often present (MORISHIMA et al. 1976; SATO et al. 1979). They included in this group lesions in which the naevus cell proliferation was localized around eccrine ducts and which were first described by MISHIMA (1973) as eccrine-centred naevi.

Finally, this entity of speckled lentiginous naevus should not be confused with cases of regional or segmental lentigines, which have recently been referred to as lentiginous mosaicism (FULK 1984).

2.7 PUVA Lentigo

Freckles (BLEEHEN 1978), and lentigines (FARBER et al. 1983; RHODES et al. 1983c) have been reported in patients treated with psoralens and ultraviolet A (PUVA), particularly in sun-protected sites. Some lesions are characterized by a lentiginous proliferation of relatively large, sometimes cytologically atypical melanocytes (RHODES et al. 1984). PUVA lentigines were found on the buttocks of 53% of psoriatic patients treated with PUVA in one series (RHODES et al. 1983c). Also of interest, is the development of melanoma in situ in two patients treated with PUVA (MARX et al. 1983).

3. Melanocytic Naevi

Descriptions of the histological features of junctional, compound and intradermal naevi can be found in standard textbooks of pathology, and will not be discussed in this review. Brief mention is made for completeness only. Interesting secondary changes are sometimes seen in naevi, and these will be considered in section 3.3.2. The following brief descriptions apply to acquired naevi. Congenital naevi will be considered in section 3.7.

3.1 Junctional Naevi

Junctional naevi are characterized by the presence of nests of naevus cells at the dermo-epidermal junction. These sometimes bulge into the underlying dermis. There is often some epidermal acanthosis and even bulbous epidermal rete ridges in some lesions. The small active junctional naevi reported recently by ENG (1983) in adolescents have some resemblance to the lesions described elsewhere in this review as lentiginous naevi.

3.2 Compound Naevi

Compound naevi have both junctional nests and an intradermal component of naevus cells. Whereas cells in the upper dermis are usually cuboidal with cytoplasmic melanin granules, deeper cells are usually smaller and contain less melanin. The cells usually lie in nests. The overlying epidermis may be flat, show some acanthosis, or have a seborrhoeic-keratosis like configuration (BENTLEY-PHILLIPS & MARKS 1976).

3.3 Intradermal Naevi

Intradermal naevi are dome-shaped, nodular or polypoid lesions which are lightly pigmented or flesh-coloured. On microscopic examination, naevus cells are confined to the dermis where they are arranged in nests and cords. Multinucleated naevus cells are often seen. The overlying epidermis may show any of the changes listed for compound naevi. In the deeper parts of the tumour the naevus cells may assume a neuroid appearance, with spindle-shaped cells and structures resembling Meissner's tactile bodies. These age-related changes are discussed further in the following section.

3.3.1 Age-related Changes

With advancing age, there is a progressive decrease in the number of naevi in a person. The average number of naevi in young adults is from 15 to 40, but this decreases markedly over the age of 50 years (STEGMAIER & BECKER 1960; NICHOLLS 1973).

MAIZE and FOSTER (1979) have reviewed the changes that occur in naevocellular naevi with increasing age of the patient. They found decreased junctional proliferation and total cellularity with age and replacement of naevus cells within the dermis by collagen, fat, elastin and ground substance. There was no tendency for naevi to assume a polypoid configuration, which would argue against the hypothesis that naevi transform into tags, which eventually fall off (STEGMAIER 1959). They concluded that the formation of cylindrical neuroid structures represented the end stage of differentiation of naevus cells (MAIZE & FOSTER 1979).

3.3.2 Secondary Changes in Naevi

Several interesting secondary changes can be found in naevocellular naevi. These were considered in some detail in my review article published in 1982, and they will be considered here only briefly, for completeness (WEEDON 1982a).

Amyloid. Small deposits of amyloid are a rare incidental finding in the upper dermis (MacDonald & Black 1980).
Bone. Naevi containing spicules of bone are called osteonaevi of Nanta (Burgdorf & Nasemann 1977). These naevi are usually found on the face (Rupec & Huck 1976). The metaplastic bone formation may follow infection or trauma. Bone has also been reported in blue naevi (Baran & Civatte 1960) and Spitz naevi (Civatte et al. 1972; Pacot et al. 1972).
Eczematous change. This refers to the presence of a subacute spongiotic change involving the epidermis overlying and adjacent to a naevus (Weedon & Farnsworth 1984). There is an underlying superficial perivascular inflammatory infiltrate, but there is no evidence of regression of the lesion. Clinically, an eczematous halo develops around one or more pigmented naevi. This clears over a period of three to ten months. The aetiology of this secondary change is unknown (Meyerson 1971; Krivanek et al. 1977).
Elastosis. Coarse fibres, with the features of solar elastosis can sometimes be seen in naevi removed from sun-damaged skin (Weedon 1982a). Elastic fibre hyperplasia may also be found in naevi (Mehregan & Staricco 1962).
Folliculitis and cysts. Cystic dilatation of a hair follicle (Haber 1952), folliculitis (Canizares 1968), abscess formation in the dermis (Saunders 1957) or epidermal cyst formation (Freeman & Knox 1962) may be found as a secondary change towards the deep edge of a naevus. These changes may produce sudden enlargement, irritation or focal colour change in a naevus. Rupture of an inflamed follicle or associated epidermal cyst usually produces a focal foreign body giant cell reaction.
Artifacts. The injection of local anaesthetic into a naevus will result in the separation of naevus cells into parallel rows (Sagebiel 1972). The formation of clefts and spaces resembling vascular or lymphatic spaces, associated with shrinkage and separation of naevus cells has been regarded as a processing artifact (Sagebiel 1972). However the author has seen a case with abundant mucopolysaccharide within these pseudoangiomatous spaces, suggesting that the change, at least in some cases, may not be an artifact.
Cockarde Naevus. This term has been applied to naevi which develop a peripheral pigmented halo with an intervening narrow zone that is non-pigmented (Mehregan & King 1972; Happle 1974; Warin 1976; James & Wells 1980). The central naevus is of compound or junctional type, while the peripheral halo is usually composed of junctional nests. The intervening non-pigmented zone is usually devoid of naevus cells.
Associated other tumours. Naevocellular naevi have been found in association with trichoepitheliomas (Rahbari & Mehregan 1975), syringomas (Schellander et al. 1974), basal cell carcinomas (Sigal & Sanders 1967), abortive hair follicle formation (Mehregan & Coskey 1972) and sweat duct proliferation (unpublished observations). Naevi have also been described in which the naevus cell proliferation was closely related to eccrine sweat ducts (Mishima 1973; Morishima et al. 1976).
Pseudomelanoma change and activation of naevi. The term 'pseudomelanoma' was coined by Kornberg and Ackerman (1975) for the worrisome changes seen in recurrent naevi, following their partial surgical removal by ablation.

These recurrent naevi have sharp circumscription of epidermal melanocytes with no lateral extension. There is some upward epidermal spread. The atypical melanocytes are confined to the epidermis, while there are mature naevus cells often seen in the dermal component. There is usually fibrosis in the papillary dermis, resulting from the previous procedure.

During pregnancy, naevocellular naevi may become 'reactivated' with the formation of renewed junctional activity (WEEDON 1982a). Similar changes have been described in naevi removed from patients with a malignant melanoma (TUCKER et al. 1980) but these changes were described before the recognition of sporadic cases of the dysplastic naevus syndrome. The changes described include marked junctional activity with lack of lateral margination, inflammation in the upper dermis, increased pigment formation and some mitotic figures (TUCKER et al. 1980).

Other changes. Other very rare changes reported include the presence of psammoma bodies (WEITZNER 1968), the development of alopecia around naevi in the scalp (YESUDIAN & THAMBIAH 1976) and the presence of focal acantholytic dyskeratosis in the adjacent epidermis (WEEDON 1982a). The author has seen massive epidermal necrosis, and another case with numerous solitary 'dyskeratotic' cells overlying an intradermal naevus. There was no apparent aetiology for these changes. Rarely, a lesion of molluscum contagiosum may overlie a naevus (MARKS & WHITE 1980).

3.4 Balloon Cell Naevus

The balloon cell naevus is a rare lesion, clinically indistinguishable from ordinary melanocytic naevi, which tends to occur in the first three decades of life (WILSON JONES & SANDERSON 1963). To qualify as a balloon cell naevus, the lesion should contain a preponderance (over 50%) of foam cells (SCHRADER & HELWIG 1967). Focal aggregations of balloon cells can be found in up to 2% of naevi, but lesions composed entirely of these cells are extremely rare (GOETTE & DOTY 1978). In addition to clear cells with a single basophilic nucleus, multinucleated balloon cells are commonly present. Sometimes transitions between naevus cells and balloon cells can be seen.

Ultrastructural studies have shown that balloon cells are formed by the progressive vacuolization of melanocytes and naevus cells brought about by the enlargement and eventual destruction of melanosomes (HASHIMOTO & BALE 1972; OKUN et al. 1974b).

Balloon cell melanomas have also been reported (GARDNER & VASQUEZ 1970; FRIEDMAN et al. 1982; HORTON & MACDONALD 1983).

3.5 Halo Naevus

The development of a depigmented halo around a naevus is most often an idiopathic phenomenon which precedes the lymphocytic destruction of the naevus cells and the clinical regression of the lesion. This change may involve one or several naevi. Halo formation has been described in patients with vitiligo and also following severe sunburn (WHIMSTER 1974). After regression of the central naevus, the depigmented halo may repigment or may remain permanently leukodermatous. Occasionally there is erythema in the depigmented halo in the early stages (BERMAN & HERSZENSON 1981). Circulating antibodies which react against melanoma cells have been found in a high proportion of cases (COPEMAN et al. 1973).

On histological examination, there is usually a dense lymphocytic infiltrate within the tumour associated with the destruction of naevus cells. There are some macrophages in the infiltrate. Skin from the depigmented halo appears normal except for the absence of melanin in the epidermis and the replacement of epidermal melanocytes by Langerhans' cells. There may be dilated vessels in the early stages with an erythematous halo. There have been cases of halo naevus reported in which the tumour itself was devoid of inflammatory cells (BERGER & VOORHEES 1971; BROWNSTEIN et al. 1977; GAUTHIER et al. 1978). No regression would occur in such cases. It should also be noted that the lymphocytic destruction of a naevus can take place without the development of a clinical halo. Ultrastructural studies have shown non-specific injury changes in some naevus cells, with destruction of other cells (HASHIMOTO 1974; GAUTHIER et al. 1975). It is possible that cell death takes place by apoptosis as well as necrosis, but this remains to be confirmed.

3.6 Spitz Naevus

The eponymous designation 'Spitz nevus' is the preferred term for the entity which is also known as 'spindle cell naevus', 'epithelioid cell naevus', 'naevus of large spindle and/or epithelioid cells' and 'benign juvenile melanoma'. Such a term gives recognition to Sophie Spitz who published for the first time criteria for the diagnosis of a specific lesion of childhood, which despite some histological resemblance to malignant melanoma was known to behave in a benign fashion (SPITZ 1948). There have been many series of cases published since that time, the most comprehensive literature review being contained in the report of 40 cases by KOPF and ANDRADE (1966). Other series include those by MCWHORTER and WOOLNER (1954) – 11 cases, DUPERRAT and DUFOURMENTEL (1959) – 40 cases, KERNEN and ACKERMAN (1960) – 27 cases, GARTMANN (1962) – 67 cases, ALLEN (1963) – 308 cases, JAKUBOWICZ (1965) – 50 cases, COSKEY & MEHREGAN (1973) – 202 cases, WEEDON and LITTLE (1977) – 211 cases, and PANIAGO-PEREIRA et al. (1978) – 200 cases. A further review of this subject has been completed recently by the author (WEEDON 1984).

3.6.1 Clinical Features

Spitz naevi account for approximately 0.5 (WEEDON 1984) to 1 per cent (KOPF & ANDRADE 1966) of surgically excised naevi of children. The annual incidence, in our material was 1.4 cases per 100,000 of the population (WEEDON & LITTLE 1977).

Table 1. Spitz naevi – Diagnostic criteria

Major Criteria	*Minor criteria*
(a) Cell type	(a) Junctional cleavage
(b) Symmetry	(b) Oedema and telangiectasia
(c) Maturation in depth	(c) Giant naevus cells
(d) Lack of single cell upward epidermal spread	(d) Absence of nuclear pleomorphism
	(e) Perivascular inflammation
(e) Coalescent eosinophilic globules	(f) Deep outlying cells
	(g) Lack of deep mitoses

The typical Spitz naevus is a pink or flesh-coloured papule or nodule, arising on the face, trunk or extremities, particularly the lower, of children or young adults. Pigmented variants and lesions in other sites or in older individuals are not unknown. Most lesions are less than 1.2 mm in diameter. Rapid clinical growth is sometimes documented. The natural history of untreated lesions remains controversial. Multiple Spitz naevi have been described either in the form of clustered (agminate) or disseminated lesions (BROWNSTEIN 1972; WALLACE 1974; CAPETANAKIS 1975; WEIMAR & ZUEHLKE 1978; LANCER et al. 1983). Agminate lesions have a predilection for the cheeks (GOULD & BLEEHEN 1980), and may follow sunburn (KRAKOWSKI et al. 1981).

3.6.2 Histological Features

The majority of Spitz naevi are compound in type although approximately 5 to 10% are junctional and 20% are intradermal lesions. No single histological feature is diagnostic, but more weight can be placed on some changes than on others (PANIAGO-PEREIRA et al. 1978). These diagnostic features may be grouped into major and minor critera (Table 1).

Cell type. Two types of Spitz naevi are found. In one form, spindle cells, sometimes quite plump, are present, while in the other type there are epithelioid cells. The diagnosis of Spitz naevus should not be considered unless the cell type is characteristic.

Symmetry. On scanning magnification, Spitz naevi are usually symmetrical, in contrast to melanoma where epidermal melanocytic activity may extend unevenly on either side of the dermal component.

Maturation in depth. This refers to the tendency of cells in the deeper parts of the tumour to become smaller, like the cells in an ordinary naevus. This change is found in less than 25% of cases, but it may be a helpful feature in borderline lesions (WEEDON & LITTLE 1977).

Upward epidermal spread. Single cell upward epidermal spread is uncommon in the Spitz naevus, although sometimes small clumps of three or more cells may be seen within the epidermis.

Eosinophilic bodies. Single or coalescent eosinophilic globules may be found at the dermo-epidermal junction in Spitz naevi, particularly if multiple step sections are examined (KAMINO et al. 1979; ARBUCKLE & WEEDON 1982). Single

globules may be found also in a small percentage of melanomas, but the presence of coalescent globules is almost diagnostic of a Spitz naevus. These globules eventually stain positively by the PAS and trichrome methods. Electron microscopy has shown these bodies to be composed of wavy bundles of filaments, situated extracellularly (ARBUCKLE & WEEDON 1982).
Minor criteria. In junctional cleavage, there is separation of the epidermis from nests of naevus cells at the dermo-epidermal junction (ALLEN 1963). Other minor criteria include superficial oedema and telangiectasia, giant naevus cells both multinucleate and uninucleate in the upper parts of the tumour, absence of nuclear pleomorphism and deep mitoses, an inflammatory infiltrate which may be perivascular in localization, and individual naevus cells up to one high power field or more below the main component of the tumour (WEEDON 1984). In Spitz naevi the cells tend to infiltrate between collagen bundles without their destruction, and the reticulin has an even pattern (BRIGGS 1980).

Neurone specific enolase, which has been used as a marker for melanoma was not found in Spitz naevi by one group (DHILLON & RODE 1982) although it has been by another (ROYDS et al. 1982). The cells are, however positive for S-100 protein (SPIEGEL et al. 1983).

3.6.3 Desmoplastic Naevus

This lesion was described by Barr et al. in 1980. It is characterized by a sclerotic dermis, sparse pigmentation, and little or no junctional activity and theque formation. The lesions may be mistaken for fibrohistiocytic lesions, both clinically and on microscopy. Well-defined intranuclear invaginations of cytoplasm are present in most cases (Barr et al. 1980).

3.6.4 Pigmented Spindle Cell Tumour

This is a rare, heavily pigmented lesion occurring particularly on the thighs of females. It is regarded by many as a distinct entity, (REED et al. 1975; GARTMANN 1981), but for convenience it can be considered as a variant of the spindle cell type of Spitz naevus. Its importance lies in its worrisome histological appearance which may be overdiagnosed as melanoma. There is usually heavy pigmentation associated with spindle-shaped melanocytes in nests, with the formation of interconnected fascicles.

3.6.5 Malignant Spitz

This term has been applied to a very rare tumour with a close histological resemblance to a Spitz naevus, but which may metastasize to the regional lymph nodes, but not beyond (REED 1980; WEEDON 1984). Because of the difficulty in distinguishing some atypical Spitz naevi from malignant melanomas it is important that this diagnosis does not become a 'waste paper basket term' for any borderline tumour. The diagnosis is often made retrospectively, after long follow up. In the cases studied by the author there was deep extension of the lesion into the lower reticular dermis or subcutaneous tissue and mitoses were usually quite prominent, sometimes at a deep level in the tumour. Otherwise the lesions closely resembled a Spitz naevus (WEEDON 1984). OKUN (1979) has highlighted the problems sometimes encountered in distinguishing between a Spitz naevus and a melanoma in his report of three cases of melanoma with histological features of a Spitz naevus.

3.7 Congenital Naevus

3.7.1 Incidence and Clinical Features

Congenital naevi are found in from 0.2–2.7% of newborn infants (ALPER et al. 1979; CASTILLA et al. 1981), although most studies have been based on clinical observations only. WALTON et al. (1976) biopsied 34 clinically discernible pigmented lesions in newborn infants and found that only 11 (1.01% of the series) were melanocytic naevi. Congenital naevi are single in at least 90% of cases (CASTILLA et al. 1981). They have a predilection for the trunk, although they may be found on the extremities, scalp (PENMAN & STRINGER 1971), or even subungually (COSKEY et al. 1983).

Small congenital naevi are approximately ten times more common than the giant or garment types (MARK et al. 1973). Seven of the 11 cases in the series of WALTON et al. (1976) were less than 1.5 cm in diameter. In another series, 29% of lesions were 1–9 mm in diameter, 63% were 10–40 mm, and the rest were larger (CASTILLA et al. 1981).

In an attempt to bring some uniformity into the literature, KOPF et al. (1979) have proposed that lesions 1.4 cm or less in diameter should be regarded as small, those 1.5–19.9 cm as medium and those 20 cm or more large (giant naevi). Acquired naevi are usually less than 1.5 cm in diameter (MARK et al. 1973).

An increased incidence of congenital deformities has been reported in association with congenital naevi (CASTILLA et al. 1981). These included various skin anomalies such as angiomas, preauricular appendages and deformities of the ear.

3.7.2 Histology

Certain histological features are said to be characteristic of congenital naevi (MARK et al. 1973). These include the presence of naevus cells in the lower two-thirds of the dermis; extension of naevus cells between collagen bundles singly or in Indian file; and extension around nerves, vessels and adnexae (Fig. 2), particularly in the lower dermis (MARK et al. 1973). The differentiation of small congenital naevi, and those removed in the first year of life, from acquired naevi is not as clear cut as suggested above (KIRSCHENBAUM 1981). Extension into the deep dermis was found in only 37% of congenital naevi

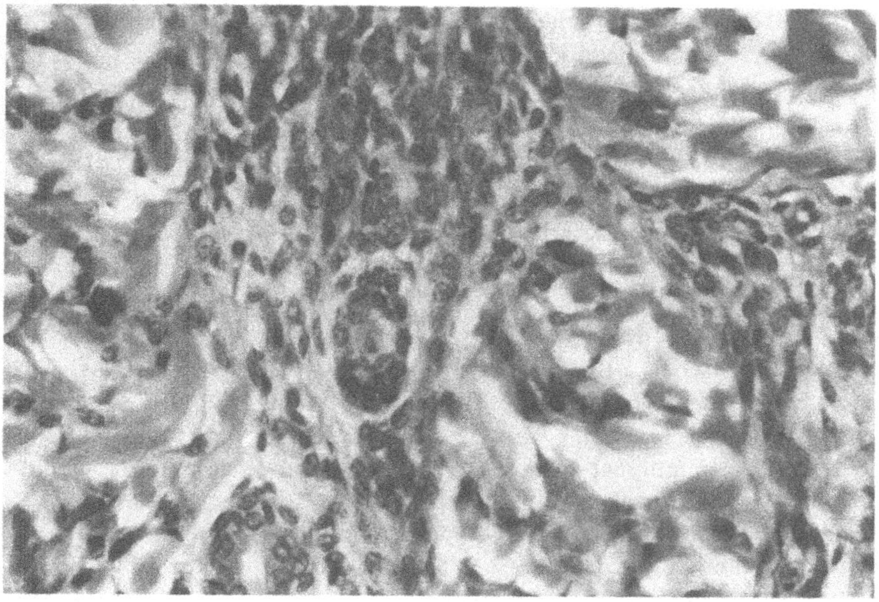

Fig. 2. Congenital naevus. Small naeval cells are arranged around a sweat gland in the lower dermis

reported recently (STENN et al. 1983). Of the 11 lesions biopsied in neonates by WALTON et al. (1976), nine were predominantly junctional in type, and only two showed the more classical features. In lesions biopsied soon after birth, melanocytic hyperplasia may be quite prominent in the epidermis and adnexal epithelium, and even atypical changes have been described (SILVERS & HELWIG 1981). In this latter study, the melanosomes in the one case studied ultrastructurally resembled those seen in the hair bulb.

3.7.3 Risk of Malignancy

Although it is accepted that there is a significant risk of malignant melanoma developing in a giant congenital naevus, there has been some controversy until recently, about the risk with small and medium-sized lesions. The incidence of melanoma in giant naevi has varied from 2–31% or more in various series, depending on the source of the material used (PERS 1963; REED et al. 1965). The Danish series by LORENTZEN et al. (1977) which found a 4.6% incidence and one from Duke University with a 6.9% incidence (LANIER et al. 1976) are probably the most reliable. RHODES et al. (1981) have estimated that the lifetime risk of developing melanoma in a giant congenital naevus is at least 6.3%. Patients with small congenital naevi who live to age 60 have an estimated cumulative risk of developing melanoma which is from three to 20 times normal (RHODES & MELSKI 1982). Other have suggested that the risk is probably smaller than this (KOPF et al. 1979). Evidence of a preexisting congenital naevus has been found in 8.1% of melanomas studied by RHODES et al. (1982), and in

1.1% of the New York University series (KOPF et al. 1979). The incidence is dependent on the number of sections studied and the criteria used for diagnosing congenital naevi.

3.7.4 Features of the Malignancy

The melanomas that arise in small congenital naevi have been said to have less aggressive growth than other melanomas (RHODES et al. 1982). They are less likely to be on the lower extremity, and more likely to be 2.25 mm or less in thickness, and of superficial spreading type (RHODES et al. 1982). In giant congenital naevi, the melanomas are often non-epidermal in origin (RHODES et al. 1981). They may have unusual morphological features which include the following patterns: – poorly differentiated round cell tumour; spindle cell differentiation; minimal deviation melanoma; and heterologous malignant mesenchymal differentiation including rhabdomyosarcoma, liposarcoma and undifferentiated spindle cell carcinoma (HENDRICKSON & ROSS 1981). A malignant blue naevus may also develop (KAPLAN 1974).

A melanoma may develop in a giant congenital naevus before 12 months of age (PENMAN & STRINGER 1971).

4. Dermal Melanocytic Lesions

4.1 Mongolian Spot

Mongolian spots are violaceous patches of discolouration occurring in the lumbosacral region of certain races. It is present at birth or soon after, but tends to disappear with increasing age (URIBE 1976).

On histological examination, there are scattered dendritic melanocytes in the lower half of the dermis.

4.2 Naevus of Ota and Ito

The naevus of Ota is a diffuse, although sometimes slightly speckled area of blue to dark brown pigmentation of the skin in the distribution of the first and second branches of the trigeminal nerve. The naevus of Ito is a similar process located in the supraclavicular, deltoid and even scapular area. Both lesions are usually unilateral and congenital. A malignant blue (Ota's) naevus was reported recently (KOPF and BART 1982).

On histological examination, there are moderate numbers of elongated melanocytes situated in the upper dermis (BURKHART & GOHARA 1981). There are sometimes nodular collections of melanocytes resembling blue naevi, with a more diffuse and less prominent infiltrate in between (Fig. 3).

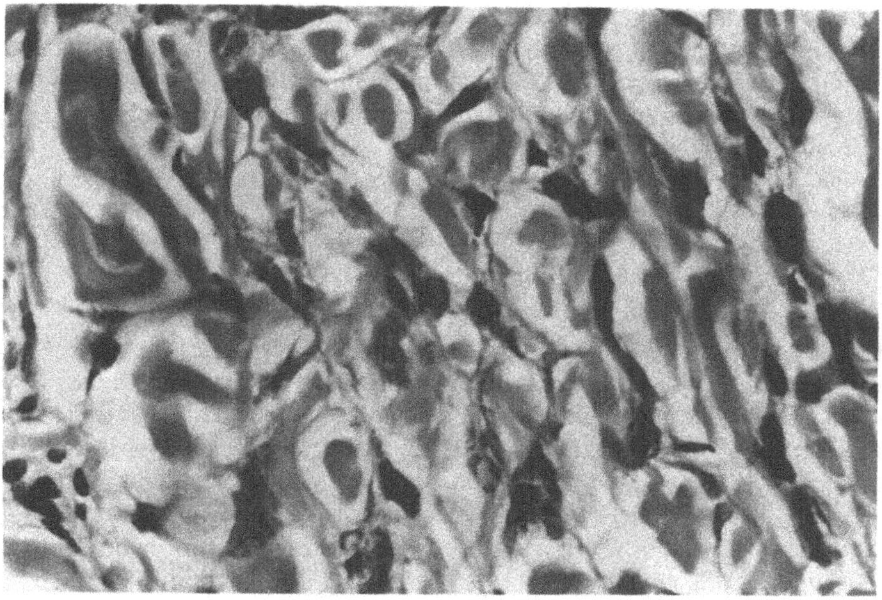

Fig. 3. Naevus of Ota. Elongate melanocytes are scattered in the dermis

4.3 Blue Naevus

The common blue naevus is a small slate-blue to blue-black macule or papule found most commonly on the dorsa of the hands and feet. The cellular variant is a much larger plaque or nodule, often found on the buttocks or sacrococcygeal region. An eruptive (HENDRICKS 1981) and target form (BONDI et al. 1983) have been described.

The histological features are well described in standard textbooks and will be mentioned only briefly. The common type is composed of slightly wavy elongated melanocytes distributed singly or in irregular bundles in the dermis. Although usually described as being in the mid and lower dermis, melanocytes often extend into the upper dermis. There are numerous melanin granules in the melanocytes and in melanophages. The collagen bundles are variably thickened and contracted. An intradermal or compound naevus may also be present ("true and blue" naevus). The cellular type is composed of spindle-shaped melanocytes as well as epithelioid cells with abundant pale cytoplasm and sometimes little pigment. There are usually numerous melanophages. The tumour often extends into the subcutaneous fat as a nodular downgrowth.

A recent ultrastructural study found some Schwannian features in cellular blue naevi, a feature that was not observed in some earlier reports (BHAWAN et al. 1980).

The presence of blue naevi in lymph node capsules has been reviewed recently (LAMBERT & BRODKIN 1984; LAMOVEC 1984). LAMOVEC (1984) favoured migration arrest over "benign metastasis" in the aetiology of this lesion.

4.4 Dermal Melanocyte Hamartoma

This refers to a diffuse, gray-blue pigmentation with darker macules present at birth, and with some similarities to the naevus of Ota and Ito (BURKHART and GOHARA 1981). A similar punctate lesion, terminating in the fifth decade in disseminated melanoma was reported by LEVENE (1979). He refers to an earlier case of MEVORAH et al. (1977).

5. Dysplastic Naevus Syndrome

The term 'dysplastic naevus syndrome' refers to the occurrence of clinically distinctive, atypical naevi with characteristic histology, in patients who have an increased risk of developing malignant melanoma (ELDER et al. 1980). Familial cases of this syndrome were described by CLARK and colleagues in 1978, under the term 'B-K mole syndrome', based on the names of two of the probands (CLARK et al. 1978; REIMER et al. 1978). This designation was changed to the 'dysplastic naevus syndrome', following the recognition of sporadic as well as familial cases (ELDER et al. 1980; RAHBARI & MEHREGAN 1981). The individual naevi with these atypical features are referred to as dysplastic naevi.

Familial cases of this syndrome have also been reported as the familial atypical mole-malignant melanoma (FAMMM) syndrome (FRICOT et al. 1977; LYNCH et al. 1978; LYNCH et al. 1981; FUSARO et al. 1983). The term large atypical naevus syndrome (LANS) was also used for a brief period (BONDI et al. 1981). MacKie has recently suggested that the term dysplastic naevus syndrome is unsatisfactory, and has proposed 'activated and expanded melanocyte syndrome' as being more appropriate (MACKIE 1982). To date, there has been no support for this view.

There are some dermatopathologists who feel that the diagnosis of dysplastic naevus syndrome is being applied indiscriminately (PELLEGRINI 1982). Furthermore, caution has been urged in accepting sporadic cases of this syndrome (PELLEGRINI 1982; FUSARO et al. 1983).

5.1 Clinical Features

Clinically, the lesions have a variegated appearance with mixtures of tan, dark brown and pink areas. They have an irregular outline and may have an indistinct border, with the persistence of macular areas in a lesion which by its size would be expected to be solely papular (ELDER et al. 1982). They are often increased both in number and size, when compared to usual naevi. Although they predominate on the trunk and upper limbs, they also occur in unusual sites such as the scalp (TUCKER et al. 1983) buttocks and female breasts (KRAEMER 1983). Patients with the dysplastic naevus syndrome usually develop an increased number of normal appearing naevi in childhood. Abnormal lesions appear in adolescence and continue to develop even in adult life.

In familial cases, the melanoma trait is inherited as an autosomal dominant with incomplete penetrance, but the dysplastic naevus trait has a more complicated inheritance, as it occurs more commonly than is usual for dominant inheritance (GREENE 1984). Recently it has been suggested that a dysplastic naevus syndrome/cutaneous melanoma susceptibility gene may be located on the short arm of chromosome 1, within 30 map units of the Rh locus (GREENE et al. 1983a). Another group has proposed a polygenic inheritance of the precursor nevi (HAPPLE et al. 1982).

Dysplastic naevi are now being recognized on a significant percentage of the population. The reported prevalence of individuals with dysplastic naevi is in the range of 2–8% (GREENE 1984). In the latter study, clinical photographs of 380 residents of Milton, New Zealand were examined, from which it was concluded that 8% of the group had at least one lesion that met the clinical criteria for the diagnosis of a dysplastic naevus, and that half of these individuals had more than one lesion (GREENE 1984). MACKIE (1981) has reported identifying four families with the familial dysplastic naevus syndrome in Scotland from June 1978 to December 1980, from a total of 560 new cases of cutaneous malignant melanoma.

Intraocular melanomas and other tumours have also been reported in families with the dysplastic naevus syndrome (LYNCH et al. 1981), although the association of intraocular tumours may be coincidental (GREEN et al. 1983b). There has also been a recent report of two families with the dysplastic naevus syndrome and coexistent multiple endocrine abnormalities (ADAMS et al. 1984).

5.2 Histological Features

The characteristic features on microscopy are basal melanocytic hyperplasia with cytological atypia. This includes nuclear hyperchromatism, and often nuclear enlargement (ELDER et al. 1980; ELDER et al. 1982). This is associated with elongation of the rete ridges. In addition, there is a superficial dermal lymphocytic infiltrate together with lamellar and concentric fibroplasia of the papillary dermis (ELDER et al. 1980). There may be some new vessel formation in the papillary dermis. These changes may occur only focally and require multiple sections for their demonstration. There is also marked variation in the degree of dysplasia in moles between and within members of families (LYNCH et al. 1980).

Two patterns of melanocyte proliferation may be seen (ELDER et al. 1980). In one, there are spindle-shaped melanocytes, sometimes arranged horizontally and often showing prominent retraction artifact. The second pattern is less common and consists of epithelioid melanocytes aggregating in nests of variable size, which fuse with those in adjacent rete ridges to produce bridging (Fig. 4). Some of the cells contain fine dusty melanin pigment. The average mean diameter of basal melanocytes in dysplastic naevi is greater than in usual naevi, but smaller than in superficial spreading melanoma (RHODES et al. 1983b).

A dermal naevus-cell component is usually present, consisting of small cells or epithelioid cells, but showing only slight evidence of maturation and with

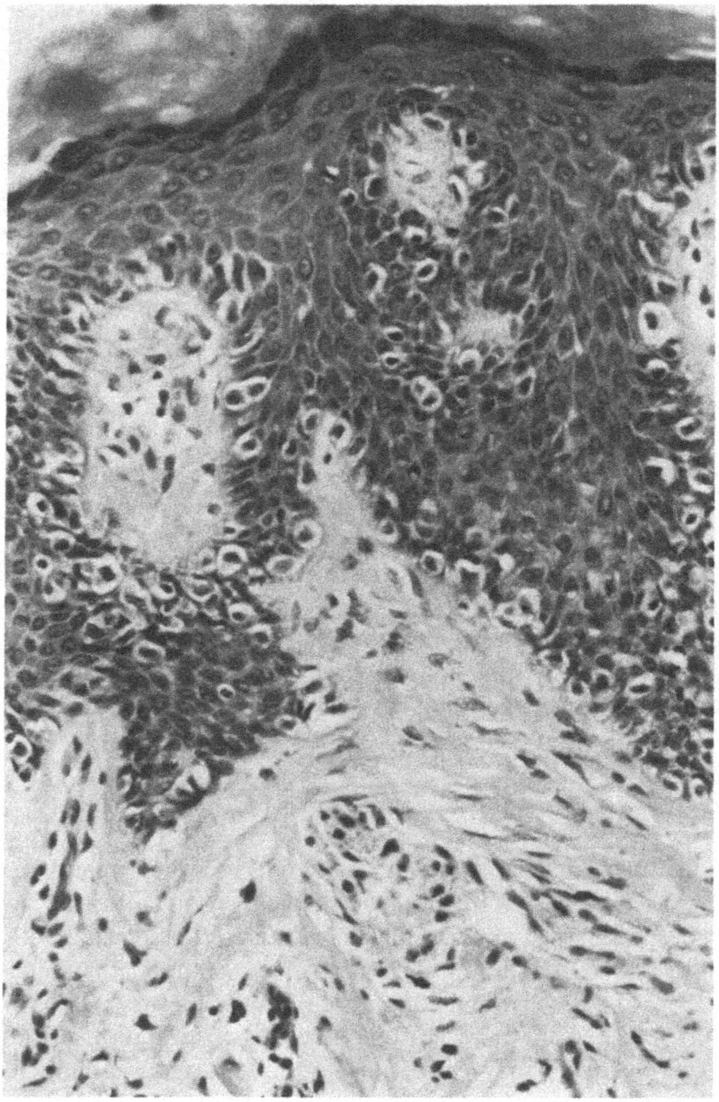

Fig. 4. Dysplastic naevus. Lentiginous proliferation of slightly atypical epithelioid melanocytes with some dermal fibroplasia. The patient had the familial dysplastic naevus syndrome

impairment of pigment synthesis (ELDER et al. 1982). In patients with the dysplastic naevus syndrome, some of the lesions that are excised prove to be typical compound or intradermal naevi (WHITE & MACDONALD 1981).

Dysplastic naevi have been found in contiguity with malignant melanoma in from 22% (RHODES et al. 1983a) to 36% (ELDER et al. 1982) of sporadic melanomas, in 69% of 105 hereditary but otherwise unselected melanomas, and in 94% of 31 prospectively diagnosed hereditary melanomas (ELDER et al. 1982). Recently, it has been suggested that as not all individuals with the dysplastic naevus syndrome are at the same high risk for developing melanoma, patients with the dysplastic naevus syndrome should be divided into putative melanoma risk categories (KRAEMER et al. 1983). In the material from the Sydney Melanoma Unit, premalignant melanocytic hyperplasia resembling that seen in dysplastic naevi was present in 39% of 723 cases of superficial spreading melanoma (McGOVERN et al. 1984). The lesions tended to be thicker and have more mitotic activity than those with adjacent melanoma in situ. The prognosis of each group was not stated (McGOVERN et al. 1984).

In determining whether a contiguous dysplastic naevus is present, it has been proposed that the atypical melanocytic hyperplasia in a lentiginous epidermal pattern should extend three or more consecutive rete beyond the most lateral margin of the intraepidermal (in situ) or invasive melanoma (RHODES et al. 1983a). This definition assumes that most pathologists will have no difficulty in distinguishing between melanoma in situ and the less atypical cytological changes of the dysplastic naevus. Lamellar fibrosis, blood vessel proliferation, a dermal naevus component, and a lymphocytic dermal infiltrate, although all often present, are not essential for the diagnosis of a contiguous dysplastic naevus (RHODES et al. 1983a). In the series from RHODES et al. (1983a), a dermal naevus cell component was present in nearly one half of the melanomas with an adjacent dysplastic naevus. The melanoma which develops in association with a dysplastic naevus is most often of superficial spreading type (RHODES et al. 1983a). It is usually thin (KRAEMER 1983) although this was not the experience of McGOVERN et al. (1984). It may have a better prognosis than melanomas without an adjacent dysplastic naevus, but further studies are required to assess this factor. McGovern has shown that although the proportion of patients diagnosed as having superficial spreading melanoma at the Sydney Melanoma Unit has more than doubled from 33% prior to 1960 to 78% during 1980–83, there appeared to be no difference in the proportion of lesions commencing de novo when compared to the number arising in a precursor dysplastic nevus (McGOVERN et al. 1984).

It has been calculated that the lifetime risk of developing a melanoma (for a Caucasian resident in the U.S.A.) is 0.6%, whereas in patients with dysplastic nevi, this risk is 10% (N.I.H. Consensus Development Conference 1983). The risk may approach 100% in patients with dysplastic naevi from melanoma-prone families.

5.3 Other Features

Fibroblasts from patients with the dysplastic naevus syndrome have enhanced sensitivity to ultraviolet irradiation in vitro (SMITH et al. 1982). They also show an abnormal response to the carcinogen 4-nitroquinolone 1-oxide (SMITH et al. 1983). It has been suggested that the results point to the possibility of an undefined metabolic anomaly that may contribute to the carcinogenic risk in some patients with the dysplastic naevus syndrome (SMITH et al. 1983).

An ultrastructural study, has shown no specific features in the melanocytes, in one case of familial dysplastic naevus syndrome (CESARINI & PUISSANT 1980).

6. Malignant Melanoma

The clinico-pathological classification of malignant melanoma has evolved into five major groups:

(1) Lentigo maligna melanoma
(2) Superficial spreading melanoma
(3) Nodular melanoma
(4) Acral lentiginous melanoma
(5) Desmoplastic melanoma, including the neurotropic variant

Amelanotic melanoma is best regarded as a poorly differentiated melanoma, rather than a special group (BHAWAN 1980). Minimal deviation melanoma has been defined as a separate group by REED (1978), and will be considered below.

The classification used above is based on that proposed 15 years ago by Clark and McGovern (CLARK et al. 1969; MCGOVERN 1970; MCGOVERN et al. 1973). The clinical and morphological features of lentigo maligna melanoma, superficial spreading melanoma and nodular melanoma are covered in standard textbooks and will be mentioned only briefly. They have also been well reviewed by SOBER et al. (1980).

ACKERMAN (1980, 1982) has rejected the classification proposed above, on the basis that all melanomas evolve in a similar way and that no single clinical or histological feature, or combination of them allows one to differentiate melanomas one from another. He advocates a diagnosis of melanoma solely with a notation as to site and thickness (ACKERMAN 1980).

The relative proportion of each type of melanoma varies somewhat in different areas. There is a higher incidence of lentigo maligna melanoma in tropical and subtropical climates (LITTLE et al. 1980; GREEN et al. 1983) than in more temperate areas (ROBERTS et al. 1981). Approximate figures based on several reports are:

Lentigo maligna melanoma	15%
Superficial spreading melanoma	50%
Nodular melanoma	30%
Acral lentiginous melanoma	5%
Desmoplastic melanoma	rare

In some reports there has been a high incidence of unclassified lesions (LARSEN & GRUDE 1978a; ROBERTS et al. 1981).

There has been some controversy in recent years about the designation that should be used for precursor lesions of melanoma in the radial growth phase. Terms such as atypical melanocytic hyperplasia have been used by some (LOPANSRI & MIHM 1979; SAGEBIEL 1979), while other have claimed that melanoma in situ should be called what it is (ACKERMAN 1983; REDMAN 1983). If multiple levels are cut from lesions initially reported as melanoma in situ, a superficial invasive component may be found in about 10% of cases (WEEDON 1982b). This is particularly so if there are features of regression present.

Several recent studies have examined the sun exposure habits of patients with melanoma and found evidence for increased light sensitivity in these patients (BEITNER et al. 1981; BERAL et al. 1983). Changes in melanoma incidence have been linked to freak sunspot activity 9–12 years earlier (HOUGHTON and VIOLA 1981). A history of painful or blistering sunburn during childhood or adolescence is sometimes obtained (LEW et al. 1983).

6.1 Lentigo Maligna Melanoma

6.1.1 Clinical Features

Lentigo maligna melanoma occurs most frequently on the face and sun-exposed skin of elderly patients. Its precursor lesion the lentigo maligna is an irregularly pigmented flat brown macule which expands very slowly. There is a great variation in colour in various areas. Amelanotic variants have been described (PAVER et al. 1981; BORKOVIC & SCHWARTZ 1983). Malignant change with invasive (vertical growth phase) tumour is recognized by thickening and the development of discrete tumour nodules. Rapid progression to deeply invasive tumour has been reported recently (MICHALIK et al. 1983). This may come about by the development of more aggressive foci, rather than by evolution of preexisting lower-grade lesions (CRAMER & KIEHN 1982). An increase in the incidence of this type of melanoma has been reported in Queensland, Australia (LITTLE et al. 1980).

6.1.2 Histological Features

On histological examination the radial growth phase is characterized by a lentiginous proliferation of atypical melanocytes, often involving adjacent adnexal epithelium (CLARK & MIHM 1969). The epidermis is often atrophic and there is usually prominent solar elastosis with a patchy lymphocytic infiltrate and some melanophages. The cells are more bloated and pleomorphic than the more uniform cells of the in-situ phase of superficial spreading melanoma (LEVENE 1980). The invasive component (vertical growth phase) may have a spindle cell appearance. On ultrastructural examination the melanosomes are usually ellipsoidal and resemble those of normal melanocytes, unlike the spheroidal and abnormal appearance of the melanosomes in superficial spreading and nodular melanoma (HUNTER et al. 1978).

6.1.3 Prognosis

Prognostic aspects will be considered in Section 6.8. However, it should be noted that MCGOVERN et al. (1980) have claimed that the better prognosis of lentigo maligna melanoma may be an inherent biological property not related to the thickness of the individual lesion.

6.2 Superficial Spreading Melanoma

6.2.1 Clinical Features

Superficial spreading melanomas may develop on any part of the body, and at any age. It has a shorter radial growth phase than lentigo maligna melanoma and is usually superficially invasive, at least, at the time of diagnosis. It has a variegated colour pattern with an irregular edge. An amelanotic variant resembling Bowen's disease has recently been reported (GOLDBERG (1983)).

6.2.2 Histological Features

Histological examination reveals a proliferation of melanocytes, singly and in nests at all levels within the epidermis and often the adnexal epithelium ('buckshot scatter'). The infiltrative component is composed of epithelioid or even nevus-like cells without evidence of maturation with descent into the dermis (PRICE et al. 1976). Ultrastructural examination shows abnormal-shaped melanosomes (HUNTER et al. 1978; MINTZIS & SILVERS 1978).

6.3 Nodular Melanoma

6.3.1 Clinical Features

Nodular melanoma may occur on any part of the body. The colour is usually uniform blue, dark brown or black. It may be amelanotic with a pink or flesh-coloured appearance. Ulceration may occur. Polypoid and even pedunculated variants occur. There is no antecedent radial growth phase of spreading pigmentation.

6.3.2 Histological Features

Nodular melanomas have no intraepidermal growth without associated dermal invasion. Any cell type or mixture of cell types may be seen.

6.4 Acral Lentiginous Melanoma

Acral lentiginous melanoma is the fourth major variant of malignant melanoma. It accounts for between 5–8% of all melanomas, although this figure is much higher in some racial groups, particularly the Japanese, where acral melanomas are the commonest type of melanoma (SEIJI et al. 1983). It is also common in blacks (COLEMAN et al. 1980). This group of lesions was first delineated by Richard Reed and colleagues (ARRINGTON et al. 1977).

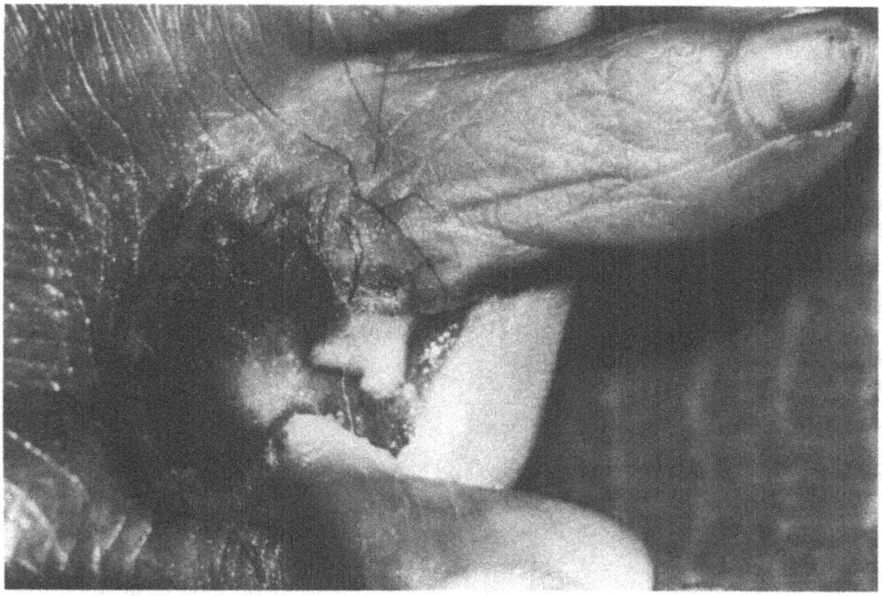

Fig. 5. Acral lentiginous melanoma. Treated for 12 months as intertrigo with delayed diagnosis

6.4.1 Clinical Features

Acral lentiginous melanomas arise on volar and subungual skin (FEIBLEMAN et al. 1980; PATTERSON & HELWIG 1980; PAPACHRISTOU & FORTNER 1982; PALADUGU et al. 1983). Similar melanomas arising on mucous surfaces such as the vagina and oral cavity have been included with acral lentiginous melanoma (MCDONALD et al. 1983), although others have stated that these mucosal tumours should be separated from the volar and subungual types at present (PALADUGU et al. 1983). Melanomas of the oral cavity and vagina (BASTABLE et al. 1980) will not be considered further. Acral lentiginous melanomas account for from 37–70% of volar-subungual melanomas (FEIBLEMAN et al. 1980; KREMENTZ et al. 1982; PALADUGU et al. 1983), most of the remainder being of superficial spreading type or unclassified. All 19 cases reported by VAZQUEZ et al. (1984) in these sites were of acral lentiginous type.

This tumour is found predominantly in elderly patients with a male preponderance, although tumours are sometimes found in the third and fourth decades (KREMENTZ et al. 1982). Typical lesions are pigmented plaques or nodules which are often ulcerated. Rare cases may mimick plantar warts (MCBURNEY & HERRON 1979) or intertrigo (Fig. 5), with consequent delay in treatment. Inadequate biopsy may also delay diagnosis as the lesions may be difficult to diagnose in the radial growth phase (SHIFFMAN et al. 1980). Patients may have regional lymph node enlargement at the time of diagnosis (VAZQUEZ et al. 1984).

6.4.2 Histological Features

The radial growth phase is characterized by atypical melanocytes in a lentiginous pattern in the basal layer (Fig. 6). There is usually some upward extension

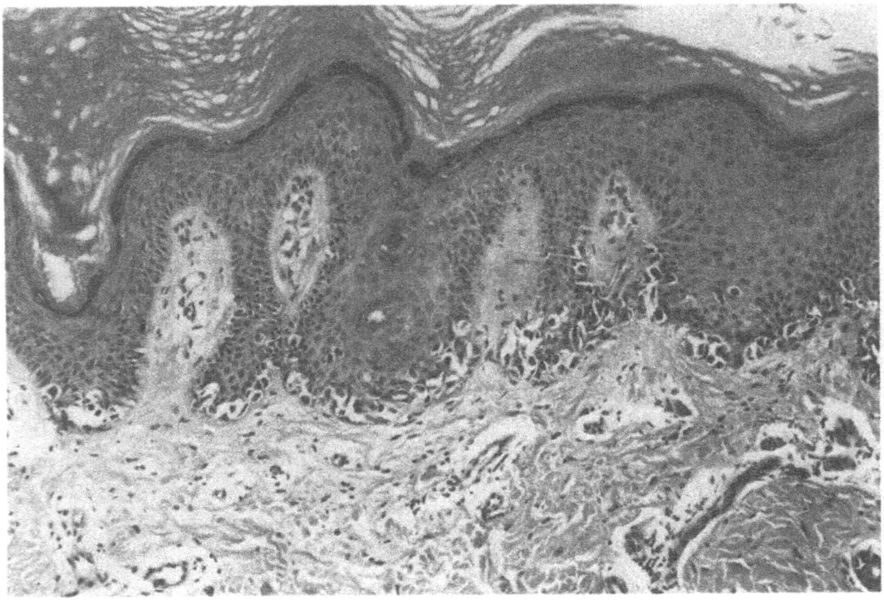

Fig. 6. Acral lentiginous melanoma. Radial growth phase. The appearances can sometimes be disarmingly bland

of melanocytes, but this is never as marked as in superficial spreading melanoma. Melanocytes may be plump with a surrounding clear area giving a lacunar appearance, or they may have heavily pigmented dendritic processes. Sometimes small junctional nests are present. The epidermis is almost invariably hyperplastic with elongated rete ridges, although ulcerated areas are not uncommon. Transitions between acral lentiginous and superficial spreading melanoma patterns have been described (SONDERGAARD & OLSEN 1980). The epidermal component may sometimes look disarmingly benign.

The invasive component (vertical growth phase) is often spindle cell in type, although it may be composed of epithelioid or naevus-like cells. Areas of regression are common. There is often a desmoplastic stromal response. Superficially, there may be a mild lymphocytic infiltrate. Most tumours are level 4 or 5 at the time of diagnosis (FEIBLEMAN et al. 1980) and lesions over 5 mm in thickness are not uncommon (VÁZQUEZ et al. 1984). Vascular invasion may be seen (ARRINGTON et al. 1977). There is usually no evidence of an antecedent naevus. The metastatic deposits in one case report were said to mimic a clear cell sarcoma of tendon sheath (WARNER et al. 1983).

6.4.3 Prognosis

This will be discussed further in Section 6.8. In brief, survival rates are usually poor, reflecting the thickness of the lesion and the clinical stage at the time of diagnosis. It has been stated that thickness and level do not have as high a predictive value for volar lesions as for melanomas on other parts of the body (FEIBLEMAN et al. 1980), although others have stated that survival is related to thickness (PALADUGU et al. 1983). SEIJI et al. (1983) reported a five year survival of 35%, and COLEMAN et al. (1980) a three year survival of 11%. Recently, it was reported that the median survival for plantar-palmar lesions was 87 months and for subungual lesions 74 months (PALADUGU et al. 1983). It has also been stated recently that the survival in acral lentiginous melanoma is essentially the same as for all acral melanomas (KREMENTZ et al. 1982).

6.5 Desmoplastic Melanoma

Desmoplastic melanoma is a rare form of malignant melanoma, first described by CONLEY et al. (1971). Although usually found on the head and neck region (CONLEY et al. 1971; MAN et al. 1981), cases have also been reported in other sites (FROLOW et al. 1975; BERRY et al. 1982). One case has been described on the upper eyelid, arising in an area of acquired mucosal melanosis, and clinically resembling a chalazion (SUTULE et al. 1982). Clinically the lesions are spreading indurated plaques or bulky firm tumefactions. The lesions are often non-pigmented, although areas of lentigo maligna like change may overlie part of the lesion (MAN et al. 1981) or be found at the periphery. Sometimes the desmoplastic pattern is only found in the recurrence or metastasis of a more usual type of melanoma. Desmoplastic melanomas are highly malignant, stubbornly recurring and often metastasizing lesions (CONLEY et al. 1971). As most reports in the literature have been limited to only a few cases, it is not possible to give meaningful five year survival rates.

6.5.1 Histological Features

Desmoplastic melanomas are composed of strands of elongate, spindle-shaped cells surrounded by mature collagen bundles (Fig. 7). Some of the spindle cells have hyperchromatic and even bizarre nuclei while others resemble normal fibroblasts (FROM et al. 1983). There may be scattered foci of lymphocytes within the tumour (CONLEY et al. 1971). There is usually extensive infiltration of the reticular dermis and sometimes extension into the subcutaneous tissue. The tumour resembles a fibrosarcoma or unusual fibrohistiocytic tumour (BRYANT et al. 1982; LABRECQUE et al. 1976). The reticulin stain has been reported as showing epithelial-like delimitation of spindle cell bundles (VALENSI 1977).

A lentigo maligna epidermal component is often present overlying part of the tumour or towards one edge (LABRECQUE et al. 1976). More or less recognizable atypical melanocytes may be seen in the dermis, usually below any epidermal component. One of the cases reported by VALENSI (1977) was thought to have developed in a congenital naevus.

The tumours are nearly always amelanotic, apart from the epidermal component. Melanin has been demonstrated in the spindle-shaped cells in at least two reports (BERRY et al. 1982; BRYANT et al. 1982). These cells are positive for S 100 protein. Malignant cells not obvious on routine H and E sections

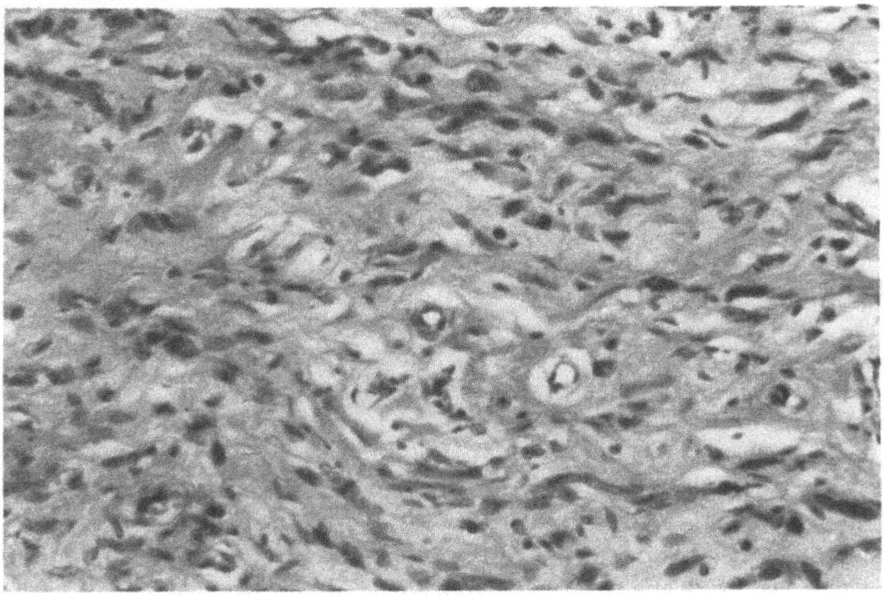

Fig. 7. Desmoplastic melanoma. Spindle cells in the dermis with background collagen

may be seen in perineural spaces in the S 100 protein preparation (FROM et al. 1983).

6.5.2 Ultrastructural Examination

On electron microscopy, the spindle-shaped cells have abundant rough endoplasmic reticulum, which may be filled with flocculent material. There may be intracytoplasmic collagen fibrils (FROM et al. 1983) and macular desmosomes (VALENSI 1979). Non-membrane bound melanin granules and premelanosomes have been recognized in some cases (BRYANT et al. 1982; FROM et al. 1983), but specifically excluded in others (DI MAIO et al. 1982). Unusual tubuloreticular intracytoplasmic inclusions have also been noted (BRYANT et al. 1982). The consensus view is that the desmoplastic component is derived from melanocytes that have undergone adaptive fibroplasia (FROM et al. 1983), although contrary views favour a fibroblastic response (LABRECQUE et al. 1976; MAN et al. 1981) or neurosarcomatous differentiation (DI MAIO et al. 1982). These latter authors reported Schwann cell differentiation in the spindle cells.

6.5.3 Neurotropic Melanoma

Neurotropic melanoma is regarded as a variant of desmoplastic melanoma (REED & LEONARD 1979). Like desmoplastic melanoma, it has a predilection for the head and neck region of middle aged to elderly patients (REED & LEONARD 1979). It has also been reported on the vulva (WARNER et al. 1982). The tumour has a propensity for local recurrence and even metastatic disease with death in approximately half the cases.

On light microscopy, it is a spindle cell tumour with atypical neuroma-like patterns and poorly defined margins (REED & LEONARD 1979). Neurotropism is a characteristic feature with loosely arranged spindle-shaped cells, often having a circumferential arrangement around small nerves in the lower dermis and subcutaneous tissue, thereby expanding the perineurium of these nerves (REED & LEONARD 1979). Interlacing bundles of cells are also seen. The cells vary in size and nuclear staining. Like desmoplastic melanoma, there is often an associated melanocyte dysplasia which includes lentigo maligna and minimal deviation melanoma (REED & LEONARD 1979). The neurotropic pattern has also been recorded in the metastatic deposits of these tumours (WARNER et al. 1981). On ultrastructural examination, it has been suggested that the cells show Schwann cell features, without evidence of premelanosomes or melanin (WARNER et al. 1981; WARNER et al. 1982).

6.6 Minimal Deviation Melanoma

The term "minimal deviation melanoma" has been proposed by Richard Reed for an uncommon nevomelanocytic tumour which is less cytologically atypical in its vertical growth phase than the more common forms of melanoma (REED 1978; MUHLBAUER et al. 1983). Recently, Reed and colleagues described two types (MUHLBAUER et al. 1983), one characterized by expansile growth in the papillary dermis with infiltration of the reticular dermis (minimal deviation type) and a second without reticular dermis invasion (borderline type). There is usually a uniform population of cells, whose cytological features deviate only minimally from naevus cells. Epithelioid or spindle cell features may be present.

In their report of 21 patients with a mean tumour thickness of 3.6 mm, only three patients had recurrent disease after a mean observation period of 57 months. Cases of metastatic minimal deviation melanoma have been reported (BECKER et al. 1980; WARNER et al. 1980b).

The concept of minimal deviation melanoma is not universally accepted. Included in this group are cases diagnosed by others as "melanomas composed of small naeval-like cells" (Fig. 8). There is danger that the diagnosis of minimal deviation melanoma may become a waste paper basket for difficult and borderline lesions.

6.7 Other Variants

6.7.1 Inflammatory Melanoma

This term was coined recently for the lesions in two patients who had extensive inflammatory involvement of the skin overlying dermal lymphatic invasion by metastatic melanoma (HAUPT et al. 1984). The lesion was similar to the inflammatory carcinoma of the breast.

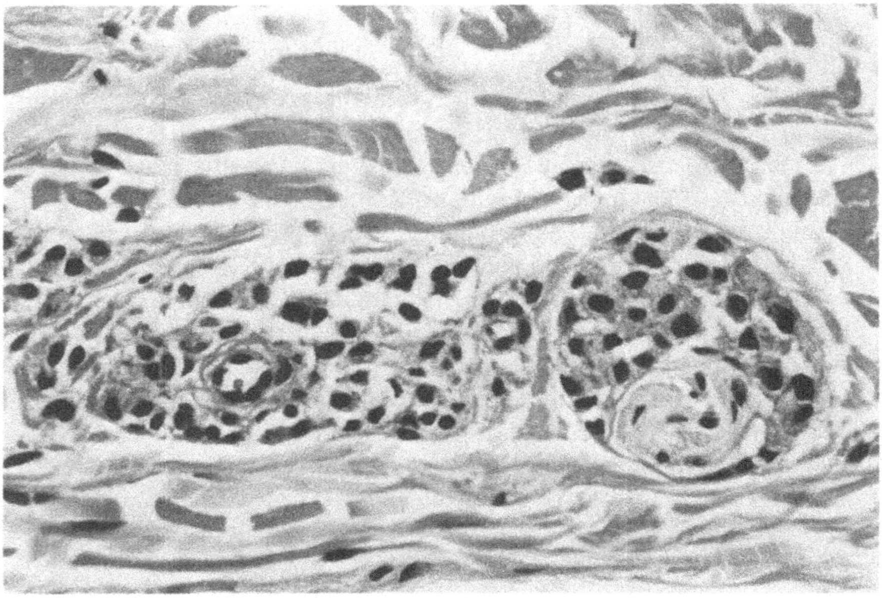

Fig. 8. Melanoma composed of small naeval-like cells surrounding vessels and a nerve in the lower dermis

6.7.2 Melanoma Originating from Intradermal Naevi

Four cases claiming to represent the malignant transformation of intradermal naevi, without the development of a junctional element, have been reported (OKUN et al. 1974a; BENISCH et al. 1980).

6.7.3 Verrucous-keratotic Melanoma

Verrucous-keratotic forms of melanoma are found most commonly in women, and favour the extremities (KUEHNL-PETZOLDT et al. 1982). They can usually be classified into one of the four major types. Their prognosis does not differ from non-verrucous melanomas matched for sex, site and thickness.

6.8 Prognostic Factors in Malignant Melanoma

A plethora of clinical and histological variables have been claimed to influence the prognosis of cutaneous melanomas (RAMPEN 1981). The comparatively recent introduction of sophisticated statistical techniques, particularly the use of multivariate analyses has allowed the delineation of dominant variables with independent predictive value with respect to prognosis. These studies have shown the dominant influence of maximum tumour thickness (Breslow) as a prognostic determinant, and the importance of cutaneous ulceration and possibly the mitotic activity, sex of the patient and location of the lesion (ELDH et al. 1978; DRZEWIECKI et al. 1980; VAN DER ESCH et al. 1981; PRADE et al. 1982; KUEHNL-PETZOLDT et al. 1983; SOBER et al. 1983b); HACENE et al. 1983; SCHMOECKEL et al. 1983c). Because there is still no uniform agreement on the significance of the parameters other than thickness and ulceration, these features will be discussed in more detail below. There is general agreement, however, that the incidence of low risk melanomas has dramatically increased in proportion to high risk melanomas in recent years (BAGLEY et al. 1981; GRIFFEL 1981; SHAFIR et al. 1982).

The five year survival rates for malignant melanoma from different centres are difficult to compare as some refer to survivals, some to disease free survivals and some for clinical stage 1 cases as opposed to all cutaneous melanomas. The five year survival for clinical stage 1 reported by BLOIS et al. (1983a) was 89% for females and 74% for males, while the 10 year figures were 71% and 55% for females and males respectively. The 5 year survival figures for the Queensland Melanoma Project are 87.7% for females and 73.6% for males.

The various clinical and histological features which may influence prognosis will be discussed in turn.

6.8.1 Tumour Thickness

It is now generally accepted that the maximum tumour thickness (measured from the granular layer to the deepest tumour cell) as proposed by BRESLOW (1970, 1975), is the most important single predictor of survival in clinical Stage 1 malignant melanoma (BALCH et al. 1978; DVIR 1980; MILTON et al. 1980; VAN DER ESCH et al. 1981; PRADE et al. 1982; MAIZE 1983). A possible caveat is for thin tumours (those less than 0.76 mm), where the level may be a more reliable predictor of low risk status (BLOIS et al. 1983a), and for thin tumours with regression where some reports, but not all, have reported significant numbers with metastases (see Section 6.8.9). The risk increases with thickness in quantum jumps, and DAY et al. (1981b) have proposed certain breakpoints on the basis of their data. They have suggested that 0.85 mm is superior to 0.75, in that all 35 patients in the NYU-MGH study between 0.75 and 0.85 mm are alive without disease (DAY et al. 1981b). Their eight year survival figures based on their proposed breakpoints were: – less than 0.85 mm ($99 \pm 1\%$), 0.85–1.69 mm ($93 \pm 2\%$), 1.70–3.60 mm ($69 \pm 5\%$), and greater than 3.60 mm ($38 \pm 6\%$). Looked at in another way, the risk of dying from malignant melanoma after 10 years has been put at less than 15% if the primary lesion is less than 1.5 mm but greater than 80% if thicker than 8 mm (JEFFREY et al. 1983). The thickness of the primary lesion is less predictive for patients with Stage 2 and 3 disease (BALCH et al. 1978).

The thickness has been found to correlate with the Clark level, the presence of ulceration, the greatest diameter, the histologic stage, age of the patient, site, and the presence of satellite deposits but not with the duration of the lesion, sex of the patient, or the clinical presence of involved regional nodes (KOPF et al. 1981).

Thin melanomas (those less than 0.76 mm, or 0.85 mm using the proposals of DAY et al. (1981b)) are increasing in overall proportion, with earlier diagnosis and treatment of malignant melanomas (BAGLEY et al. 1981; GRIFFEL 1981; BALCH et al. 1983). Thin melanomas are more common in high incidence populations than low incidence ones, probably because of earlier recognition in areas with a high incidence (LEMISH et al. 1983). The proportion of thin melanomas has been as high as 35 to 57% in some reports (SHAFIR et al. 1982; LEMISH et al. 1983; TRAU et al. 1983b; BALCH et al. 1984). Serial sectioning will increase the measured maximal thickness, and approximately 20% will move out of the category of a thin melanoma by this procedure (SOLOMON et al. 1983). In a number of series, the 5 year survival for thin lesions has been 100% (BALCH et al. 1978; BRESLOW & MACHT 1978; DAY et al. 1981b; LEMISH et al. 1983; JEFFREY et al. 1983) although several have recorded a small number of deaths, particularly for those more than level 2 (ELDH et al. 1978; BLOIS et al. 1983b; WOODS et al. 1983), and for those with regression (see Section 6.8.9).

6.8.2 Level of Invasion

The introduction of the concept of levels of invasion into the reporting of melanomas was a significant step forward in the prognostication of malignant melanoma (CLARK et al. 1969; MCGOVERN 1970; MCGOVERN et al. 1973). The levels introduced were level 1 (in situ, confined to the epidermis), level 2 (invading the papillary dermis), level 3 (expanding the papillary dermis and extending to the papillary-reticular interface), level 4 (into the reticular dermis), and level 5 (extension into subcutaneous fat). The five year disease free survival was 100% for level 1, 98–100% for level 2, 88–90% for level 3, 60% for level 4 and 15% for level 5 (WANEBO et al. 1975). Although most authors now agree that the prognostic significance of the level is derived from its secondary correlation with tumour thickness (BALCH et al. 1978; MAIZE 1983), a knowledge of the Clark level does have significance under certain circumstances. The level appears to be a more reliable predictor of low risk status than thickness (BLOIS et al. 1983a). In one series, there were only four deaths out of 247 patients at risk, over a five year period, for level 2 tumours. No women died (BLOIS et al. 1983b). The level of invasion was one of two variables found to be useful in predicting the death of patients with tumours from 0.76–1.69 mm in thickness (DAY et al. 1982d).

ALTMEYER et al. (1980) have claimed that the Clark level provided a better prognostic guide than tumour thickness. They also found that the probability of node metastases was directly proportional to the level of invasion.

6.8.3 Ulceration

Ulceration has long been regarded as an adverse prognostic feature in primary cutaneous melanomas (ALLEN & SPITZ 1953; MCGOVERN 1970; HUVOS et al. 1974; LIESTØL et al. 1982). In one series of clinical Stage 1 melanomas, the

5 year survival was 80% for non-ulcerated lesions and 55% in the presence of ulceration (BALCH et al. 1980). Ulcerated lesions are usually much thicker than non-ulcerated tumours (JEFFREY et al. 1983; BALCH et al. 1984), but this does not completely explain the poor prognosis of these cases. Many different groups have now shown that ulceration has prognostic value even after accounting for primary tumour thickness (ELDH et al. 1978; BALCH et al. 1980; VAN DER ESCH et al. 1981; DAY et al. 1982b; MCGOVERN et al. 1982; PRADE et al. 1982; KUEHNL-PETZOLDT et al. 1983). Although ulceration was shown to be predictive of metastases when the primary lesion was 1.51–3.39 mm in thickness (DAY et al. 1982b), it was not a useful prognostic feature for those greater than 3.65 mm (DAY et al. 1982a). COX et al. (1980) have reported that ulceration provided no significant added prognostic information.

Ulceration width greater than 3 mm is superior to ulceration per se as a prognostic variable (SOBER et al. 1983a; DAY et al. 1984). Depth of ulceration is not a significant feature (BALCH et al. 1980).

Ulceration has been found in 23% of superficial spreading melanomas, 49% of nodular melanomas and 74% of polypoid lesions (BALCH et al. 1980). It was present in 12.5% of lesions less than 0.76 mm in thickness, but in 72.5% of those over 4 mm (BALCH et al. 1980).

6.8.4 Site

The anatomical subsite of a melanoma has been claimed to be the best prognostic indicator after the thickness of the lesion has been taken into account (DAY 1982). This has been confirmed by a study using the Cox proportional hazards analysis, where it was found that the grouping of lesions by anatomical risk location had prognostic value in a model of eight other known predictive variables (ROGERS et al. 1983). High risk sites include the trunk (ARIEL 1982), parts of the head and neck (BLOIS et al. 1983a), the hands and feet, and the genitalia (ROGERS et al. 1983). Specific studies related to some of these sites will be detailed below. Day and colleagues have proposed the concept of the BANS area (Back, posterior upper Arm, posterior Neck and Scalp) as a prognostically unfavourable site (DAY et al. 1982d), although BLOIS et al. (1983b) were unable to confirm a site dependent difference in mortality for the BANS area. For melanomas 0.76–1.69 mm in thickness (DAY et al. 1982d), 11 of the 12 deaths recorded had primary lesions removed from the BANS area. The five year survival rates for different sites, reported by ELDH et al. (1978) were arms, hands and legs (88.9%), head and neck (83.7%), trunk (77.2%) and feet (51.1%).

Lesions on the upper trunk have a worse prognosis than those on the lower trunk, for the same thickness (DAY & LEW 1983a). Location on the upper trunk is one of four independent risk factors (along with thickness, mitotic rate and absent or minimal lymphocytes at the base) for lesions between 1.70 and 5.49 mm (DAY et al. 1981d). In this latter study midline lesions did not have a worse prognosis than lateral lesions, although midline trunk was an unfavourable site in another study (ROGERS et al. 1983). Location on the trunk was one of four variables that best predicted bony or visceral metastases for patients with lesions greater than or equal to 3.65 mm in thickness (DAY et al. 1982a).

Patients with tumours on the hands and feet have a much worse prognosis than those with lesions on the thigh, leg, arm and forearm (DAY & LEW 1983a). Lesions on the feet have a higher incidence of metastases to regional lymph nodes, and may have a worse prognosis at five years than for those on the hands (KEYHANI 1977). However FEIBLEMAN et al. (1980) reported that the five year survival for plantar melanomas was 43%, compared to 19% for palmar and subungual lesions. Location on the foot is an independent prognostic factor for Stage 1, lesions of the lower extremity (DAY et al. 1981c). All nine patients with lesions thicker than 3.65 mm, and situated on the hands or feet died in one series (DAY et al. 1982a). Thickness and level may not have as high a predictive value for volar lesions as for melanomas on other parts of the body (FEIBLEMAN et al. 1980).

The clinical diagnosis of subungual melanomas is often delayed (PATTERSON & HELWIG 1980; PAPACHRISTOU & FORTNER 1982). Most are deep lesions. Females have been reported to have a relatively good prognosis as opposed to the poor prognosis in males (PATTERSON & HELWIG 1980), although in one series the five year survival for palmar and subungual melanomas was only 19% (FEIBLEMAN et al. 1980).

In a large series of melanomas on the ear, the survival correlated with the patient's sex, clinical appearance of the lesion, subsite, thickness, level, presence of node metastases and treatment (BYERS et al. 1980).

6.8.5 Mitoses

Several studies have confirmed that the mitotic rate in a primary melanoma is an independent prognostic variable (ELDH et al. 1978; PRADE et al. 1980; VAN DER ESCH et al. 1981; HACENE et al. 1983). A mitotic count greater than $6/mm^2$ has been found to be an independent variable for trunk lesions 1.70–5.49 in thickness (DAY et al. 1981d), and predictive of metastases for lesions 1.51–3.39 mm thick (DAY et al. 1982b). It also correlated with death of the patient in under two years (SOBER et al. 1983a). The mitotic count was also an independent risk factor for recurrent disease in patients with clinical stage 1 lesions of the lower extremity (DAY et al. 1981C). Whereas the five year survival rate for patients with melanomas having a mitotic count of 5 or less mitoses per 10 high power fields was 90.6%, it was only 59.1% when the count exceeded 10/10 H.P.F. (ELDH et al. 1978).

SCHMOECKEL and BRAUN-FALCO (1978) have stated that the best prognostic information is derived from the product of the thickness in mm and the number of $mitoses/mm^2$. They called this the prognostic index (SCHMOECKEL et al. 1983a). The mitotic rate alone when low, was also of value in establishing a group with a low incidence of metastases (SCHMOECKEL & BRAUN-FALCO 1978).

Two other studies have found that the mitotic count correlated with survival, but that the prognostic significance was derived from correlation with tumour thickness (McGovern et al. 1979; Jeffrey et al. 1983). Several other reports have suggested that the mitotic rate was of neglible or no prognostic value (Beardmore et al. 1970; Drzewiecki et al. 1980; Liestøl et al. 1982).

6.8.6 Microscopic Satellites

This term refers to the presence of discrete tumour nests more than 0.05 mm in diameter, that are separated from the main body of the tumour by normal reticular dermal collagen or subcutaneous fat (Day et al. 1981a). The presence of microscopic satellites is associated with a poor prognosis (Sober et al. 1983a), and this is an independent variable for lesions 1.51–3.39 mm in thickness (Day et al. 1982b). In an earlier report, Day and colleagues noted that the five year survival for patients with microscopic satellites was $36 \pm 6\%$ compared to $89 \pm 2\%$ for those without (Day et al. 1981a).

The presence of microscopic satellites is a better indicator of occult regional lymph node metastases in clinical Stage 1 melanoma than is tumour thickness (Harrist et al. 1984).

6.8.7 Histological Type

The earlier studies of Clark and McGovern (Clark et al. 1969; McGovern 1970) showed that the histological type had important prognostic implications. Whereas patients with nodular melanoma had a poor prognosis, and those with lentigo maligna melanoma a good prognosis, patients with superficial spreading melanoma were at an intermediate level. The five year survivals in McGovern's series were lentigo maligna (80%), superficial spreading melanoma (70%) and nodular melanoma 53% (McGovern 1970). More recent figures were 79.1% for superficial spreading melanoma and 69.3% for nodular lesions (MgGovern et al. 1979), while in a comparable series of melanomas of lentigo maligna type it was 90.2% (McGovern et al. 1980).

It is generally agreed that there is no survival difference between superficial spreading and nodular melanomas when these are corrected for thickness (Wanebo et al. 1975; Eldh et al. 1978; McGovern et al. 1979; Van der Esch et al. 1981; Blois et al. 1983a). The same has been stated recently for acral lentiginous melanoma (Krementz et al. 1982; Sondergaard 1983). In the case of lentigo maligna melanoma, although there is agreement that these lesions have a generally favourable prognosis, (Ironside et al. 1977; Balch et al. 1978), this has usually been attributed to their being thinner lesions (Balch et al. 1978; Eldh et al. 1978). Other reports have specifically excluded lentigo maligna melanoma, because of inadequate numbers. In a large series of cases McGovern et al. (1980) have presented evidence that lentigo maligna melanoma is often thicker than other types of melanoma. The overall prognosis for lentigo maligna melanoma patients was significantly better, this being particularly so for women, none of whom died of melanoma. There was no close correlation between the prognosis and thickness of the lesions (McGovern et al. 1979).

Finally, one of the reports of Day and colleagues noted that for lesions 3.65 mm in thickness or more, histological type other than superficial spreading melanoma was predictive of metastases (DAY et al. 1982a).

6.8.8 Lymphocytic Infiltrate

Although there have been several reports suggesting a better survival for patients with melanomas having a lymphocytic infiltrate at the base (HANSEN & McCARTEN 1974; BRESLOW & MACHT 1978), and one study suggesting a worse prognosis for deep nodular melanomas with such an infiltrate (LARSEN & GRUDE 1978b), most reports have shown that the inflammatory cell reaction is not prognostically significant when other variables are taken into consideration (BALCH et al. 1978; SCHMOECKEL & BRAUN-FALCO 1978; DRZEWIECKI et al. 1980; VAN DER ESCH et al. 1981; HACENE et al. 1983; JEFFREY et al. 1983). However Day and colleagues have found that absence of a lymphocytic infiltrate results in a worse prognosis for lesions greater than 3.65 mm thick (DAY et al. 1982a), and is an independent variable leading to a worse prognosis for trunk lesions 1.7 mm–5.49 mm in thickness (DAY et al. 1981d). A lymphocytic infiltrate is much more common in thin melanomas (WANEBO et al. 1975).

6.8.9 Regression

Other studies have looked at the prognostic significance of partial regression, rather than a lymphocytic infiltrate per se. Active regression is characterized by the presence of a heavy lymphocytic infiltrate with loss or degeneration of tumour cells, while previous regression can be recognized by the presence of vascular fibrous tissue with or without melanin-containing macrophages and perhaps a scanty lymphocytic infiltrate (McGOVERN 1975). The incidence of partial regression has varied considerably from series to series, probably depending on the criteria used for mild cases. BALCH et al. (1978) reported it in 10%, LITTLE (1972) in 13%, TRAU et al. (1983a) in 24.6% and McGOVERN et al. (1979) in 32%. Regression is more likely to be found in lesions that are level 3 or less and greater than 10 mm in diameter, have solar elastosis, are on sites other than the head and neck, and that show white areas clinically (TRAU et al. 1983a). Several studies have found quite a high incidence of partial regression in thin melanomas. GROMET et al. (1978) noted regression in 19% of their 121 thin melanomas, PALADUGU and YONEMOTO (1983) in 30%, McGOVERN et al. (1983b) in 58%, DAY et al. (1982d) in 53%, and TRAU et al. (1983b) in 36.3% of cases.

In none of the recent reports on melanoma has partial regression been an independent risk factor (DAY et al. 1982d; TRAU et al. 1983a). The prognostic significance of partial regression found in some earlier reports was derived from the close correlation with tumour thickness, there being a higher incidence of regression in thin lesions (McGOVERN et al. 1979; SHAW et al. 1980a).

There has been considerable controversy regarding the role of regression in thin melanomas. GROMET et al. (1978) suggested that regression was a poor prognostic sign. They found that five of 23 thin melanomas with regression metastasized (21.7%), while only two of 98 lesions without regression (2%) did. Their findings have been confirmed recently by another group (PALADUGU & YONEMOTO 1983). In this study of 36 cases, 11 had features of partial regression and five of these (45.5%) metastasized, whereas only three of the remaining 25 lesions (12%) without regression metastasized (PALADUGU & YONEMOTO 1983). Of the 11 cases with regression, two were Clark level 3 and nine were level 2.

Contrary views have been expressed by TRAU et al. (1983b) and McGOVERN et al. (1983b) who found that the presence or absence of regression did not significantly influence the incidence of metastases (McGOVERN et al. 1983b; TRAU et al. 1983b) or the cumulative 10 year survival (McGOVERN et al. 1983b). Furthermore the presence or absence of regression in thin lesions did not appear to influence the site of first recurrence (McGOVERN et al. 1983b).

6.8.10 Metastases and Stage

Although the prognostic correlations of clinical stage 1 disease have been well studied, less is known about the prognostic parameters in patients with recurrent disease. In patients with recurrent melanoma, the clinical stage appears to be the strongest determinant of the subsequent survival (BALCH et al. 1981; KARAKOUSIS et al. 1983; DAY & LEW 1984). The pathological stage also has an independent influence on survival (BALCH et al. 1978).

Several studies have looked at clinical stage 1 with incidental metastases found in the regional lymph nodes. Positive nodes were a poor prognostic feature in clinical stage 1 patients with lesions greater than 3.65 mm in thickness (DAY et al. 1982a). In another study the risk became significant if more than 20% of the regional nodes were involved on microscopic examination (DAY et al. 1981e). However attempts to detect occult secondary deposits in lymph nodes by routine serial sectioning does not appear to be of practical applicability (REICHERT et al. 1981). Microstaging still retains prognostic significance in patients with clinical stage 1 disease with metastases found in regional lymph nodes (DAY et al. 1981e). Such patients have five year survivals of approximately 50% (DAY et al. 1981e).

Node palpability is an unfavourable risk factor for death from melanoma, independent of other variables tested (OLSON et al. 1981; DAY & LEW 1984). Five year survival rates for clinical stage 2 were similar for males and females in one study, but there was female superiority if cases were matched for age and thickness (SHAW et al. 1982). Another report has noted better female survival after the first evidence of distant metastases (RAMPEN 1980).

The probability of node metastases is directly related to the Clark level (WANEBO et al. 1975; HOLMES et al. 1976; ALTMEYER et al. 1980) and the thickness of the tumour (BALCH et al. 1979; LEE 1980). ROSES et al. (1982) noted that no patients with lesions less than 1 mm in thickness had nodal micrometastases, and there was no appreciable increase in incidence of nodal metastases until the lesions reached 4 mm in thickness, in which case the incidence of metastases was 50%. Lymph node metatases have been reported in 4% of level 2 lesions, 7% of level 3, 25% of level 4, and 70% of level 5 cases (WANEBO et al. 1975). Using the Breslow thickness, it was 0% for those less than 0.76 mm, 25% for lesions 0.76–1.50 mm, 51% for 1.50 to 3.99 mm and 62% for those greater than 4 mm in thickness (BALCH et al. 1979).

In stage 4 disease, the number of initial distinct metastatic lesions appears important. Those with a single metastatic nodule do better than those with two or more nodules (KARAKOUSIS et al. 1983). The site of the metastasis does not appear to influence survival (FEUN et al. 1982). There is some controversy whether the time interval from excision to relapse correlates with the subsequent survival of the patient (YARNOLD & COCHRANE 1980; KARAKOUSIS et al. 1983).

MILTON et al. (1980) reported that thicker lesions first recurred predominantly in the vicinity of the scar of the primary whilst very thin lesions first recurred within the regional lymph nodes or at remote sites. Local or regional recurrences may sometimes develop more than 20 years after the removal of the primary (BRIELE et al. 1983).

Finally, lymph node morphology has also been studied recently. In one report, patients treated with surgery alone whose regional lymph nodes had hyperplastic germinal centres had a significantly shorter survival than those without (PIHL et al. 1982). Another study provided a possible explanation by finding that ulceration of the primary tumour resulted in a progressive increase in the number and area of lymph node germinal centres (WEIDNER et al. 1982). Germinal centre activity was found to increase as melanoma progressively invaded the node (LEWIS et al. 1979).

6.8.11 Size and Shape

Although patients with melanomas greater than 1–2 cm in diameter (the upper limit varies in the different reports) have a worse prognosis than patients with smaller lesions (HUVOS et al. 1974; EPSTEIN & BRAGG 1980; KOPF et al. 1982), the size of a lesion does not appear to be an independent prognostic variable. Smaller lesions tend to be in younger patients, particularly females and be thinner lesions, often on the lower extremity (KOPF et al. 1982).

It is generally held that the prognosis of polypoid lesions is poor, but this appears to be due to their being generally thick and ulcerated lesions (MANCI et al. 1981; MCGOVERN et al. 1983a). A polypoid configuration was present in 21.5% of the 2296 cases studied by MCGOVERN et al. (1983a), although the incidence quoted in the literature varies from 2–43% (BEARDMORE 1977; VAN DER ESCH et al. 1981). Pedunculated lesions have often been confused or included with polypoid melanomas (SIMINOVITCH et al. 1980). Pedunculated lesions may not have the poor prognosis of polypoid lesions, but too few cases have been studied to draw any definite conclusions (BEN HUR et al. 1981; ROSENBERG et al. 1981). Metastases had developed to regional nodes by the time of surgery in another pedunculated lesion, although tumour cells were only in the pedunculated mass (NIVEN & LUBIN 1975).

By studying clinical photographs, DAY et al. (1982c) found that melanomas without a nodule had the lowest incidence of metastases, the rate increasing with nodule diameter.

6.8.12 Cell Type

Most recent studies have not found the cell type to be an independent prognostic variable (DRZEWIECKI et al. 1980), although VAN DER ESCH et al. (1981) found that the cell type did affect prognosis when adjusted for tumour thickness. LARSEN AND GRUDE (1978a) found a good prognosis related to spindle-shaped cells, but a bad one for epithelioid lesions. Giant tumour cells have been found to indicate a poor survival (HUVOS et al. 1974) but not in multivariate analyses. Tumours composed of small "lymphocytic-like" cells were found to have a high metastatic rate by SCHMOECKEL et al. (1983c).

6.8.13 Presence of Coexisting Naevus

The incidence of coexisting benign intradermal naevi in malignant melanomas has varied considerably from series to series. In part, it depends on the number of sections examined. LITTLE (1972) reported an incidence of 40% but included lentigos and junctional naevi in this figure. Although there was a higher mortality for those with coexisting intradermal naevi, it was lower when a lentigo was also present (LITTLE 1972). CRUCIOLI and STILLWELL (1982) found naevi in 10.8% of their cases of melanoma.

In a series of 349 melanomas at the NYU cooperative group, 18.4% of melanomas were associated with naevi, of which 17.3% were ordinary naevi and 1.1% congenital naevi (KOPF et al. 1979). Features of a congenital naevus were present in 8.1% of melanomas reported by RHODES et al. (1982). They suggested that such melanomas had less aggressive growth. Recently FRIEDMAN et al. (1983) have reported acquired melanocytic naevi in 23% of 557 melanomas. They reported a more favourable prognosis for these melanomas, which was independent of the thickness of the melanoma and six other variables (FRIEDMAN et al. 1983). One of their photomicrographs would probably be interpreted by some as representing a coexistent dysplastic naevus. Another report has suggested that melanomas arising in dysplastic naevi may also have a better prognosis (RHODES et al. 1983a). There is a need for further studies to elucidate this problem. SCHMOECKEL et al. (1983c) and HUVOS et al. (1974) did not find any prognostic significance for a coexistent nevocellular naevus.

6.8.14 Pigmentation

Multivariate analysis has not shown the pigmentation of a tumour to be a significant prognostic variable, thus confirming some of the earlier studies (BEARDMORE et al. 1970; MCGOVERN 1970). However LARSEN & GRUDE (1978a) did report a poorer prognosis for tumours with little pigment, but these cases were not corrected for thickness. Comparable survival figures have also been found for pigmented and amelanotic lesions in stage 2 disease (GUILIANO et al. 1982).

6.8.15 Vascular Invasion

The incidence of vascular invasion varies from series to series. It was present in 5.8% in one report (LARSEN & GRUDE 1979). Although angioinvasion has been shown to be an adverse prognostic feature (LARSEN & GRUDE 1979; SCHMOECKEL et al. 1983c), this has not always been so when corrections are made for the thickness of the tumour (VAN DER ESCH et al. 1981).

6.8.16 Sex

It is well established that females with clinical Stage 1 melanoma have superior survival rates to males (McGOVERN 1970; LIESTØL et al. 1982). Factors which appear to contribute to this better survival include the occurrence of lesions in prognostically favourable sites such as the lower extremity, and the development of less invasive (that is, thinner) tumours (SHAW et al. 1980b; BLOIS et al. 1983a). After allowing for these factors, SHAW et al. (1980b) concluded that factors other than thickness and site appeared to be operative in premenopausal women. Female patients had more favourable lesions than males in all five microstaging categories (type, site, level, thickness and stage) in another report (DANFORTH et al. 1982).

Although sex did not appear in any of the multivariate analyses of Day and colleagues as an independent prognostic variable when subsite and thickness breakpoints were used (DAY 1982), a recent prospective study from the German melanoma group found that sex, along with thickness and ulceration was a dominant variable affecting the eight year survival of 1191 patients with clinical stage 1 disease (KUEHNL-PETZOLDT et al. 1983). Sex and ulceration were independent of each other. The sex of a patient can also be used to develop a prognostic model, along with other variables (HACENE et al. 1983).

ALTMEYER et al. (1980) found that the five year survival rate was higher in females than males with stage 1 disease, for level 4 and level 5 lesions or for those greater than 2.25 mm in thickness, while BLOIS et al. (1983a) found no deaths in any of the 114 female patients with level 2 tumours in their series, regardless of site or thickness.

Although the overall five year survival in males and females with clinical stage 2 disease was similar in one study (SHAW et al. 1982), if patients were matched for thickness and age, a female superiority did exist for young patients with very thick lesions.

6.8.17 Age

Younger patients have a significantly better prognosis than older patients (ELDH et al. 1978). It has been suggested that this effect arises largely from the superior survival of young females, although this was not confirmed in a recent study (BLOIS et al. 1983). Another group has found a significant correlation between age and thickness of the lesion, and proposed this as the explanation for the better prognosis (LEVINE et al. 1981). PALANGIE et al. (1981) showed that age was the variable that added most to information on prognosis, supplied by thickness, although it has not been an independent variable in most studies.

6.8.18 Duration

A recent study of patients with superficial spreading melanoma found no correlation between the time to diagnosis and the biological state, as reflected by the thickness of the lesion (CASSILETH et al. 1982).

6.8.19 Vitiligo

A recent study of 27 patients with melanomas and vitiligo, together with a review of a further 24 cases from the literature revealed that the presence of vitiligo in patients with metastatic melanoma portends a longer survival than expected (NORDLUND et al. 1983). In most cases, the depigmentation commenced after the diagnosis of melanoma. Of the 51 patients studied, 49 had metastases, although 35 survived five year and 25 survived 10 year (NORDLUND et al. 1983). KOH et al. (1983) have confirmed the better prognosis in these patients. They preferred the term leukoderma to vitiligo because the clinical and ultrastructural features were somewhat varied (KOH et al. 1983).

6.8.20 Pregnancy

There are at least two studies which have shown that pregnancy has an adverse effect on the course of patients with malignant melanoma (SHIU et al. 1976; HOUGHTON et al. 1981), although the earlier study (SHUI et al. 1976) showed an adverse effect only on Stage 2 patients but not those with Stage 1. Whereas the five year survival for 12 patients whose melanoma developed during pregnancy was 55%, compared to 83%, for a control group, this difference was not significant when patients were matched for age, site of lesion and stage at diagnosis (HOUGHTON et al. 1981). Lesions in pregnancy tended to be found on the trunk and at an advanced stage (HOUGHTON et al. 1981).

6.8.21 Smoking

In a study of 1908 patients, SHAW et al. (1979) showed that smoking rendered men, but not women, more susceptible to developing metastases. Although attempts were made to ensure that these differences were not due to some imbalance of other prognostically important factors, these cases were not subjected to proper multivariate analysis.

6.8.22 Surgical Margins

It is generally agreed that arbitrary wide margins of excision are not justified (SCHMOECKEL et al. 1983b; COSIMI et al. 1984). BALCH et al. (1979) found no local recurrences for lesions less than 0.76 mm regardless of the surgical margin, while DAY and LEW (1983b) found that narrow margins of excision for melanomas less than 0.85 mm thick, neither shortened survival nor increased local recurrences. Similarly, narrow margins for lesions greater than 0.85 mm, did not effect survival, although local recurrence rates increased when the surgical margin was less than 3 cm (DAY & LEW 1983b; SCHMOECKEL et al. 1983b). For limb melanomas less than 1 mm in thickness, and Clark level 2 or 3, there was no difference in disease recurrence or survival whether they were treated by wide local excision, with or without lymph node dissection or chemotherapy (MCBRIDE et al. 1981).

6.8.23 Incisional Biopsy

Although there is some experimental evidence in mice that incisional biopsy of a tumour increased the risk of dissemination (RAMPEN 1981), only RAMPEN et al. (1980) in recent years have claimed that survival is reduced after incisional biopsy of primary cutaneous melanoma. However, their numbers were small, which may have influenced the results. Other studies have shown that incisional biopsy followed later by adequate excision, carries no increased risk of local recurrence, nodal metastases or death (EVERALL & DOWD 1977; BAGLEY et al. 1981). This has also been confirmed after a follow up period of 25 years (EPSTEIN & BRAGG 1980).

Small biopsies may of course preclude a diagnosis of melanoma because of sampling problems (MACY-ROBERTS & ACKERMAN 1982).

6.8.24 Multiple Primary Lesions

Patients with multiple primary lesions have been found to have an improved survival when compared to patients with a single primary, with both Stage 1 and 2 disease (MOSELEY et al. 1979). This study was done before the recognition of the sporadic dysplastic naevus syndrome, and this may have been relevant in some of the cases. Multiple primary lesions develop in about 4% of patients (BEARDMORE & DAVIS 1975), although it may be difficult sometimes to distinguish epidermotropic metastases (WARNER et al. 1980a; UNGER et al. 1981). This whole subject needs review in the light of the dysplastic naevus syndrome.

6.9 Special Techniques in Diagnosis

A number of special techniques can be used to help confirm the diagnosis of malignant melanoma in amelanotic or oligomelanotic lesions (VAN DUINEN et al. 1984). These include the identification of premelanosomes on electron microscopy, the DOPA reaction on frozen sections, a modified Warthin Starry technique on either paraffin or epoxy sections (WARKEL et al. 1980; VAN DUINEN et al. 1983), and the use of various immunohistochemical techniques, often with immunoperoxidase labelling.

The intermediate-sized filament vimentin has been identified in naevi and melanomas (MIETTINEN et al. 1983; RAMAEKERS et al. 1983). It has also been found in a metastatic amelanotic deposit of melanoma in the lung (HUSZAR et al. 1983). S-100 protein has also been found in naevi and melanomas (NAKAJIMA et al. 1982; STEFANSSON et al. 1982; PENNEYS et al. 1984), including the spindle cell elements of neurotropic melanoma (WARNER et al. 1984). It was negative in one fibrosarcoma of skin (GAYNOR et al. 1981). This has been shown to be a sensitive method when used on amelanotic and oligomelanotic secondary deposits, with a false negative rate of only 4%, compared with 45% using a monoclonal antibody against a cell membrane fraction, and 50% with a fluorescence method (PALMER 1983). S 100 protein will also stain epidermal melanocytes and Langerhans cells as well as cutaneous neural tumours (KAHN et al. 1983).

Neurone specific enolase has been found in melanomas (DHILLON & RODE 1982), including the neurotropic variant (WARNER et al. 1984). DHILLON and RODE (1982) found a progressive increase in staining for neurone specific enolase from benign to malignant lesions. Although they did not find it in the Spitz naevus, another group using enolase isoenzymes reported positive results (ROYDS et al. 1982). They found strong staining with alpha enolase for naevi and melanomas but weaker staining for neurone specific enolase with dedifferentiation of the melanoma.

Myelin basic protein has been detected in neurofibromas and neurilemmomas, but not in a variety of intradermal and compound naevi, nor in melanoma (PENNEYS et al. 1984). Neurofilaments, desmin and glial fibrillary protein were not found in one study of naevi and melanomas (MIETTINEN et al. 1983).

The monoclonal antibody NK1/C-3 has been found to have high sensitivity for melanomas, but not specificity (VAN DUINEN et al. 1984). This was confirmed in another study which showed it to stain stronger than S-100 protein and neurone specific enolase (MACKIE et al. 1984). Furthermore, the antigen recognized is not denatured by formaldehyde. Using this antibody, positive tests were obtained in 3 of 14 Spitz naevi and in all 13 dysplastic naevi tested (MACKIE et al. 1984).

The demonstration of fluorescence in unstained sections from formalin-fixed, paraffin-embedded tissue from cases of malignant melanoma may prove to be a valuable ancillary test for differentiating melanoma cells from other cutaneous tumour cells (INOSHITA & YOUNGBERG 1982). A proportion of benign naevi will also give positive fluorescence. This technique has also proved useful in diagnosing amelanotic melanomas using touch preparations (MORISHIMA & NAGASHIMA 1983).

Fine needle aspiration biopsy cytology has been reported to be a valuable tool for the diagnosis of metastatic and primary melanoma (KLINE & KANNAN 1982). Melanin could be verified in the preparations using the Masson-Fontana method. Additional features which were noted were anisocytosis, cell isolation, multinucleation, eosinophilic nucleoli and intranuclear inclusions (KLINE & KANNAN 1982).

Monoclonal antibodies have been used to measure the human melanoma-associated antigen of molecular weight 100,000, to monitor tumour burden in patients with malignant melanoma (MORGAN et al. 1984). Monoclonal antibodies have also been used in experimental situations to stain early human melanoma colonies grown in vitro (NAKANO et al. 1984).

The measurement of the urinary excretion of 5-S-cysteinyldopa has been undertaken in an attempt to detect the presence of metastatic melanoma (AGRUP et al. 1979). Although this test shows good sensitivity and specificity it is not absolutely reliable in diagnosing metastatic melanoma (AGRUP et al. 1979).

Finally, frozen sections are now being used less often in the management of malignant melanoma. The technique has proved to be reliable in experienced hands (LITTLE & DAVIS 1974; BRAUN-FALCO et al. 1981; SHAFIR et al. 1983).

References

Ackerman AB (1980) Malignant melanoma: A unifying concept. Human Pathol 11:591–595

Ackerman AB (1982) Disagreements about classification of malignant melanomas. Am J Dermatopathol 4:447–452

Ackerman AB (1983) Macular and patch lesions of malignant melanoma: malignant melanoma in situ. J Dermatol Surg Oncol 9:615–618

Ackerman AB, Ragaz A (1984) The lives of lesions. Chronology in dermatopathology. Masson Publishing USA, New York

Adams SJ, Rustin MHA, Robinson TWE, Munro DD (1984) The dysplastic naevus syndrome and endocrine disease. Br Med J 288:1790–1791

Agrup G, Agrup P, Andersson T, Hafstrom L, Hansson C, Jacobsson S, Jönsson P-E, Rorsman H, Rosengren A-M, Rosengren E (1979) 5 years experience of 5-S-cysteinyldopa in melanoma diagnosis. Acta Derm Venereol 59:381–388

Allen AC (1963) Juvenile melanomas. Ann NY Acad Sci 100:29–46

Allen AC, Spitz S (1953) Malignant melanoma. A clinico-pathological analysis of the criteria for diagnosis and prognosis. Cancer 6:1–45

Alper J, Holmes LB, Mihm MC (1979) Birthmarks with serious medical significance: nevocellular nevi, sebaceous nevi, and multiple café au lait spots. J Pediatr 95:696–700

Altmeyer P, Nodl F, Merkel H (1980) [Lymphogene metastasierungsbereitschaft des maligene melanomas]. Dtsch Med Wochenschr 105:1769–1772

Arbuckle S, Weedon D (1982) Eosinophilic globules in the Spitz nevus. J Am Acad Dermatol 7:324–327

Ariel IM (1982) Malignant melanoma of the trunk: A retrospective review of 1128 patients. Cancer 49:1070–1078

Arrington JH, Reed RJ, Ichinose H, Krementz ET (1977) Plantar lentiginous melanoma: A distinctive variant of human cutaneous malignant melanoma. Am J Surg Pathol 1:131–143

Bagley FH, Cady B, Lee A, Legg MA (1981) Changes in clinical presentation and management of malignant melanoma. Cancer 47:2126–2134

Balch CM, Murad TM, Soong SJ, Ingalls AL, Halpern NB, Maddox WA (1978) A multifactorial analysis of melanoma: Prognostic histopathological features comparing Clark's and Breslow's staging methods. Ann Surg 188:732–742

Balch CM, Murad TM, Soong SJ, Ingalls AL, Richards PC, Maddox WA (1979) Tumor thickness as a güide to surgical management of clinical stage 1 melanoma patients. Cancer 43:883–888

Balch CM, Wilkerson JA, Murad TM, Soong SJ, Ingalls AL, Maddox WA (1980) The prognostic significance of ulceration of cutaneous melanoma. Cancer 45:3012–3017

Balch CM, Soong SJ, Murad TM, Ingalls AL, Maddox WA (1981) A multifactorial analysis of melanoma. III. Prognostic factors in melanoma patients with lymph node metastases (stage II). Ann Surg 193:377–388

Balch CM, Soong SJ, Milton GW, Shaw HM, McGovern VJ, McCarthy WH, Murad TM, Maddox WA (1983) Changing trends in cutaneous melanoma over a quarter century in Alabama, USA, and New South Wales, Australia. Cancer 52:1748–1753

Balch CM, Karakousis C, Mettlin C, Natarajan N, Donegan WL, Smart CR, Murphy GP (1984) Management of cutaneous melanoma in the United States. Surg Gynecol Obstet 158:311–318

Baran LR, Civatte J (1960) Un osteonevus de Nanta aux caractères inusités. B de la Soc Fr de Dermatol et de Syphil 67:109–110

Barr RJ, Morales RV, Graham JH (1980) Desmoplastic nevus. A distict histologic variant of mixed spindle cell and epithelioid cell nevus. Cancer 46:557–564

Bastable JH, Gompel C, Verhest A (1980) Malignant melanoma of the vulva. Diagn Gynecol Obstet 2:55–62

Beardmore GL (1977) Primary cutaneous polypoidal non-stageable melanomas in Queensland. Australas J Dermatol 18:73–76

Beardmore GL, Davis NC (1975) Multiple primary cutaneous melanomas. Arch Dermatol 111:603–609

Beardmore GL, Quinn RL, Little JH (1970) Malignant melanoma in Queensland: Pathology of 105 fatal cutaneous melanomas. Pathology 2:277–286

Becker DW, Miller CJ, Keller HB (1980) Metastatic minimal-deviation melanoma. Ann Plast Surg 4:230–237

Beitner H, Ringborg U, Wennersten G, Lagerlof B (1981) Further evidence for increased light sensitivity in patients with malignant melanoma. Br J Dermatol 104:289–294

Ben-Hur N, Golan J, Rosenberg L, Baruchin A (1981) Pedunculated malignant melanoma. J Dermatol Surg Oncol 7:127–129

Benisch B, Person B, Kannerstein M, Spivack J (1980) Malignant melanoma originating from intradermal nevi. A clinicopathologic entity. Arch Dermatol 116:696–698

Bentley-Phillips CB, Marks R (1976) The epidermal component of melanocytic naevi. J Cutan Pathol 3:190–194

Beral V, Evans S, Shaw H, Milton G (1983) Cutaneous factors related to the risk of melanoma. Br J Dermatol 109:165–172

Berger RS, Voorhees JJ (1971) Multiple congenital giant nevocellular nevi with halos. Arch Dermatol 104:515–521

Berman A, Herszenson S (1981) Vascular response in halo of recent halo nevus. J Am Acad Dermatol 4:537–540

Berry RB, Subbuswamy SG, Hackett MEJ (1982) Desmoplastic malignant melanoma: the first British report. Br J Plast Surg 35:324–327

Bhawan J (1980) Amelanotic melanoma or poorly differentiated melanoma? J Cutan Pathol 7:55–56

Bhawan J, Chang WH, Edelstein LM (1980) Cellular blue nevus. An ultrastructural study. J Cutan Pathol 7:109–122

Bleehen SS (1978) Freckles induced by PUVA treatment. Br J Dermatol 99 (suppl 16):20

Blois MS, Sagebiel RW, Abarbanel RM, Caldwell TM, Tuttle MS (1983a) Malignant melanoma of the skin. 1. The association of tumor depth and type, and patient sex, age and site with survival. Cancer 52:1330–1341

Blois MS, Sagebiel RW, Tuttle MS, Caldwell TM, Taylor HW (1983b) Judging prognosis in malignant melanoma of the skin. A problem of inference over small data sets. Ann Surg 198:200–206

Bondi EE, Clark WH, Elder D, Guerry D, Greene MH (1981) Topical chemotherapy of dysplastic melanocytic nevi with 5% fluorouracil. Arch Dermatol 117:89–92

Bondi EE, Elder D, Guerry D, Clark WH (1983) Target blue nevus. Arch Dermatol 119:919–920

Borkovic SP, Schwartz RA (1983) Amelanotic lentigo maligna melanoma manifesting as a dermatitislike plaque. Arch Dermatol 119:423–425

Braun-Falco O, Korting HC, Konz B (1981) Histological and cytological criteria in the diagnosis of malignant melanomas by cryostat sections. Virchows Arch [Pathol Anat] 393:115–121

Breslow A (1970) Thickness, cross-sectional area and depth of invasion in the prognosis of cutaneous-melanoma. Ann Surg 172:902–908

Breslow A (1975) Tumor thickness, level of invasion and node dissection in Stage 1 cutaneous melanoma. Ann Surg 182:572–575

Breslow A, Macht SD (1978) Evaluation of prognosis in stage 1 cutaneous melanoma. Plast Reconstr Surg 61:342–346
Briele HA, Beattie CW, Ronan SG, Chaudhuri PK, Das Gupta TK (1983) Late recurrence of cutaneous melanoma. Arch Surg 118:800–803
Briggs JC (1980) Reticulin impregnation in the diagnosis of malignant melanoma. Histopathology 4:507–516
Brownstein MH, Kazam BB, Hashimoto K (1977) Halo congenital nevus. Arch Dermatol 113:1572–1575
Brownstein WE (1972) Multiple agminated juvenile melanoma. Arch Dermatol 106:89–91
Bryant E, Ronan SG, Felix EL, Manaligod JR (1982) Desmoplastic malignant melanoma: a study by conventional and electron microscopy. Am J Dermatopathol 4:467–474
Burgdorf W, Nasemann T (1977) Cutaneous osteomas: A clinical and histopathologic review. Arch Dermatol Res 260:121–135
Burkhart CG, Gohara A (1981) Dermal melanocyte hamartoma. A distinctive new form of dermal melanocytosis. Arch Dermatol 117:102–104
Byers RM, Smith JL, Russell N, Rosenberg V (1980) Malignant melanoma of the external ear. Review of 102 cases. Am J Surg 140:518–521
Canizares O (1968) Subnevic folliculitis resembling melanoma. Arch Dermatol 97:363
Capetanakis J (1975) Juvenile melanoma disseminatum. Br J Dermatol 92:207–211
Cassileth BR, Clark WH, Heiberger RM, March V, Tenaglia A (1982) Relationship between patients' early recognition of melanoma and depth of invasion. Cancer 49:198–200
Castilla EE, Dutra MDG, Orioli-Parreiras IM (1981) Epidemiology of congenital pigmented naevi: 1. Incidence rates and relative frequencies. Br J Dermatol 104:307–315
Cesarini JP, Puissant A (1980) Ultrastructure of normal and abnormal melanocytes in one case of familial B-K mole syndrome. J Cutan Pathol 7:186
Civatte J, Tsoitis G, Barrau-Fusade C (1972) Ostéo-melanome juvenile. B de la Soc Fr de Dermatol et de Syphil 78:609–611
Clark WH, Mihm MC (1969) Lentigo maligna and lentigo-maligna melanoma. Am J Pathol 53:39–67
Clark WH, From L, Bernadino EA, Mihm MC (1969) The histogenesis and biologic behavior of primary human malignant melanomas of the skin. Cancer Res 29:705–727
Clark WH, Reimer RR, Greene M, Ainsworth AM, Mastrangelo MJ (1978) Origin of familial malignant melanomas from heritable melanocytic lesions. 'The B-K mole syndrome'. Arch Dermatol 114:732–738
Cohen HJ, Minkin W, Frank SB (1970) Nevus spilus. Arch Dermatol 102:433–437
Coleman WP, Loria PR, Reed RJ, Krementz ET (1980) Acral lentiginous melanoma. Arch Dermatol 116:773–776
Conley J, Lattes R, Orr W (1971) Desmoplastic malignant melanoma. Cancer 28:914–936
Copeman PWM, Lewis MG, Phillips TM, Elliott PG (1973) Immunological associations of the halo naevus with cutaneous malignant melanoma. Br J Dermatol 88:127–137
Cosimi AB, Sober AJ, Mihm MC, Fitzpatrick TB (1984) Conservative surgical management of superficially invasive cutaneous melanoma. Cancer 53:1256–1259
Coskey RJ, Mehregan A (1973) Spindle cell nevi in adults and children. Arch Dermatol 108:535–536
Coskey RJ, Magnell TD, Bernacki EG (1983) Congenital subungual nevus. J Am Acad Dermatol 9:747–751
Cox E, Shingleton WW, Martell J, Nicholson E, Seigler HF (1980) Specific active immunization in melanoma: Prognostic factors. Proc Am Assoc Cancer Res: p 521
Cramer SF, Kiehn CL (1982) Sequential histologic study of evolving lentigo maligna melanoma. Arch Pathol Lab Med 106:121–125
Crucioli V, Stilwell J (1982) The histogenesis of malignant melanoma in relation to pre-existing pigmented lesions. J Cutan Pathol 9:396–404
Danforth DN, Russell N, McBride CM (1982) Hormonal status of patients with primary malignant melanoma: A review of 313 cases. South Med J 75:661–664
Day CL (1982) Subsite concept for metastases in clinical stage 1 melanoma. Lancet 2:154
Day CL, Lew RA (1983a) Malignant melanoma prognostic factors 2: The subsite concept. J Dermatol Surg Oncol 9:525–526
Day CL, Lew RA (1983b) Malignant melanoma prognostic factors 3: Surgical margins. J Dermatol Surg Oncol 9:797–801

Day CL, Lew RA (1984) Malignant melanoma prognostic factors 5: Clinical staging. J Dermatol Surg Oncol 10:351–353

Day CL, Sober AJ, Fitzpatrick TB, Lew RA, Mihm MC (1980) Prognosis in malignant melanoma. J Am Acad Dermatol 3:525–526

Day CL, Harrist TJ, Gorstein F, Sober AJ, Lew RA, Friedman RJ, Pasternack BS, Kopf AW, Fitzpatrick TB, Mihm MC (1981a) Malignant melanoma. Prognostic significance of 'microscopic satellites' in the reticular dermis and subcutaneous fat. Ann Surg 194:108–112

Day CL, Lew RA, Mihm MC, Harris MN, Kopf AW, Sober AJ, Fitzpatrick TB (1981b) The natural break points for primary-tumor thickness in clinical stage 1 melanoma. N Engl J Med 305:1155

Day CL, Sober AJ, Kopf AW, Lew RA, Mihm MC, Golomb FM, Hennessey P, Harris MN, Gumport SL, Raker JW, Malt RA, Cosimi AB, Wood WC, Roses DF, Gorstein F, Fitzpatrick TB, Postel A (1981c) A prognostic model for clinical stage 1 melanoma of the lower extremity. Location on foot as independent risk factor for recurrent disease. Surgery 89:599–603

Day CL, Sober AJ, Kopf AW, Lew RA, Mihm MC, Golomb FM, Postel A, Hennessey P, Harris MN, Gumport SL, Raker JW, Malt RA, Cosimi AB, Wood WC, Roses DF, Gorstein F, Fitzpatrick TB (1981d) A prognostic model for clinical stage 1 melanoma of the trunk. Location near the midline is not an independent risk factor for recurrent disease. Am J Surg 142:247–251

Day CL, Sober AJ, Lew RA, Mihm MC, Fitzpatrick TB, Kopf AW, Harris MN, Gumport SL, Raker JW, Malt RA, Golomb FM, Cosimi AB, Wood WC, Casson P, Lopransi S, Gorstein F, Postel A (1981e) Malignant melanoma patients with positive nodes and relatively good prognoses: Microstaging retains prognostic significance in clinical stage 1 melanoma patients with metastases to regional nodes. Cancer 47:955–962

Day CL, Lew RA, Mihm MC, Sober AJ, Harris MN, Kopf AW, Fitzpatrick TB, Harrist TJ, Golomb FM, Postel A, Hennessey P, Gumport SL, Raker JW, Malt RA, Cosimi AB, Wood WC, Roses DF, Gorstein F, Rigel D, Friedman RJ, Mintzis MM, Grier RW (1982a) A multivariate analysis of prognostic factors for melanoma patients with lesions greater than or equal to 3.65 mm in thickness. The importance of revealing alternative Cox models. Ann Surg 195: 44–49

Day CL, Mihm MC, Lew RA, Harris MN, Kopf AW, Fitzpatrick TB, Harrist TJ, Golomb FM, Postel A, Hennessey P, Gumport SL, Raker JW, Malt RA, Cosimi AB, Wood WC, Roses DF, Gorstein R, Rigel D, Friedman RJ, Mintzis MM, Sober AJ (1982b) Prognostic factors for patients with clinical stage 1 melanoma of intermediate thickness (1.51–3.39 mm). A conceptual model for tumor growth and metastasis. Ann Surg 195:35–43

Day CL, Mihm MC, Sober AJ, Fitzpatrick TB, Malt RA, Kopf AW, Lew RA, Harrist TJ (1982c) Skin lesions suspected to be melanoma should be photographed. Gross morphological features of primary melanoma associated with metastases. JAMA 248:1077–1081

Day CL, Mihm MC, Sober AJ, Harris MN, Kopf AW, Fitzpatrick TB, Lew RA, Harrist TJ, Golomb FM, Postel A, Hennessey P, Gumport SL, Raker JW, Malt RA, Cosimi AB, Wood WC, Roses DF, Gorstein F, Rigel D, Friedman RJ, Mintzis MM (1982d) Prognostic factors for melanoma patients with lesions 0.76–1.69 mm in thickness. An appraisal of 'thin' level IV lesions. Ann Surg 195:30–34

Day CL, Lew RA, Harrist TJ (1984) Malignant melanoma prognostic factors 4: Ulceration width. J Dermatol Surg Oncol 10:23–24

Dhillon AP, Rode J (1982) Patterns of staining for neurone specific enolase in benign and malignant melanocytic lesions of the skin. Diagn Histopathol 5:169–174

Di Maio SM, Mackay B, Smith JL, Dickersin GR (1982) Neurosarcomatous transformation in malignant melanoma. An ultrastructural study. Cancer 50:2345–2354

Drzewiecki KT, Christensen HE, Ladefoged C, Poulsen H (1980) Clinical course of cutaneous malignant melanoma related to histopathological criteria of primary tumour. Scand J Plast Reconstr Surg 14:229–234

Duperrat M, Dufourmentel C (1959) Etude du mélanome juvénile d'apres 40 cas personnels. Minerva Derm 34:190–193

Dvir E, Gellei B, Hirshowitz B (1980) Measurement of tumor thickness as a prognostic tool in primary malignant melanoma of the skin. Ann Plast Surg 5:216–221

Elder DE, Goldman LI, Goldman SC, Greene MH, Clark WH (1980) Dysplastic nevus syndrome. A phenotypic association of sporadic cutaneous melanoma. Cancer 46:1787–1794

Elder DE, Green MH, Guerry D, Kraemer KH, Clark WH (1982) The dysplastic nevus syndrome. Our definition. Am J Dermatopathol 4:455–460

Eldh J, Boeryd B, Peterson LE (1978) Prognostic factors in cutaneous malignant melanoma in stage 1. A clinical, morphological and multivariate analysis. Scand J Plast Reconstr Surg 12:243–255

Eng AM (1983) Solitary small active junctional nevi in juvenile patients. Arch Dermatol 119:35–38

Epstein E, Bragg K (1980) Curability of melanoma: a 25-year retrospective study. Cancer 46:818–821

Everall JD, Dowd PM (1977) Diagnosis, prognosis, and treatment of melanoma. Lancet 2:286–289

Farber EM, Abel EA, Cox AJ (1983) Long-term risks of psoralen and UV-A therapy for psoriasis. Arch Dermatol 119:426–431

Feibleman CE, Stoll H, Maize JC (1980) Melanomas of the palm, sole, and nailbed: A clinocopathologic study. Cancer 46:2492–2504

Feun LG, Gutterman J, Burgess MA, Hersh EM, Mavligit G, McBride CM, Benjamin RS, Richman SP, Murphy WK, Bodey GP, Brown BW, Mountain CF, Leavens ME, Freireich EJ (1982) The natural history of resectable metastatic melanoma (Stage IVA melanoma). Cancer 50:1656–1663

Freeman RG, Knox JM (1962) Epidermal cysts associated with pigmented nevi. Arch Dermatol 85:590–594

Frichot BC, Lynch HT, Guirgis HA, Harris RE, Lynch JF (1977) New cutaneous phenotype in familial malignant melanoma. Lancet 1:864–865

Friedman M, Rao U, Fox S (1982) The cytology of metastatic balloon cell melanoma. Acta Cytol 26:39–43

Friedman RJ, Rigel DS, Kopf AW, Lieblich L, Lew R, Harris MN, Roses DF, Gumport SL, Ragaz A, Waldo E, Levine J, Levenstein M, Koenig R, Bart RS, Trau H (1983) Favorable prognosis for malignant melanomas associated with acquired melanocytic nevi. Arch Dermatol 119:455–462

Frolow GR, Shapiro L, Brownstein MH (1975) Desmoplastic malignant melanoma. Arch Dermatol 111:753–754

From L, Hanna W, Kahn HJ, Gruss J, Marks A, Baumal R (1983) Origin of the desmoplasia in desmoplastic malignant melanoma. Hum Pathol 14:1072–1080

Fulk CS (1984) Primary disorders of hyperpigmentation. J Am Acad Dermatol 10:1–16

Fusaro RM, Lynch HT, Kimberling WJ (1983) Familial atypical multiple mole melanoma syndrome (FAMM). Arch Dermatol 119:2–3

Gardner AW, Vazquez DM (1970) Balloon cell melanoma. Arch Pathol 89:470–472

Gartmann H (1962) Das sog. juvenile Melanom. Munchen Med Wschr 104:587–592

Gartmann H (1981) Der pigmentierte Spindelzellentumor. Z Hautkr 56:862–876

Gauthier Y, Surleve-Bazeille JE, Gauthier O, Texier L (1975) Ultrastructure of halo nevi. J Cutan Pathol 2:71–81

Gauthier Y, Surleve-Bazeille JE, Texier L (1978) Halo nevi without dermal infiltrate. Arch Dermatol 114:1718

Gaynor R, Herschman HR, Irie R, Jones P, Morton D, Cochran A (1981) S 100 protein: a marker for human malignant melanomas? Lancet 1:869–871

Glinick SE, Alper JC, Bogaars H, Brown JA (1983) Becker's melanosis: Associated abnormalities. J Am Acad Dermatol 9:509–514

Goette DK, Doty RD (1978) Balloon cell nevus. Summary of the clinical and histologic characteristics. Arch Dermatol 114:109–111

Goldberg DJ (1983) Amelanotic melanoma presenting as Bowen's disease. J Dermatol Surg Oncol 9:902–904

Gould DJ, Bleehen SS (1980) Multiple agminate juvenile melanoma. Clin Exp Dermatol 5:63–65

Green A, Little JH, Weedon D (1983) The diagnosis of Hutchinson's melanotic freckle (lentigo maligna) in Queensland. Pathology 15:33–35

Greene MH (1984) Dysplastic nevus syndrome. Hosp Pract 19:91–103, 107–108

Greene MH, Goldin LR, Clark WH, Lovrien E, Kraemer KH, Tucker MA, Elder DE, Fraser MC, Rowe S (1983a) Familial cutaneous malignant melanoma: Autosomal dominant trait possibly linked to the Rh locus. Proc Natl Acad Sci USA 80:6071–6075

Greene MH, Sanders RJ, Chu FC, Clark WH, Elder DE, Cogan DG (1983b) The familial occurrence

of cutaneous melanoma, intraocular melanoma and the dysplastic nevus syndrome. Am J Ophthalmol 96:238–245
Griffel M (1981) Survival of cutaneous malignant melanoma patients at University of Iowa Hospitals: 1950–1974. Cancer 47:176–183
Gromet MA, Epstein WL, Blois MS (1978) The regressing thin melanoma. A distinctive lesion with metastatic potential. Cancer 42:2282–2292
Guiliano AE, Cochran AJ, Morton DL (1982) Melanoma from unknown primary site and amelanotic melanoma. Semin Oncol 9:442–447
Haber H (1962) Some observations on common moles. Br J Dermatol 74:224–228
Hacene K, Le Doussal V, Brunet M, Lemoine F, Guerin P, Hebert H (1983) Prognostic index for clinical Stage 1 cutaneous malignant melanoma. Cancer Res 43:2991–2996
Hansen MG, McCarten AB (1974) Tumor thickness and lymphocytic infiltration in malignant melanoma of the head and neck. Am J Surg 128:557–561
Happle R (1974) Kokardennaevus. Hautarzt 25:594–596
Happle R, Traupe H, Vakilzadeh F, Macher E (1982) Arguments in favor of a polygenic inheritance of precursor nevi. J Am Acad Dermatol 6:540–543
Harrist TJ, Rigel DS, Day CL, Sober AJ, Lew RA, Rhodes AR, Harris MH, Kopf AW, Friedman RJ, Golomb FM, Cosimi AB, Gorstein F, Malt RA, Wood WC, Postel A, Hennessey P, Gumport SL, Roses DF, Mintzis MM, Raker JW, Fitzpatrick TB, Mihm MC (1984) "Microscopic satellites" are more highly associated with lymph node metastases than is primary melanoma thickness. Cancer 53:2183–2187
Hashimoto K (1974) Ultrastructural studies of halo nevus. Cancer 34:1653–1666
Hashimoto K, Bale GF (1972) An electron microscopic study of balloon cell nevus. Cancer 30:530–540
Haupt HM, Hood AF, Cohen MH (1984) Inflammatory melanoma. J Am Acad Dermatol 10:52–55
Hendricks WM (1981) Eruptive blue nevi. J Am Acad Dermatol 4:50–53
Hendrickson MR, Ross JC (1981) Neoplasms arising in congenital giant nevi. Morphologic study of seven cases and a review of the literature. Am J Surg Pathol 5:109–135
Holmes EC, Clark W, Morton DL, Eilber FR, Bochow AJ (1976) Regional lymph node metastases and the level of invasion of primary melanoma. Cancer 37:199–201
Horton JJ, MacDonald DM (1983) Balloon cell melanoma: A case report. Br J Dermatol 108:617–619
Houghton AN, Viola MV (1981) Solar radiation and malignant melanoma of the skin. J Am Acad Dermatol 5:477–483
Houghton AN, Flannery J, Viola MV (1981) Malignant melanoma of the skin occurring during pregnancy. Cancer 48:407–410
Hunter JAA, Zaynoun S, Paterson WD, Bleehen SS, MacKie R, Cochran AJ (1978) Cellular fine structure in the invasive nodules of different histogenetic types of malignant melanoma. Br J Dermatol 98:255–272
Huszar M, Halkin H, Herczeg E, Bubis J, Geiger B (1983) Use of antibodies to intermediate filaments in the diagnosis of metastatic amelanotic malignant melanoma. Hum Pathol 14:1006–1008
Huvos AG, Shah JP, Mike V (1974) Prognostic factors in cutaneous malignant melanoma. A comparative study of long term and short term survivors. Hum Pathol 5:347–357
Inoshita T, Youngberg GA (1982) Fluorescence of melanoma cells. A useful diagnostic tool. Am J Clin Pathol 78:311–315
Ironside P, Pitt TTE, Rank BK (1977) Malignant melanoma: Some aspects of pathology and prognosis. Aust NZ J Surg 47:70–75
Ito M, Hamada Y (1952) Nevus spilus en nappe. Tohuku J Exper Med 55:44
Jakubowicz K (1956) Über die Zugehörigkeit des sogenannten juvenilen Melanoms zur Gruppe des aktiven Naevuzellnaevus. Hautarzt 16:411–417
James MP, Wells RS (1980) Cockade naevus: An unusual variant of the benign cellular naevus. Acta Derm Venereol 60:360–363
Jeffrey I, Royston P, Sowter C, Slavin G, Price A, Pomerance A, Goolamali S, Pinto D (1983) Prognostic value of tumour thickness in cutaneous malignant melanoma. J Clin Pathol 36: 51–56
Kahn HJ, Marks A, Thom H, Baumal R (1983) Role of antibody to S 100 protein in diagnostic pathology. Am J Clin Pathol 79:341–347

Kamino H, Misheloff E, Ackerman AB, Flotte TJ, Greco MA (1979) Eosinophilic globules in Spitz's nevi. New findings and a diagnostic sign. Am J Dermatopathol 1:319–324
Kaplan EN (1974) The risk of malignancy in large congenital nevi. Plast Reconstr Surg 53:421–428
Karakousis CP, Temple DF, Moore R, Ambrus JL (1983) Prognostic parameters in recurrent malignant melanoma. Cancer 52:575–579
Kernen JA, Ackerman LV (1960) Spindle cell nevi and epithelioid cell nevi (so-called juvenile melanomas) in children and adults. A clinicopathological study of 27 cases. Cancer 13:612–625
Keyhani A (1977) Comparison of clinical behavior of melanoma of the hands and feet. A study of 238 patients. Cancer 40:3168–3173
Kirschenbaum MB (1981) Congenital melanocytic nevi. Arch Dermatol 117:379
Kline TS, Kannan V (1982) Aspiration biopsy cytology and melanoma. Am J Clin Pathol 77:597–601
Koh HK, Sober AJ, Nakagawa H, Albert DM, Mihm MC, Fitzpatrick TB (1983) Malignant melanoma and vitiligo-like leukoderma. An electron microscopic study. J Am Acad Dermatol 9:696–708
Kopf A, Andrade R (1966) Benign juvenile melanoma. In Baer R & Kopf A (eds) Yearbook of dermatology (1965–1966), Yearbook Medical Publishers, Chicago, pp 7–52
Kopf AW, Bart RS (1982) Malignant Blue (Ota's?) nevus. J Dermatol Surg Oncol 8:442–445
Kopf AW, Bart RS, Hennessey P (1979) Congenital nevocytic nevi and malignant melanoma. J Am Acad Dermatol 1:123–130
Kopf AW, Rigel D, Bart RS, Mintzis MM, Hennessey P, Harris MN, Ragaz A, Trau H, Friedman RJ, Esrig B (1981) Factors related to thickness of melanoma. Multifactorial analysis of variables correlated with thickness of superficial spreading malignant melanoma in man. J Dermatol Surg Oncol 7:645–650
Kopf AW, Rodriguez-Sains RS, Rigel DS, Friedman RJ, Bart RS, Grier WR, Mintzis MM, Postel AH (1982) Small melanomas: relation of prognostic variables to diameter of primary superficial spreading melanomas. J Dermatol Surg Oncol 8:765–770
Kornberg R, Ackerman AB (1975) Pseudomelanoma. Recurrent melanocytic nevus following partial surgical removal. Arch Dermatol 111:1588–1590
Kraemer K (1983) Dysplastic nevi as precursors to hereditary melanoma. J Dermatol Surg Oncol 9:619–622
Kraemer KH, Greene MH, Tarone R, Elder DE, Clark WH, Guerry D (1983) Dysplastic naevi and cutaneous melanoma risk. Lancet 2:1076–1077
Krakowski A, Tur E, Brenner S (1981) Multiple agminated juvenile melanoma: A case with a sunburn history, and a review. Dermatologica 163:270–275
Krementz ET, Reed RJ, Coleman WP, Sutherland CM, Carter RD, Campbell M (1982) Acral lentiginous melanoma. A clinicopathologic entity. Ann Surg 195:632–645
Krivanek JFC, Cains GD, Paver K (1977) Halo eczema and junctional naevi: A case report. Australas J Dermatol 18:81–83
Kuehnl-Petzoldt C, Berger H, Wiebelt H (1982) Verrucous-keratotic variations of malignant melanoma. A clinicopathological study. Am J Dermatopathol 4:403–410
Kuehnl-Petzoldt C, Wiebelt H, Berger H (1983) Prognostic groups of patients with stage 1 melanoma. Arch Dermatol 119:816–819
Labrecque PG, Hu C-H, Winkelmann RK (1976) On the nature of desmoplastic melanoma. Cancer 38:1205–1212
Lambert WC, Brodkin RH (1984) Nodal and subcutaneous cellular blue nevi. A pseudometastasizing pseudomelanoma. Arch Dermatol 120:367–370
Lamovec J (1984) Blue nevus of the lymph node capsule. Report of a new case with review of the literature. Am J Clin Pathol 81:367–372
Lancer HA, Muhlbauer JE, Sober AJ (1983) Multiple agminated spindle cell nevi: Unique clinical presentation and review. J Am Acad Dermatol 8:707–711
Lanier VC, Pickrell KL, Georgiade NG (1976) Congenital giant nevi: Clinical and pathological considerations. Plast Reconstr Surg 58:48–54
Larsen TE, Grude TH (1978a) A retrospective histological study of 669 cases of primary cutaneous malignant melanoma in clinical stage 1. 2. The relation of cell type, pigmentation, atypia and mitotic count to histological type and prognosis. Acta Path Microbiol Scand [A] 86:513–522
Larsen TE, Grude TH (1978b) A retrospective histological study of 669 cases of primary cutaneous malignant melanoma in clinical stage 1. 3. The relation between the tumour-associated lymphocyte

infiltration and age and sex, tumour cell type, pigmentation, cellular atypia, mitotic count, depth of invasion, ulceration, tumour type and prognosis. Acta Path Microbiol Scand [A] 86:523–530

Larsen TE, Grude TH (1979) A retrospective histological study of 669 cases of primary cutaneous malignant melanoma in clinical stage 1. 4. The relation of cross-sectional profile, level of invasion, ulceration and vascular invasion to tumour type and prognosis. Acta Path Microbiol Scand [A] 87:131–138

Lee YTN (1980) Diagnosis, treatment and prognosis of early melanoma. The importance of depth of microinvasion. Ann Surg 191:87–97

Lemish WM, Heenan PJ, Holman CDJ, Armstrong BK (1983) Survival from preinvasive and invasive malignant melanoma in Western Australia. Cancer 52:580–585

Levene A (1979) Disseminated dermal melanocytosis terminating in melanoma. Br J Dermatol 101:197–205

Levene A (1980) On the histological diagnosis and prognosis of malignant melanoma. J Clin Pathol 33:101–124

Levine J, Kopf AW, Rigel DS, Bart RS, Hennessey P, Friedman RJ, Mintzis MM (1981) Correlation of thicknesses of superficial spreading malignant melanomas and ages of patients. J Dermatol Surg Oncol 7:311–316

Lew RA, Sober AJ, Cook N, Marvell R, Fitzpatrick TB (1983) Sun exposure habits in patients with cutaneous melanoma: A case control study. J Dermatol Surg Oncol 9:981–986

Lewis MG, Phillips TM, Noble PB, Hartmann DP (1979) Immune derangement in patients with malignant melanoma. J Cutan Pathol 6:201–207

Liestøl K, Larsen TE, Grude TH (1982) A retrospective histological study of 669 cases of primary cutaneous malignant melanoma in clinical stage I. 8. The relative prognostic value of various clinical and histological features evaluated by Cox's regression model. Acta Pathol Microbiol Immunol Scand [A] 90:449–454

Little JH (1972) Histology and prognosis in cutaneous malignant melanoma. In Melanoma and Skin Cancer, ed WH McCarthy, New South Wales Government Printer, Syndney, pp 107–119

Little JH, Davis NC (1974) Frozen section diagnosis of suspected malignant melanoma of the skin. Cancer 34:1163–1172

Little JH, Holt J, Davis N (1980) Changing epidemiology of malignant melanoma in Queensland. Med J Aust 1:66–69

Lopansri S, Mihm MC (1979) Clinical and pathological correlation of malignant melanoma. J Cutan Pathol 6:180–194

Lorentzen M, Pers M, Bretteville-Jensen G (1977) The incidence of malignant transformation in giant pigmented nevi. Scand J Plast Reconstr Surg 11:163–167

Lynch HT, Frichot BC, Lynch JF (1978) Familial atypical multiple mole-melanoma syndrome. J Med Genet 15:352–256

Lynch HT, Fusaro RM, Pester J, Lynch JF (1980) Familial atypical multiple mole melanoma (FAMMM) syndrome: Genetic heterogeneity and malignant melanoma. Br J Cancer 42:58–70

Lynch HT, Fusaro RM, Pester J, Oosterhuis JA, Went LN, Rumke P, Neering H, Lynch JF (1981) Tumour spectrum in the FAMMM syndrome. Br J Cancer 44:553–560

MacDonald DM, Black MM (1980) Secondary localized cutaneous amyloidosis in melanocytic naevi. Br J Dermatol 103:553–556

MacKie RM (1981) Which moles matter? The association between melanocytic naevi and malignant melanomata. Br J Dermatol 105:607–609

MacKie RM (1982) Multiple melanoma and atypical melanocytic naevi – evidence of an activated and expanded melanocytic system. Br J Dermatol 107:621–629

MacKie RM, Campbell I, Turbitt ML (1984) Use of NK1 C3 monoclonal antibody in the assessment of benign and malignant melanocytic lesions. J Clin Pathol 37:367–372

Macy-Roberts E, Ackerman AB (1982) A critique of techniques for biopsy of clinically suspected malignant melanomas. Am J Dermatopathol 4:391–398

Maize JC (1983) Primary cutaneous malignant melanoma. An analysis of the prognostic value of histologic characteristics. J Am Acad Dermatol 8:857–863

Maize JC, Foster G (1979) Age-related changes in melanocytic naevi. Clin Exp Dermatol 4:49–58

Man D, Weiner LJ, Reiman HM (1981) Desmoplastic malignant melanoma: a case report. Br J Plast Surg 34:79–82

Manci EA, Balch CM, Murad TM, Soong SJ (1981) Polypoid melanoma, a virulent variant of the nodular growth pattern. Am J Clin Pathol 75:810–815

Mark GJ, Mihm MC, Liteplo MG, Reed RJ, Clark WH (1973) Congenital melanocytic nevi of the small and garment type. Clinical, histologic, and ultrastructural studies. Hum Pathol 4:395–418

Marks JG, White JW (1980) Molluscum contagiosum in a halo nevus. Int J Dermatol 19:258–259

Marx JL, Auerbach R, Possick P, Myrow R, Gladstein AH, Kopf AW (1983) Malignant melanoma in situ in two patients treated with psoralens and ultraviolet A. J Am Acad Dermatol 9:904–911

Matsudo H, Reed WB, Homme D, Bartok W, Horowitz R (1973) Zosteriform lentiginous nevus. Arch Dermatol 107:902–905

McBride CM, Smith JL, Brown BW (1981) Primary malignant melanoma of the limbs: a re-evaluation using microstaging techniques. Cancer 48:1463–1468

McBurney EI, Herron CB (1979) Melanoma mimicking plantar wart. J Am Acad Dermatol 1:144–146

McDonald JS, Miller RL, Wagner W, Giammara B (1983) Acral lentiginous melanoma of the oral cavity. Head Neck Surg 5:257–262

McGovern VJ (1970) The classification of melanoma and its relationship with prognosis. Pathology 2:85–98

McGovern VJ (1975) Spontaneous regression of melanoma. Pathology 7:91–99

McGovern VJ, Mihm MC, Bailly C, Booth JC, Clark WH, Cochran AJ, Hardy EG, Hicks JD, Levene A, Lewis MG, Little JH, Milton GW (1973) The classification of malignant melanoma and its histologic reporting. Cancer 32:1446–1457

McGovern VJ, Shaw HM, Milton GW, Farago GA (1979) Prognostic significance of the histological features of malignant melanoma. Histopathology 3:385–393

McGovern VJ, Shaw HM, Milton GW, Farago GA (1980) Is malignant melanoma arising in a Hutchinson's melanotic freckle a separate disease entity? Histopathology 4:235–242

McGovern VJ, Shaw HM, Milton GW, McCarthy WH (1982) Ulceration and prognosis in cutaneous malignant melanoma. Histopathology 6:399–407

McGovern VJ, Shaw HM, Milton GW (1983a) Prognostic significance of a polypoid configuration in malignant melanoma. Histopathology 7:663–672

McGovern VJ, Shaw HM, Milton GW (1983b) Prognosis in patients with thin malignant melanoma: influence of regression. Histopathology 7:673–680

McGovern VJ, Shaw HM, Milton GW (1984) Histogenesis of malignant melanoma with an adjacent component of superficial spreading type. Pathology (to be published)

McWhorter HE, Wooner LB (1954) Pigmented nevi, juvenile melanomas, and malignant melanomas in children. Cancer 7:564–585

Mehregan AH, Coskey RJ (1972) Pigmented nevi of sole. A report of two cases with histologic evidence of hair follicle formation. Arch Dermatol 106:886–887

Mehregan AH, King JR (1972) Multiple target-like pigmented nevi. Arch Dermatol 105:129–130

Mehregan AH, Staricco RG (1962) Elastic fibers in pigmented nevi. J Invest Dermatol 38:271–276

Mevorah B, Frenk E, Delacretaz J (1977) Dermal melanocytosis. Report of an unusual case. Dermatologica 154:107–114

Meyerson LB (1971) A peculiar papulosquamous eruption involving pigmented nevi. Arch Dermatol 103:510–512

Michalik EE, Fitzpatrick TB, Sober AJ (1983) Rapid progression of lentigo maligna to deeply invasive lentigo maligna melanoma. Report of two cases. Arch Dermatol 119:831–835

Miettinen M, Lehto VP, Virtanen I (1983) Presence of fibroblast-type intermediate filaments (vimentin) and absence of neurofilaments in pigmented nevi and malignant melanomas. J Cutan Pathol 10:188–192

Milton GW, Shaw HM, Farago GA, McCarthy WH (1980) Tumour thickness and the site and time of first recurrence in cutaneous malignant melanoma (stage 1). Br J Surg 67:543–546

Mintzis MM, Silvers DN (1978) Ultrastructural study of superficial spreading melanoma and benign simulants. Cancer 42:502–511

Mishima Y (1973) Eccrine-centered nevus. Arch Dermatol 107:59–61

Montagna W, Hu F, Carlisle K (1980) A reinvestigation of solar lentigines. Arch Dermatol 116:1151–1154

Morgan AC, Crane MM, Rossen RD (1984) Measurement of a monoclonal antibody-defined, melanoma-associated antigen in human sera: correlation of circulating antigen levels with tumour burden. JNCI 72:243–249

Morishima T, Nagashima N (1983) Formaldehyde-induced fluorescence method for touch preparations from amelanotic melanoma tissues: a simple and rapid method for the demonstration of melanogenic activities of amelanotic melanoma cells. Acta Derm Venereol 63:418–421

Morishima T, Endo M, Imagawa I, Morioka S (1976) Clinical and histopathological studies on spotted grouped pigmented nevi with special reference to eccrine-centered nevus. Acta Derm Venereol 56:345–351

Moseley HS, Giuliano AE, Storm FK, Clark WH, Robinson DS, Morton DL (1979) Multiple primary melanoma. Cancer 43:939–944

Muhlbauer JE, Margolis RJ, Mihm MC, Reed RJ (1983) Minimal deviation melanoma: A histologic variant of cutaneous malignant melanoma in its vertical growth phase. J Invest Dermatol 80 Suppl: 63s–65s

Nakajima T, Watanabe S, Sato Y, Kameya T, Shimosato Y, Ishihara K (1982) Immunohistochemical demonstration of S 100 protein in malignant melanoma and pigmented nevus, and its diagnostic application. Cancer 50:912–918

Nakano GM, Natale RB, Lobuglio AF, Hughton AN (1984) Immunoperoxidase staining of early human melanoma colonies with monoclonal antibodies. A new method for in vitro antigenic-morphologic correlation. Am J Pathol 114:380–386

National Institutes of Health Consensus Development Conference (1983) Precursors to malignant melanoma. Volume 4, No. 9.

Nicholls EM (1973) Development and elimination of pigmented moles, and the anatomical distribution of primary malignant melanoma. Cancer 32:191–195

Niven J, Lubin J (1975) Pedunculated malignant melanoma. Arch Dermatol 111:755–756

Nordlund JJ, Kirkwood JM, Forget BM, Milton G, Albert DM, Lerner AB (1983) Vitiligo in patients with metastatic melanoma: a good prognostic sign. J Am Acad Dermatol 9:689–696

Okun MR (1979) Melanoma resembling spindle and epithelioid cell nevus. Report of three cases. Arch Dermatol 115:1416–1420

Okun MR, Di Mattia A, Thompson J, Pearson SH (1974a) Malignant melanoma developing from intradermal nevi. Arch Dermatol 110:599–601

Okun MR, Donellan B, Edelstein L (1974b) An ultrastructural study of balloon cell nevus. Cancer 34:615–625

Olson RM, Woods JE, Soule EH (1981) Regional lymph node management and outcome in 100 patients with head and neck melanoma. Am J Surg 142:470–473

Pacot C, Noury G, Umbert P (1972) Mélanome juvénile de Spitz et ostéome. Bde la Soc Fr de Dermatol et de Syphil 78:611–612

Paladugu RR, Yonemoto RH (1983) Biologic behavior of thin malignant melanomas with regressive changes. Arch Surg 118:41–44

Paladugu RR, Winberg CD, Yonemoto RH (1983) Acral lentiginous melanoma. A clinicopathologic study of 36 patients. Cancer 52:161–168

Palangie A, Lassau F, Moreau T, Noury-Duperrat G, Cottenot F (1981) [Stage 1 malignant melanoma of the skin. Prognostic value of thickness and level]. Nouv Presse Med 10:2337–2341

Palmer AA (1983) Recent methods for identifying amelanotic melanoma. Paper presented at the Conference on Malignant Melanoma, November 26, 1983, Sydney.

Paniago-Pereira C, Maize JC, Ackerman AB (1978) Nevus of large spindle and/or epithelioid cells (Spitz's nevus). Arch Dermatol 114:1811–1823

Papachristou DN, Fortner JG (1982) Melanoma arising under the nail. J Surg Oncol 21:219–222

Patterson RH, Helwig EB (1980) Subungual malignant melanoma. A clinical-pathologic study. Cancer 46:2074–2087

Paver K, Stewart M, Kossard S, Krivanek J (1981) Amelanotic lentigo maligna. Australas J Dermatol 22:106–108

Pellegrini AE (1982) The dysplastic nevus syndrome: What is it? Am J Dermatopathol 4:453–454

Penman HG, Stringer HCW (1971) Malignant transformation in giant congenital pigmented nevus. Arch Dermatol 103:428–432

Penneys NS, Mogollon R, Kowalczyk A, Nadji M, Adachi K (1984) A survey of cutaneous neural lesions for the presence of myelin basic protein. An Immunohistochemical study. Arch Dermatol 120:210–213

Pers M (1963) Naevus pigmentosus giganticus. Ugeskr Laeger 125:613–619
Person JR, Longcope C (1984) Becker's nevus: An androgen-mediated hyperplasia with increased androgen receptors. J Am Acad Dermatol 10:235–238
Peterson LL, Serrill WS (1984) Lentiginosis associated with left atrial myxoma. J Am Acad Dermatol 10:337–340
Pihl E, Jansson B, Schwartz MA, Malahy MA, Smith JL, Gutterman JV, Hersh EM (1982) Germinal centre hyperplasia: an unfavourable immune response in recurrent malignant melanoma. Pathology 14:13–16
Port M, Courniotes J, Podwal M (1978) Zosteriform lentiginous naevus with ipsilateral rigid cavus foot. Br J Dermatol 98:693–698
Prade M, Bognel C, Charpentier P, Gadenne C, Duvillard P, Sancho-Garnier H, Petit JY (1982) Malignant melanoma of the skin: Prognostic factors derived from a multifactorial analysis of 239 cases. Am J Dermatopathol 4:411–412
Price NM, Rywlin AM, Ackerman AB (1976) Histologic criteria for the diagnosis of superficial spreading malignant melanoma formulated on the basis of proven metastatic lesions. Cancer 38:2434–2441
Rahbari H, Mehregan AH (1975) Trichoepithelioma and pigmented nevus. A combined malformation. J Cutan Pathol 2:225–231
Rahbari H, Mehregan AH (1981) Sporadic atypical mole syndrome. A report of five nonfamilial B-K mole syndrome-like cases and histopathologic findings. Arch Dermatol 117:329–331
Ramaekers FC, Puts JJ, Moesker O, Kant A, Vooijs GP, Jap PH (1983) Intermediate filaments in malignant melanoma. Identification and use as a marker in surgical pathology. J Clin Invest 71:635–643
Rampen F (1980) Malignant melanoma. Sex differences in survival after evidence of distant metastasis. Br J Cancer 42:52–57
Rampen F (1981) Changing concepts in melanoma management. Br J Dermatol 104:341–348
Rampen FHJ, Van Houten WA, Hop WCJ (1980) Incisional procedures and prognosis in malignant melanoma. Clin Exp Dermatol 5:313–320
Redman JC (1983) Calling malignant melanoma in situ what it is. Finding from a recent survey may make this possible. Am J Dermatopathol 5:297–298
Reed RJ (1978) Consultation case. Am J Surg Pathol 2:215–220
Reed RJ (1980) Malignant Spitz naevus. Case presented at the Clinicopathology Conference, American Academy of Dermatology Meeting, New York, December 1980
Reed RJ, Leonard DD (1979) Neurotropic melanoma. A variant of desmoplastic melanoma. Am J Surg Pathol 3:301–311
Reed RJ, Ichinose H, Clark WH, Mihm MC (1975) Common and uncommon melanocytic nevi and borderline melanomas. Semin Oncol 2:119–147
Reed WB, Becker SW Jr, Becker SW, Nickel WR (1965) Giant pigmented nevi, melanoma, and leptomeningeal melanocytosis: A clinical and histopathological study. Arch Dermatol 91:100–119
Reichert CM, Rosenberg SA, Weber BL, Costa J (1981) Malignant melanoma; a search for occult lymph node metastases. Hum Pathol 12:449–451
Reimer RR, Clark WH, Greene MH, Ainsworth AM, Fraumeni JF (1978) precursor lesions in familial melanoma. A New genetic preneoplastic syndrome. JAMA 239:744–746
Rhodes AR, Melski JW (1982) Small congenital nevocellular nevi and the risk of cutaneous melanoma. J Pediatr 100:219–224
Rhodes AR, Wood WC, Sober AJ, Mihm MC (1981) Non epidermal origin of malignant melanoma associated with a giant congenital nevocellular nevus. Plast Reconstruct Surg 67:782–790
Rhodes AR, Sober AJ, Day CL, Melski JW, Harrist TJ, Mihm MC, Fitzpatrick TB (1982) The malignant potential of small congenital nevocellular nevi. An estimate of association based on a histologic study of 234 primary cutaneous melanomas. J Am Acad Dermatol 6:230–241
Rhodes AR, Harrist TJ, Day CL, Mihm MC, Fitzpatrick TB, Sober AJ (1983a) Dysplastic melanocytic nevi in histologic association with 234 primary cutaneous melanomas. J Am Acad Dermatol 9:563–574
Rhodes AR, Melski JW, Sober AJ, Harrist TJ, Mihm MC, Fitzpatrick TB (1983b) Increased intraepidermal melanocyte frequency and size in dysplastic melanocytic nevi and cutaneous melanoma. A comparative quantitative study of dysplastic melanocytic nevi, superficial spreading melanoma, nevocellular nevi, and solar lentigines. J Invest Dermatol 80:452–459

Rhodes AR, Stern RS, Melski JW (1983c) The PUVA lentigo: An analysis of predisposing factors. J Invest Dermatol 81:459–463

Rhodes AR, Harrist TJ, Momtaz-TK (1984) The PUVA-induced pigmented macule: A lentiginous proliferation of large, sometimes cytologically atypical, melanocytes. J Am Acad Dermatol 9:47–58

Roberts G, Martyn AL, Dobson AJ, McCarthy WH (1981) Tumour thickness and histological type in malignant melanoma in New South Wales, Australia, 1970–76. Pathology 13:763–770

Rogers GS, Kopf AW, Rigel DS, Friedman RJ, Levine JL, Levenstein M, Bart RS, Mintzis MM (1983) Effect of anatomical location on prognosis in patients with clinical stage 1 melanoma. Arch Dermatol 119:644–649

Rosenberg L, Goldstein J, Ben-Yakar Y, Mahler D (1981) The pedunculated malignant melanoma: A misunderstood and neglected variant. J Dermatol Surg Oncol 7:123–126

Roses DF, Harris MN, Hidalgo D, Valensi QJ, Dubin N (1982) Primary melanoma thickness correlated with regional lymph node metastases. Arch Surg 117:921–923

Royds JA, Parsons MA, Rennie IG, Timperley WR, Taylor CB (1982) Enolase isoenzymes in benign and malignant melanocytic lesions. Diagn Histopathol 5:175–181

Rupec M, Huck HJ (1976) Zur Frage des sogenannten osteo-Naevus Nanta. Dermatologische Monatsschrift 162:730–737

Ruth WK, Shelburne JD, Jegasothy BV (1980) Zosteriform lentiginous nevus. Arch Dermatol 116:478

Sagebiel RW (1972) Histologic artifacts of benign pigmented nevi. Arch Dermatol 106:691–693

Sagebiel RW (1979) Histopathology of borderline and early malignant melanomas. Am J Surg Pathol 3:543–552

Sato S, Kato H, Hidano A (1979) Divided nevus spilus and divided form of spotted grouped pigmented nevus. J Cutan Pathol 6:507–512

Saunders TS (1957) Abscess formation in pigmented nevi. Report of three cases. Arch Dermatol 76:189–192

Schellander F, Mark R, Wilson Jones E (1974) Basal cell hamartoma and cellular naevus. An unusual combined malformation. Br J Dermatol 90:413–419

Schmoeckel C, Braun-Falco O (1978) Prognostic index in malignant melanoma. Arch Dermatol 114:871–873

Schmoeckel C, Bockelbrink A, Bockelbrink H, Braun-Falco O (1983a) Low-and high-risk malignant melanoma-II. Multivariate analyses for a prognostic classification. Eur J Cancer Clin Oncol 19:237–243

Schmoeckel C, Bockelbrink A, Bockelbrink H, Kistler H, Braun-Falco O (1983b) Low-and high-risk malignant melanoma-III. Prognostic significance of the resection margin. Eur J Cancer Clin Oncol 19:245–249

Schmoeckel C, Bockelbrink A, Bockelbrink H, Koutsis J, Braun-Falco O (1983c) Low-and high-risk malignant melanoma-I. Evaluation of clinical and histological prognosticators in 585 cases. Eur J Cancer Clin Oncol 19:227–235

Schrader WA, Helwig EB (1967) Balloon cell nevi. Cancer 20:1502–1514

Seiji M, Takematsu H, Hosokawa M, Obata M, Tomita Y, Kato T, Takahashi M, Mihm MC (1983) Acral melanoma in Japan. J Invest Dermatol 80 Suppl: 56s–60s

Shafir R, Hiss J, Tsur H, Bubis JJ (1982) The thin malignant melanoma: Changing patterns of epidemiology and treatment. Cancer 50:817–819

Shafir R, Hiss J, Tsur H, Bubis JJ (1983) Pitfalls in frozen section diagnosis of malignant melanoma. Cancer 51:1168–1170

Shaw HM, Milton GW, McCarthy WH, Farago GA, Dilworth P (1979) Effect of smoking on the recurrence of malignant melanoma. Med J Aust 1:208–209

Shaw HM, McGovern VJ, Milton GW, Farago GA, McCarthy WH (1980a) Histologic features of tumors and the female superiority in survival from malignant melanoma. Cancer 45:1604–1608

Shaw HM, McGovern VJ, Milton GW, Farago GA, McCarthy WH (1980b) Malignant melanoma: Influence of site of lesion and age of patient in the female superiority in survival. Cancer 46:2731–2735

Shaw HM, McGovern VJ, Milton GW, Farago GA, McCarthy WH (1982) The female superiority in survival in clinical stage II cutaneous malignent melanoma. Cancer 49:1941–1944

Shiffman N, Arndt KA, Noe JM (1980) Acral lentiginous melanoma. Ann Plast Surg 5:232–235

Shiu MH, Schottenfeld D, Maclean B, Fortner JG (1976) Adverse effect of pregnancy on melanoma. A reappraisal. Cancer 37:181–187

Sigal C, Saunders TS (1967) Basal cell epithelioma and nevus pigmentosus, their simultaneous occurrence. Arch Dermatol 96:520–523

Silvers DN, Helwig EB (1981) Melanocytic nevi in neonates. J Am Acad Dermatol 4:166–175

Siminovitch JM, Bergfeld W, Dinner M (1980) Exophytic (pedunculated) malignant melanoma – Cleveland Clinic experience. Ann Plast Surg 5:432–435

Simões GA (1981) Speckled zosteriform lentiginous nevus. J Am Acad Dermatol 4:236–238

Smith PJ, Greene MH, Devlin DA, McKeen EA, Paterson MC (1982) Abnormal sensitivity to UV-radiation in cultured skin fibroblasts from patients with hereditary cutaneous malignant melanoma and dysplastic nevus syndrome. Int J Cancer 30:39–45

Smith PJ, Greene MH, Adams D, Paterson MC (1983) Abnormal responses to the carcinogen 4-nitroquinoline 1-oxide of cultured fibroblasts from patients with dysplastic nevus syndrome and hereditary cutaneous malignant melanoma. Carcinogenesis 4:911–916

Sober AJ, Fitzpatrick TB, Mihm MC (1980) Primary melanoma of the skin: Recognition and management. J Am Acad Dermatol 2:179–197

Sober AJ, Day CL, Fitzpatrick TB, Lew RA, Kopf AW, Mihm MC (1983a) Early death from clinical stage 1 melanoma. J Invest Dermatol 80: Supl:50s–52s

Sober AJ, Day CL, Fitzpatrick TB, Lew RA, Kopf AW, Mihm MC (1983b) Factors associated with death from melanoma from 2 to 5 years following diagnosis in clinical stage 1 patients. J Invest Dermatol 80 Suppl:53s–55s

Solomon AR, Ellis CN, Headington JT (1983) An evaluation of vertical growth in thin superficial spreading melanomas by sequential serial microscopic sections. Cancer 52:2338–2341

Sondergaard K (1983) Histological type and biological behavior of primary cutaneous malignant melanoma. 2. An analysis of 86 cases located on so-called acral region as plantar, palmar and sub-/parungual areas. Virchows Arch [A] 401:333–343

Sondergaard K, Olsen G (1980) Malignant melanoma of the foot. A clinicopathological study of 125 primary cutaneous malignant melanomas. Acta Pathol Microbiol Scand [A] 88:275–283

Spiegel J, Nadji M, Penneys NS (1983) Fibrous papule: An immunohistochemical study with an antibody to S-100 protein. J Am Acad Dermatol 9:360–362

Spitz S (1948) Melanomas of childhood. Am J Pathol 24:591–609

Stefansson K, Wollmann R, Jerkovic M (1982) S-100 protein in soft-tissue tumors derived from Schwann cells and melanocytes. Am J Pathol 106:261–268

Stegmaier OC (1959) Natural regression of the melanocytic nevus. J Invest Dermatol 32:413–419

Stegmaier OC, Becker SW (1960) Incidence of melanocytic nevi in young adults. J Invest Dermatol 34:125–128

Stenn KS, Arons M, Hurwitz S (1983) Patterns of congenital nevocellular nevi. A histologic study of thirty-eight cases. J Am Acad Dermatol 9:388–393

Stewart DM, Altman J, Mehregan AH (1978) Speckled lentiginous nevus. Arch Dermatol 114:895–896

Sutula FC, Dortzbach RK, Bolles JC (1982) Desmoplastic malignant melanoma of the upper eyelid. Ann Ophthalmol 14:141–143

Thompson GW, Diehl AK (1980) Partial unilateral lentiginosis. Arch Dermatol 116:356

Trau H, Kopf AW, Rigel DS, Levine J, Rogers G, Levenstein M, Bart RS, Mintzis MM, Friedman RJ (1983a) Regression in malignant melanoma. J Am Acad Dermatol 8:363–368

Trau H, Rigel DS, Harris MN, Kopf AW, Friedman RJ, Gumport SL, Bart RS, Grier WRN (1983b). Metastases of thin melanomas. Cancer 51:553–556

Tucker MA, Greene MH, Clark WH, Kraemer KH, Fraser MC, Elder DE (1983) Dysplastic nevi on the scalp of prepubertal children from melanoma-prone families. J Pediatr 103:65–69

Tucker SB, Horstmann JP, Hertel B, Aranha G, Rosai J (1980) Activation of nevi in patients with malignant melanoma. Cancer 46:822–827

Unger SW, Wanebo HJ, Cooper PH (1981) Multiple cutaneous malignant melanomas with features of primary melanoma. Ann Surg 193:245–250

Uribe MGA (1976) The Mongoloid spot. Australas J Dermatol 17:61–64

Valensi QJ (1977) Desmoplastic malignant melanoma. A report on two additional cases. Cancer 39:286–292

Valensi QJ (1979) Desmoplastic malignant melanoma. A light and electron microscopic study of two cases. Cancer 43:1148–1155

Van der Esch EP, Cascinelli N, Preda F, Morabito A, Bufalino R (1981) Stage 1 melanoma of the skin: Evaluation of prognosis according to histologic characteristics. Cancer 48:1668–1673
Van Duinen SG, Ruiter DJ, Scheffer E (1983) A staining procedure for melanin in semithin and ultrathin epoxy sections. Histopathology 7:35–48
Van Duinen SG, Ruiter DJ, Hageman P, Vennegoor C, Dickersin GR, Scheffer E, Rumke P (1984) Immunohistochemical and histochemical tools in the diagnosis of amelanotic melanoma. Cancer 53:1566–1573
Vázquez M, Ramos FA, Sánchez JL (1984) Melanomas of volar and subungual skin in Puerto Ricans. A clinicopathologic study. J Am Acad Dermatol 10:39–45
Wallace HJ (1974) Eruptive juvenile melanomata. Br J Dermatol 91 (Suppl 10):37–38
Walton RG, Jacobs AH, Cox AJ (1976) Pigmented lesions in newborn infants. Br J Dermatol 95:389–396
Wanebo HJ, Woodruff J, Fortner JG (1975) Malignant melanoma of the extremities: A clinicopathologic study using levels of invasion (microstage). Cancer 35:666–676
Warin AP (1976) Cockarde naevus. Clin Exp Dermatol 1:221–224
Warkel RL, Luna LG, Helwig EB (1980) A modified Warthin-Starry procedure at low pH for melanin. Am J Clin Pathol 73:812–815
Warner TFCS, Gilbert EF, Ramirez G (1980a) Epidermotropism in melanoma. J Cutan Pathol 7:50–54
Warner TFCS, Seo IS, Bennett JE (1980b) Minimal deviation melanoma with epidermotropic metastases arising in a congenital nevus. Am J Surg Pathol 4:175–183
Warner TFCS, Hafez GR, Finch RE, Brandenberg JH (1981) Schwann cell features in neurotropic melanoma. J Cut Pathol 8:177–187
Warner TFCS, Hafez GR, Buchler DA (1982) Neurotropic melanoma of the vulva. Cancer 49:999–1004
Warner TFCS, Hafez GR, Padmalatha C, Lange TA (1983) Acral lentiginous melanoma simulating clear cell sarcoma of tendon and aponeuroses. J Cut Pathol 10:193–200
Warner TFCS, Lloyd RV, Hafez GR, Angevine JM (1984) Immunocytochemistry of neurotropic melanoma. Cancer 53:254–257
Weedon D (1982a) Unusual features of nevocellular nevi. J Cutan Pathol 9:284–292
Weedon D (1982b) A reappraisal of melanoma in situ. J Dermatol Surg Oncol 8:774–775
Weedon D (1984) The Spitz naevus. Clin Oncol 3:(in press)
Weedon D, Farnsworth J (1984) Spongiotic changes in melanocytic nevi. Am J Dermatopathol 6 (suppl):257–259
Weedon D, Little JH (1977) Spindle and epithelioid cell nevi in children and adults. A review of 211 cases of the Spitz nevus. Cancer 40:217–225
Weidner F, Schroll S, Schonberger A (1982) The influence of lymph node metastasis and ulceration of primary melanoma on germinal centers within draining lymph nodes: a histomorphometric study. Arch Dermatol Res 272:155–161
Weimar VM, Zuehlke RL (1978) Multiple agminate spindle and epithelioid cell nevi in an adult. Arch Dermatol 114:1383–1384
Weitzner S (1968) Intradermal nevus with psammoma body formation. Arch Dermatol 98:287–289
Whimster IW (1974) The halo naevus and cutaneous malignant melanoma. Br J Dermatol 90:111–113
White IR, MacDonald DM (1981) Familial multiple melanocytic naevi – the B-K mole syndrome. Clin Exp Dermatol 6:549–553
Wilson Jones E, Sanderson KV (1963) Cellular naevi with peculiar foam cells. Br J Dermatol 74:47–54
Woods JE, Soule EH, Creagan ET (1983) Metastasis and death in patients with thin melanomas (less than 0.76 mm). Ann Surg 198:63–64
Yarnold JR, Cochrane JP (1980) Malignant melanoma: Significance of disease-free interval. Br J Radiol 53:1068–1070
Yesudian P, Thambiah AS (1976) Perinevoid alopecia. An unusual variant of alopecia areata. Arch Dermatol 112:1432–1434

Addendum: Since the preparation of this manuscript a special supplement of the American Journal of Dermatopathology (1984, Volume b) has been published with various articles dealing with some aspect of malignant melanoma, melanoma in situ, displastic naevi and the management of congenital naevi.

Cutaneous Vasculitis

T.J. RYAN and S.M. BURGE

Over the course of two centuries the problem of cutaneus vasculitis has been recognised, discussed *ad nauseam* and it has evolved into a relatively clear picture of a disease process or reaction pattern. The physical signs which are recognised by the clinician now include urticaria, purpura, vesiculation and infarction and affect the skin with varied intensity, depth or distribution creating a number of named syndromes. Terms such as erythema nodosum, Henoch Schonlein purpura, or Wegener's granulomatosus are used for communication between the physicians and any colleague who knows the language. Complete understanding of the language requires definitions and therein is the greatest difficulty because reaction patterns are varied and the grouping of physical signs show overlap. The more these patterns are artifically separated from one another, so the more complicated their classification becomes and the more uncertain the appropriateness of the definitions (RYAN 1976; RYAN and WILKIN-

Table 1. Vascular injury

Vascular injury is a combination of:		
Noxious trigger, e.g.		Constitutional defect
Immune complexes		Altered reactivity
Infective agents	plus	Prepared site
Drugs		The anatomy of stasis
Food		Pathergic tissue
		Locus minores resistentiae

SON 1985; WOLFF and WINKELMANN 1980; CUPPS and FAUCI 1981; ALARCON-SEGOVIA 1980; BRAVERMAN 1981; WINKELMANN 1980; COPEMAN 1983).

In this chapter we will begin by using the broad definition of vasculitis, *microvascular injury* (RYAN 1976). We will describe what happens when small vessels are injured and what this looks like under the microscope. In the final section we will apply this knowledge to certain disease entities described by the physician and point to how the pathologist, looking at a skin biopsy makes a diagnosis which tallies with the views of the physician and may be a guide to prognosis and treatment. The physician and pathologist usually come to their conclusions in partnership. The purpose of this chapter is to prevent this conclusion being based on a false interpretation of what is observed.

Our view of vasculitis differs from that of some previous authors in the following respects. We believe that vasculitis is not solely due to immune complexes or solely due to anything else. It is not synonymous with immunologically induced inflammation (WINKELMANN 1980). Vasculitis is not what is left when other causes of vessel injury such as thrombosis, embolus or adjacent inflammation have been excluded (BORRIE and STANSFELD 1966). Vasculitis is not synonymous with arteritis, but it is the same as angiitis or 'the vasculitides' (CUPPS and FAUCI 1981). As it is a reaction to injury, (RYAN 1980) it is by definition an inflammation of vessels. We do not exclude from our definition, inflammation of the vessel secondary to other disease processes in adjacent tissues, but identification of such processes should always be attempted.

The vascular injury is often due to some noxious circulating agent and usually there is some failure of the tissues to detoxicate it. This may be a systemic or local constitutional defect that is in itself the primary raison d'etre of the vasculitis (Table 1).

1. Identification of Vessels

Injury may disturb the vascular pattern and repair may alter normal vascular morphology (RYAN 1980). The vessels in the skin are typically distributed in a so called candelabra pattern, illustrated in Fig. 1a. Blood drains into a succession of horizontal or more characteristically, diagonally disposed venules (MORETTI 1968; YEN and BRAVERMAN 1976; BRAVERMAN and YEN 1977; RYAN 1983), which are found in greatest density near the epidermis and the adnexa (Fig. 1b). However, within a few days of injury, inflammation and repair, new vessel

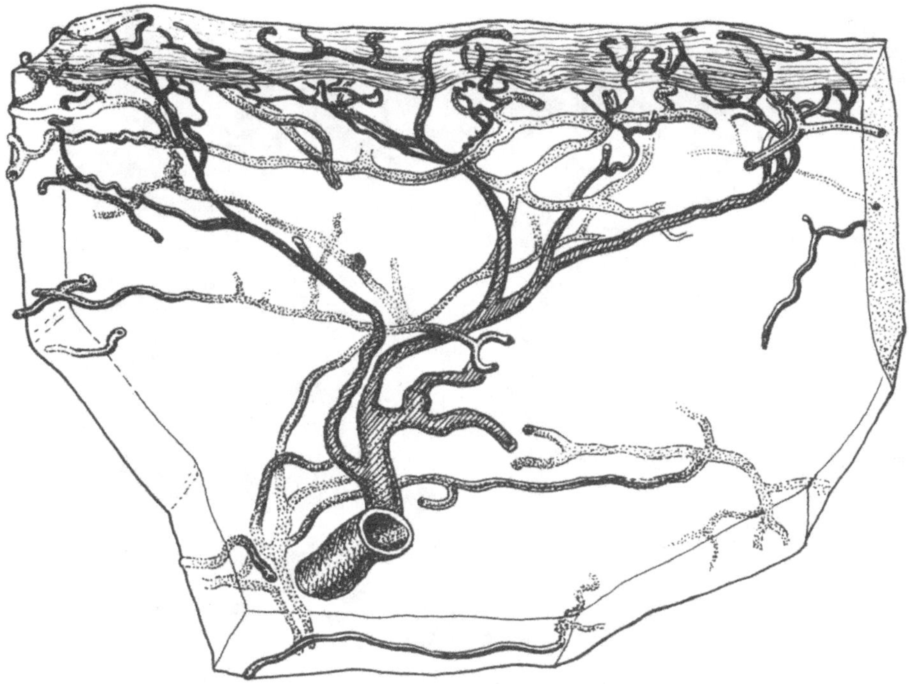

Fig. 1a. The vessels in the skin are distributed in a candelabra pattern. A central arteriole feeds horizontal vessels which supply the capillaries of the papillae. Blood drains via one or more diagonally disposed or horizontal venules which are the primary sites of most dermal vascular pathology

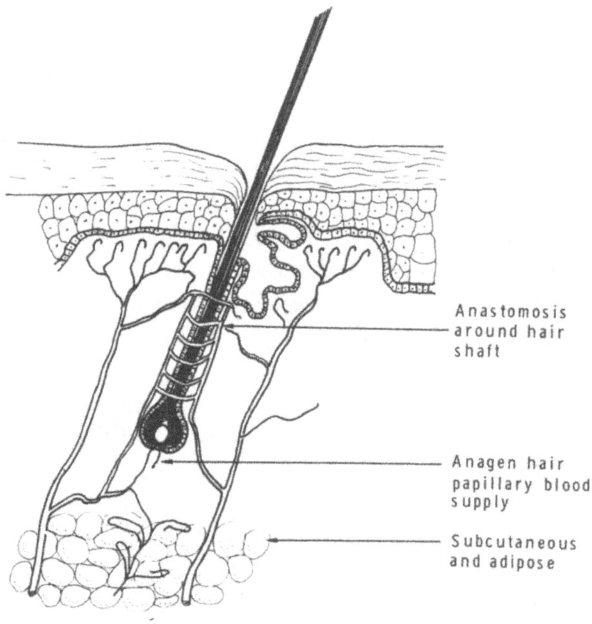

Fig. 1b. Capillaries and venules are distributed in greatest density near the epidermis and adnexa

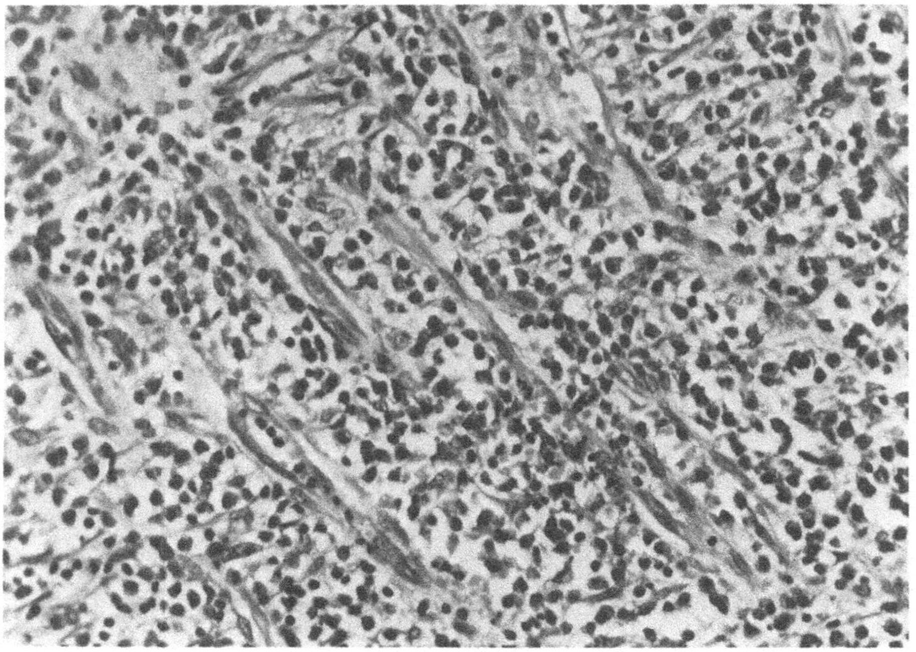

Fig. 2. Healing with granulation tissue in pyoderma gangrenosum. New vessel formation occurring after injury upsets the normal vascular pattern and provides a more vulnerable vasculature which may become the site of persistent or recurrent vascular disease. HE ×380

formation can occur at any site in the dermis, adding granulation tissue and upsetting the vascular pattern (Fig. 2).

It is important to know where one might expect to see venules or small arteries. The papillary dermis, for instance, has no arteries and hence pathology therein cannot be labelled as arteritis however thick-walled a superficial vessel may become in inflammation.

Venules are the commonest vascular target for injury by circulating agents, e.g. immune complexes, while arteries are more vulnerable to ischaemic injury. Venulitis rather than arteriolitis is usually a more appropriate sub-classification of vasculitis in upper and mid-dermal disease (COPEMAN 1975) (Fig. 3). In the deep dermis it is helpful to look for a neurovascular bundle, as here an artery can be distinguished more readily from a vein. It is the vein which is usually affected by pathology (COPEMAN and RYAN 1970; BEACHAM et al. 1980).

Lymphatics are invariably involved in any inflammatory process (FOLDI and CASLEY-SMITH 1983) and inflamed lymphatics must be distinguished from inflamed venules. While thin-walled terminal lymphatics can be identified in the mid dermis (MORTIMER et al. 1983), lymphatic trunks tend to run along the undersurface of the deep dermis and in the legs these deep lymphatics may have thicker walls. Identification of deep dermal lymphatics and blood vessels is often best in a neurovascular bundle (Fig. 4a, b).

The diameter of the lumen of dermal papillary vessels is variable, it is commonly around 2.5 μm and is rarely more than the diameter of a neutrophil,

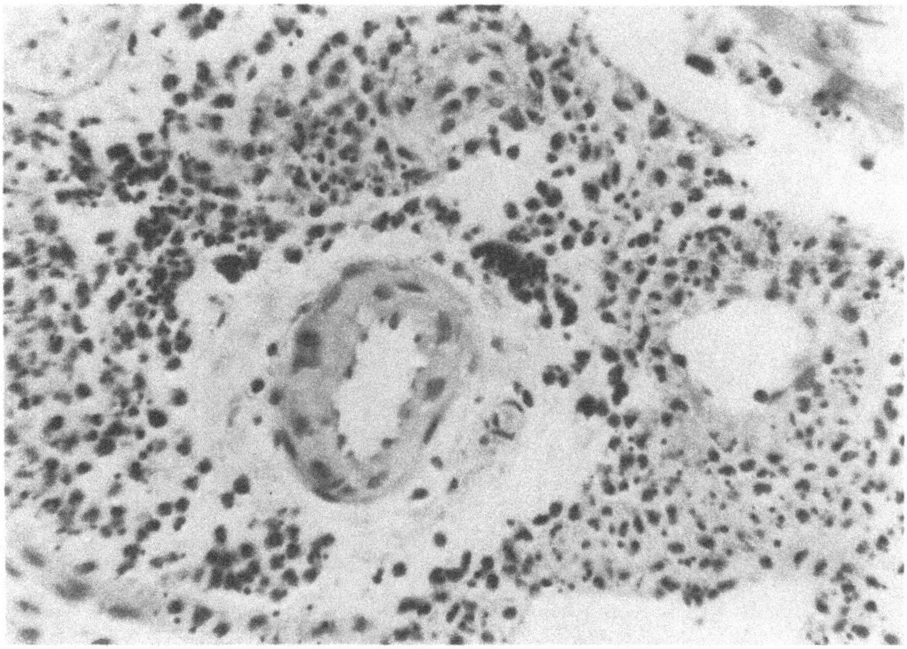

Fig. 3. Leukocytoclastic vasculitis affecting a venule but sparing an adjacent arteriole. Circulating agents are preferentially precipitated in venules where flow is slow and the vessel wall is leaky so it is the vein not the artery which is the target in most forms of vasculitis. HE ×605

i.e. 10 μm. The outside diameter is about twice that of the lumen, i.e. 8–15 μm. In the mid and deep dermis, the ascending arterioles and collecting venules have an outside diameter of 20–30 μm (HIGGINS and EADY 1981).

The vessels at the dermal subcutaneous junction are the most difficult to identify (Fig. 4). First it must be realised that, especially in the lower leg, there are fewer arterial vessels than veins and that arteries take a more direct course, so are unlikely to be sectioned in such a way that they appear duplicated. Veins, on the other hand, pursue a tortuous course both horizontally and vertically and may be sectioned repeatedly, although there may only be five or six such vessels in each 3 mm biopsy (BRAVERMAN and KEH-YEN 1984). The diameter of the lumen of these veins lies between 70–120 μm, and they may be round, oval or convoluted. The walls can be up to 25 μm thick containing several layers of smooth muscle. Older textbooks, basing their information on animal studies believed that elastic fibres were not a feature of veins smaller than 200 μm, but elastin is often plentiful lying in the mid to peripheral parts of the vascular wall (BRAVERMAN and KEH-YEN 1984). Usually but not invariably there is no sub-endothelial elastin. The presence of valves is possibly the most certain marker of veins but only to distinguish them from arteries. Even in the upper dermis valves are frequent in lymphatics (Fig. 5). In the lower leg which is preferentially affected by vasculitis, venous hypertension and arteriole vasoconstriction are normal physiological features which contribute to thickening of the walls of all small vessels.

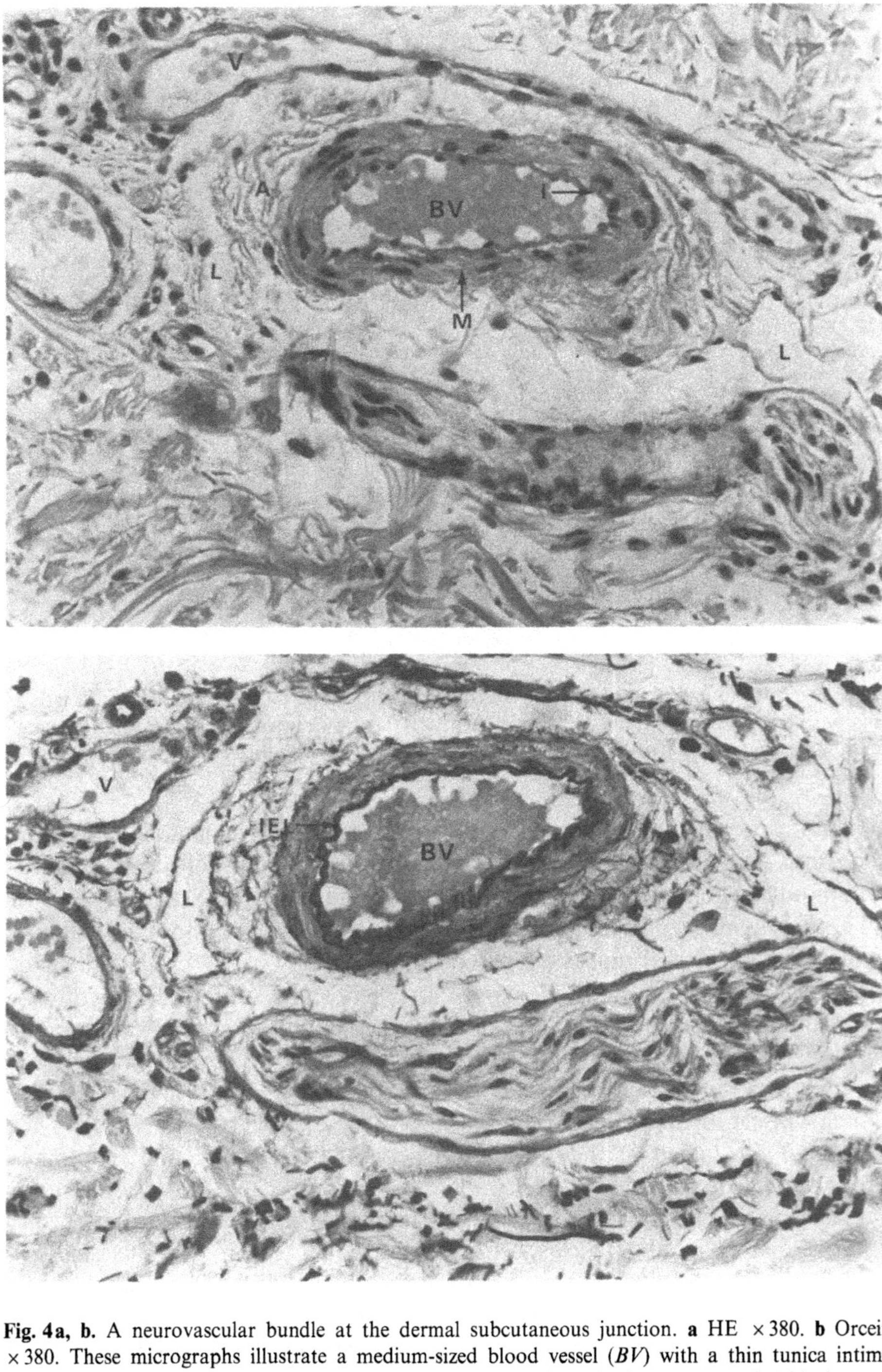

a

b

Fig. 4a, b. A neurovascular bundle at the dermal subcutaneous junction. **a** HE ×380. **b** Orcein ×380. These micrographs illustrate a medium-sized blood vessel (*BV*) with a thin tunica intima (*I*); tunica media (*M*) and loose tunica adventitia (*A*). Orcein stain demonstrates the thin internal elastic lamina (*IEL*) but no external elastic lamina. This vessel could either be a vein or a large arteriole. Small veins (*V*) are characterised by thin walls and a relatively wide lumen. In some areas this vessel has a poorly developed internal elastic lamina. Elastin may be plentiful in the mid and peripheral parts of the vascular wall. Lymphatics (*L*) may be identified more easily using an orcein stain since elastin is a normal component of the walls of healthy dermal lymphatics

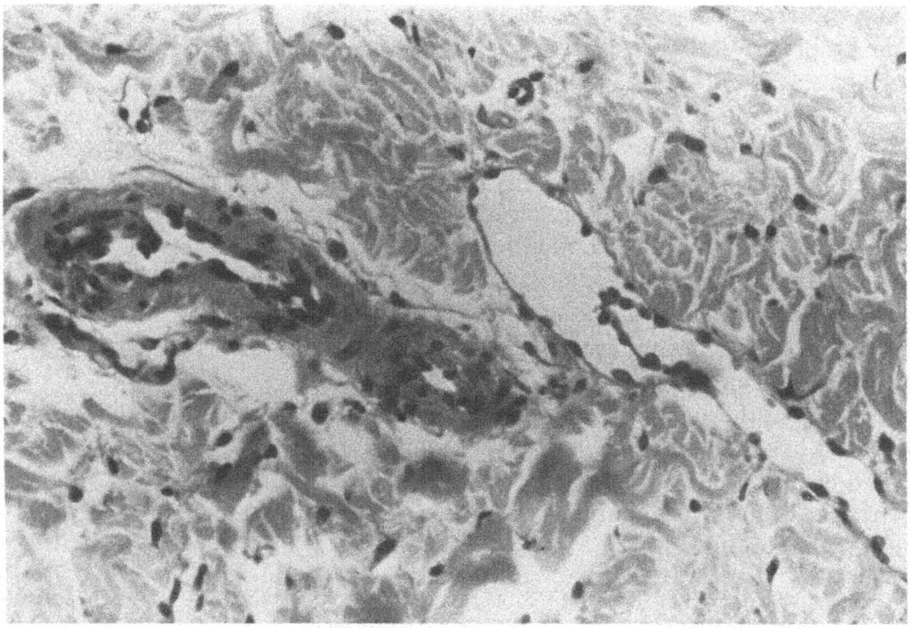

Fig. 5. Pigskin section demonstrated a thin-walled lymphatic with a valve. In subcutaneous tissue valves are found in both lymphatics and veins but it is only the lymphatic that shows this feature in the mid dermis. The thin attenuated wall of the lymphatic can be compared to the plumper endothelium of the adjacent blood vessels (RYAN 1983). HE ×420 (Courtesy of R.J. JONES, Slade Hospital, Oxford)

1.1 Functions of Endothelium – Disrupted by Injury

It is important to recognise that blood vessels are not simply containers but are lined by endothelial cells which have numerous functions and enormous potential for taking up new functions (FISHMAN 1982; WOOLF 1983). The endothelial cell normally secretes plasminogen activator and manufactures lipoxygenases which between them control surface coagulation and platelet aggregation. The endothelial cell has various systems for detoxicating serotonin, angiotensin, adrenalin, kinins or oxygen-radicals. In addition, there are receptors for Ia antigen and C_3B so that endothelium is a target for immunologically mediated injury.

A principle function of all endothelial cells is control of vessel wall permeability. This is especially the case in lymphatics in the skin. The permeability depends on transport across cytoplasm or between cells. It is altered by agents such as platelets, fibrinogen or albumin (SCHNEEBERGER 1982) lying on the surface of the cell or by changes in the immediate extracellular environment.

Normal blood vessels in the skin have tightly applied endothelial cells with no gaps. Fenestrated endothelial cells only occur at sites close to the epidermis or within the dermal papilla of the hair follicle (HIGGINS and EADY 1981). Control of permeability or leakiness is fine and depends not solely on the apparent tightness of junctions or on vesicular transport but possibly also on the function of the capillary wall as a charge barrier.

The mapping of charge distribution on the endothelial cell surface reveals the existence of sites that are anionic and may repulse anionic macromolecules while other sites may favour their transport. Fenestrated endothelium may possess anionic sites which do not favour the transport of protein (SIMIONESCU et al. 1982). In the rabbit's ear, the only skin preparation so far studied, anionic dextrans cross the vessel wall less readily than neutral or cationic dextrans. Studies in the kidney, not yet repeated in the skin, suggest that the charge on the surface of agents, such as immune complexes, determines where they alight if the vessel wall is undamaged (CAULIN-GLASER et al. 1983). Macrovesicles, so often equated with injury (see below), may be a transport system which is not dependent on charge.

Normal endothelial cells, show great functional variability in different species and sites, while damaged and repairing endothelium may take on new roles. The skin has been little studied in this respect. However, any theorising about the effect of endothelial injury in cutaneous vasculitis should not forget the pluri-potential of this cell.

1.2 Local Factors Which Alter Endothelial Cell Function

Stasis, high blood pressure, warming and cooling all alter vascular function in the skin (RYAN 1976) (Fig. 6). Vessels affected by these factors such as those around the ankle, cannot be regarded as similar, anatomically or physiologically

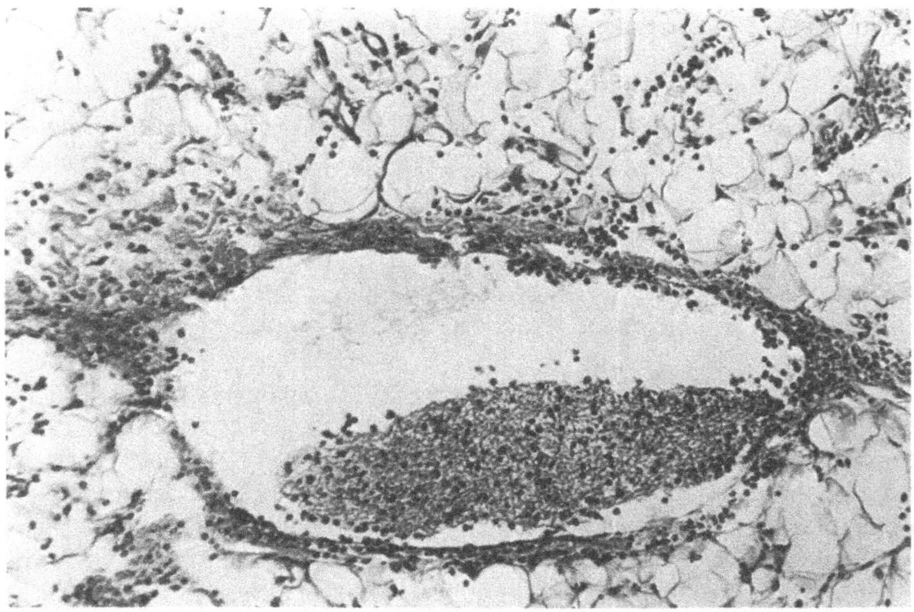

Fig. 6. An experimentally induced dependent skin flap with features of stasis. Venules of the hypodermis show endothelial damage and stickiness of blood cells. HE ×160

in their pathologic responses, to vessels found anywhere else. This may be relevant in vasculitis since these local factors influence the capacity to produce plasminogen activator (DODMAN et al. 1973) prostacyclin, Factor VIII and angiotensin converting enzyme or to control the kallikrein kinin system. In areas of venous hypertension e.g. the leg, the pH and pO_2 are low and the cells vulnerable to injury.

Membrane bound H_2 receptors are found at venular sites, in particular those especially rich in filaments and near endothelial cell junctions. Histamine may stimulate endothelial cell contraction, open gap junctions and increase leakiness. This may point to reasons for localisation of disease in the venular compartment of the legs where mast cells are especially prominent.

The integrity of the vessel wall is important in determining its interaction with other cells such as platelets. Viruses, toxins, complement or shear stress alter such integrity and encourage platelets to release vasoactive agents, mitogens, cationic proteins and leucotactic materials.

2. Consequences of Injury

The theoretical consequences of injury include changes in permeability or leakiness, loss of integrity with respect to platelet or leucocyte interaction; release and exhaustion of secretions such as plasminogen activator; impairment of supply and disposal of waste; repair with changes in identity and pattern (RYAN 1980).

Arteries and arterioles carry blood to the site, the capillaries supply the tissue and the venules take away blood. Lymphatics in partnership with macrophages take away waste, especially macromolecules. These functions are disrupted by disease. In acute vascular injury supply may cease or drainage may be impaired. Protein in the tissues may be washed away into neighbouring sites, enter blood vessels instead of lymphatics or build up and concentrate in pockets of oedema with chronic inflammation and fibrosis (CASLEY-SMITH and GAFFNEY 1981).

Small veins, because they are already permeable and slow flowing, are especially vulnerable to injury but they recover well without irreparable damage to their wall. They seem to survive ischaemia since they are normally hypoxic (RYAN 1980). Arteries are normally well perfused with oxygen and suffer disproportionately on the rare occasion in which this perfusion is impaired especially if reperfusion at high pressure occurs after a period of ischaemia (TILTON et al. 1983). Perfusion is impaired by vasoconstriction, thrombosis and coagulation or embolism, as well as by projection of endothelial cells into the lumen, or plugging of distal vessels by haemoconcentrated blood as may occur in inflammation.

2.1 Ischaemia

There is a spectrum of vascular responses to injury ranging from the exudative to the obstructive (Fig. 7). At some stage in inflammatory lesions ischaemia

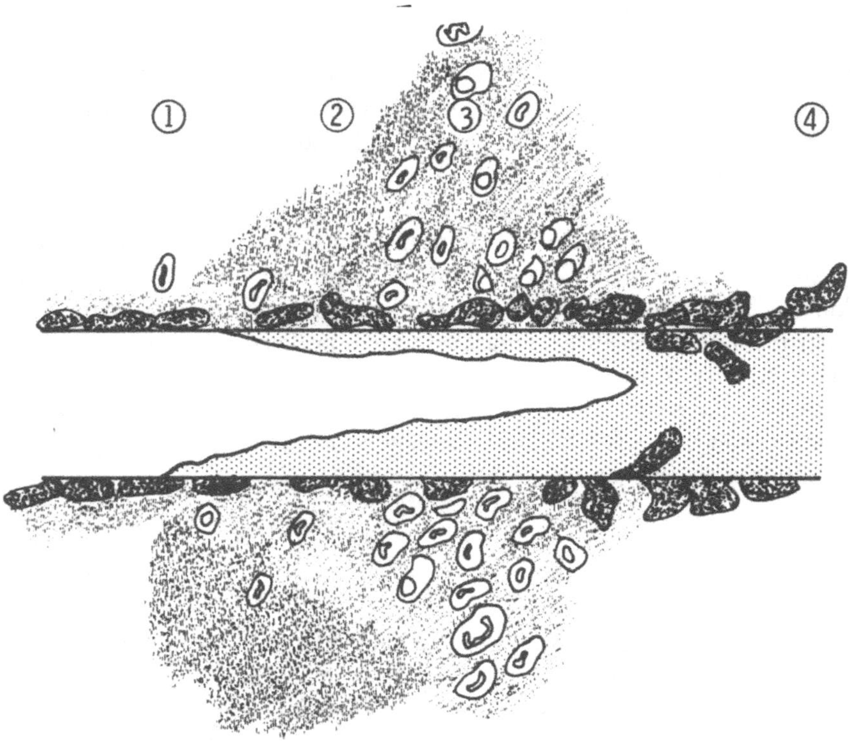

Fig. 7. Spectrum of injury suggested by a study of mechanisms (RYAN 1976). (*1*) No pathology. (*2*) Gross increase in permeability. (*3*) Numerous leucocytes. (*4*) Total ischaemic necrosis and endothelial proliferation

is inevitable. It is the most neglected aspect of the pathogenesis of vasculitis ignored by almost all previous authors and particularly relevant to the problem of acute necrosis. The term ischaemia denotes a deficient blood supply and hypoxia is an important consequence. The respiratory enzymes and mitochondria within cells are damaged within minutes of hypoxia. Functions of endothelial cells, such as the release of coagulation or fibrinolytic enzymes or prostacyclin, are affected. This may be quickly followed by the interaction of platelets and leucocytes or leakiness. The endothelial cell may survive such short term hypoxia, but smooth muscle and fat cells recover less well (WILMS-KRETCHMER and MAJNO 1969). Studies of vessel walls after tourniquet ischaemia and reperfusion after meniscectomy (ZAHAVI et al. 1980) have drawn attention to endothelial damage, exhaustion of prostacyclins and platelet embolisation.

In decubitus ulcers or in experimental skin flaps (RYAN et al. 1976) the consequences of ischaemia can be studied. The earliest sign of pressure induced ischaemia is a blanchable erythema, associated with swelling of the endothelial cells and dilatation of vessels nearest the epithelium (WITKOWSKI and PARISH 1982). There is oedema and the occasional fibrin clot in vessels of the deep dermis. Neutrophils appear wherever epithelial cells begin to degenerate, especially around sweat glands and fat cells. Slightly severer injury with non-a 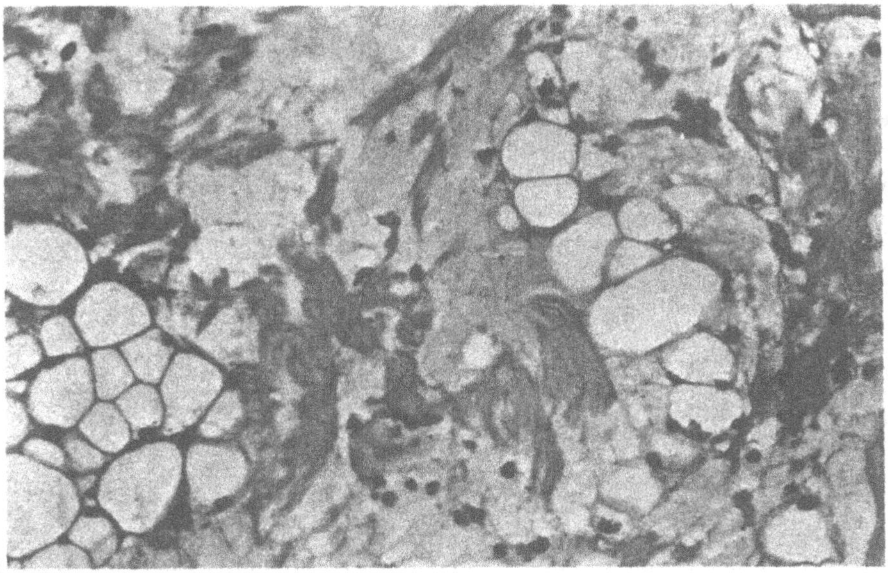

b 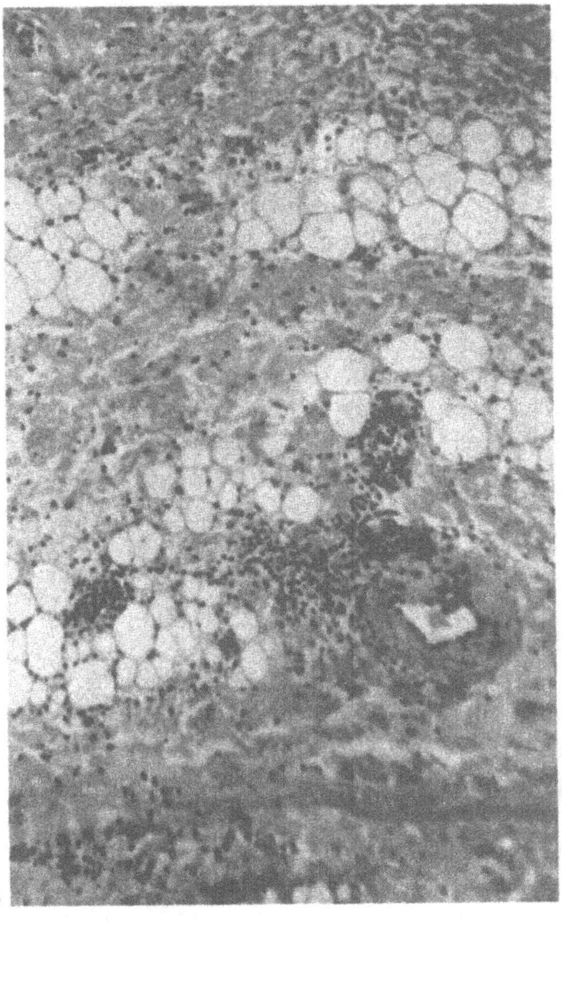

Fig. 8a, b. Reperfusion after a period of ischaemia may cause further tissue damage, bringing platelets, neutrophils, activated complement and oxygen derived free radicals to a site that is no longer equipped to deal with them. **a** Marked thickening of interlobular fat septa due to transudation of fluid and plasma proteins after repersuion of an ill-prepared vascular bed. Such protein induces further inflammation and subsequent fibrosis. HE ×105. **b** Hypodermal venules engorged with neutrophils, some of which have extravasated into surrounding tissues. HE ×42 blanchable erythema may cause vessel engorgment, platelet aggregation and red cell extravasation.

Ischaemia occurs whenever either inflow or outflow is obstructed. In the granulomatous vasculitides, the angiocentric infiltrate is more destructive when it causes obliteration of the lumen, e.g. Wegener's granulomatosis. Ischaemia is a feature of arterial vasospasm or embolus, intravascular coagulation and thrombosis; and severe inflammation engorging the capillary bed. These are all phenomenon which occur in vasculitis and hence it should be emphasised that ischaemia is part of the pathology of vasculitis (RYAN et al. 1976).

The role of reperfusion is even less studied than ischaemia. There is evidence that the restoration of blood supply to ischaemic tissue, brings oxygen to a vascular bed which is ill-prepared for it and it is actually damaged by it (CHERRY and RYAN 1976; TILTON et al. 1983). Fig. 8a, b are taken from studies of ischaemia and reperfusion of pig skin (RYAN et al. 1976).

2.2 Lymphoedema

The role of lymphoedema as part of the pathology of vasculitis has been ignored. The lymphatics clear macromolecules with the help of macrophages. Their involvement in inflammation is inevitable; their damage by inflammation is to be expected. Damaged lymphatics are dilated, filled with blood and fibrin and surrounded by inflammatory cells (ALTORFER et al. 1977). Their function is impaired and the tissues therefore suffocate from the effects of a protein (inflammatory) oedema (CASLEY-SMITH and GAFFNEY 1981). Histopathological identification of these damaged lymphatics becomes very difficult.

In experimental lymphoedema certain recognisable histological features which are also seen in many chronic forms of vasculitis, have been identified (ALTORFER et al. 1977). They include fibrosis, increased macrophage activity and the formation of lymphoid aggregates. There is focal accumulation of mononuclear cells around blood vessels. Increased pinocytosis and macromolecular transport by vacuoles in the endothelial cell is also well recognised.

3. Diagnosis of Vasculitis

3.1 The Endothelial Cell as a Marker for Vasculitis

Swelling and shrinkage are two signs of endothelial damage. RUSSELL JONES and EADY (1984) drew attention to large rounded pale nuclei with prominant nucleoli as an early feature of hypertrophy seen in 1 μm Epon embedded sections. Swollen endothelial cells project into the lumen and obliterate it. WILMS-KRETCHMER and MAJNO (1969) and HAMMERSEN (1972) have shown that endothelial swelling is an early sign of ischaemic injury. Microbleeding occurs after two hours of ischaemia and can take place with little experimental evidence

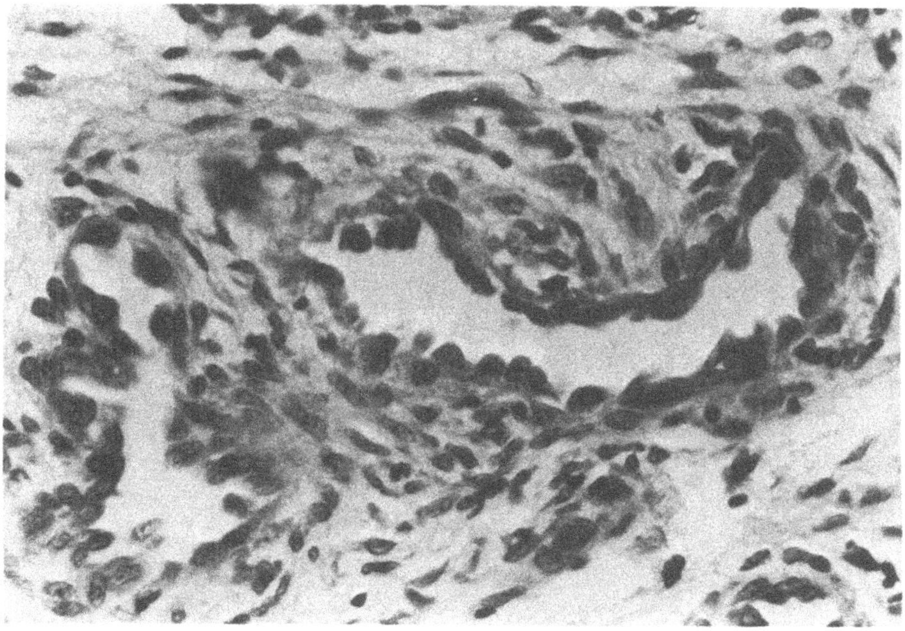

a

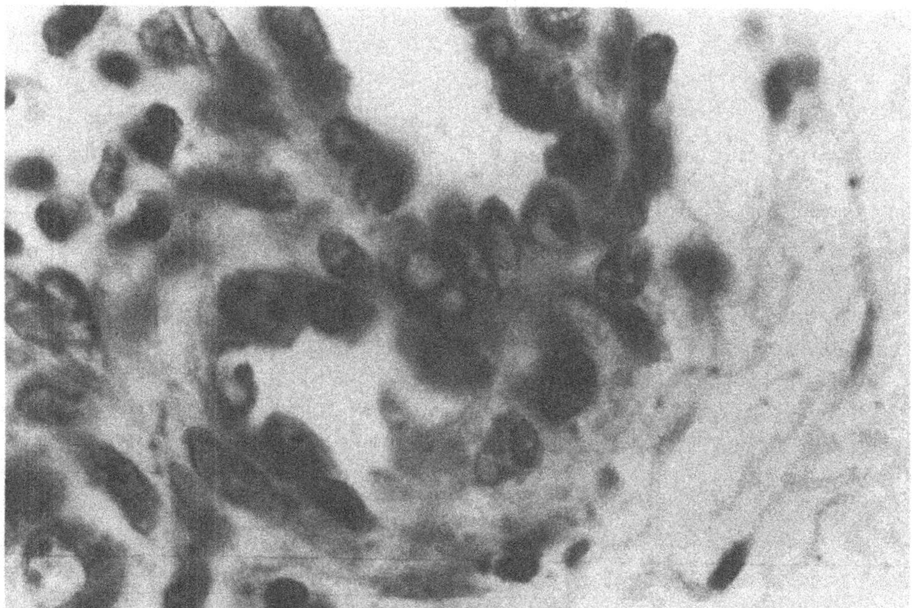

b

Fig. 9. a Blood vessels with swollen endothelial cells (high endothelium) protruding into the lumen in pseudopyogenic granuloma (angiolymphoid hyperplasia with eosinophilia). HE $\times 605$. **b** There is vacuolation of some endothelial cells. HE $\times 1{,}470$. High endothelium is a feature of post capillary venules in the lymph node, but also occurs in lymphoedema and chronic inflammation in the dermis of disruption of the endothelial lining (SKALAK et al. 1970). Such an appearance is an early feature of decubitus ulcers and it is also a feature of lymphoedema.

Endothelial cell blebs are also a feature blamed as a fixation artefact by HIGGINS and EADY (1981), but are well recognised by others as either a sign of endothelial disruption or as macropinocytosis whereby there is bulk transport of cells or macromolecules, as in the canal of Schlemm and arachnoid cells (TRIPATHI and TRIPATHI 1984). BLEBBING is also a feature in angiolymphoid hyperplasia (EADY and WILSON JONES 1977) (Fig. 9). The phenomenon of high endothelium which contains such blebs is well known as a response to macrophage lymphocyte interaction (GOWANS and KNIGHT 1964), neoplasia (FREEMONT 1982) and chronic inflammation (GRAHAM et al. 1972).

Early endothelial cell necrosis is difficult to identify but the extruded nucleus stained deeply with haematoxylin is one identifiable feature (STALKER et al. 1969). SCHWARTZ (1982) has suggested that uptake of IgG in the cytoplasm of endothelial cells is a marker of loss of integrity. This has been noted in vasculitis where it may be a useful early sign of endothelial cell injury.

3.2 Leucocytoclasia

Neutrophil derived nuclear debris (nuclear dust) is often equated with vasculitis (WINKELMANN and DITTO 1964), and in combination with a rich neutrophilic perivascular infiltrate of the vessel wall and its immediate surrounds, red cell extravasation and the deposition of fibrinoid material, the diagnosis of vasculitis is secure (Fig. 3). One cause of these features is activation of the complement cascade by immunological processes. It is however important to realise that leucocytoclasia is also seen in healthy humans after 6 h of ischaemia, as has been demonstrated in one Swedish study (ROMANUS et al. 1978).

C5a is a powerful chemotactant which also causes degranulation of leukocytes. The oxygen radical (superoxide) also produced by complement activation of neutrophils can injure endothelium. Other agents that attract neutrophils include fibrinopeptides and products of the lipoxygenase system.

The production of nuclear dust is most marked when the infiltrate is predominately neutrophilic. Mixed infiltration with lymphocytes and macrophages is associated with correspondingly little nuclear disruption, while plasma cells are rarely associated with nuclear dust. Leucocytoclasia often accompanies clinically palpable purpura. Haemorrhage is seen with leucocytoclasia in early lesions whereas skin necrosis and fibrinoid are features of older lesions in which leucocytoclasia is not a notable feature.

3.2.1 Lymphocytic Angiitis

Lymphocytes are recruited to all inflammatory sites non-selectively since they adhere to inflamed endothelium. So-called committed lymphocytes mediating cellular hypersensitivity may be selectively recruited. Vessels lined by high endothelium (Fig. 9) cuboidal and projecting into the lumen, appear to select lymphocytes both in the lymph node post capillary venule and possibly also in the skin in T-cell diseases such as mycosis fungoides and other disorders in which there are lymphoid aggregates such as pseudo pyogenic granuloma (Fig. 9) (EADY and WILSON JONES 1977). *In vitro* blast transformation of lymphocytes encourages penetration through the endothelial lining of the vessels. A necrotising vasculitis has been described within the cutaneous lesions of mycosis fungoides, possibly induced by malignant T lymphocytes (GRANSTEIN et al. 1983). DE BONO (1983) suggested that there is a mechanism of non-specific adhesiveness which is related to the spreading of activated endothelium such as is observed in vessel repair. In which case it should be no surprise to see lymphocytes in a late but healing phase of vasculitis.

Immunoglobulins and complement are detected in about two-thirds of vasculitic lesions showing a leucocytoclasia and in about 40% of those showing a lymphocytic picture (ANDREWS et al. 1979). There is little correlation with blood levels and immune complexes.

3.2.2 Immunofluorescent Studies

For more than two decades mixed cryoglobulins have been distinguished from monoclonal types as a cause of leucocytoclasia. Their exact role remains the subject of debate (LEVINKSY 1981). Early studies of localisation were too dogmatic in their interpretation (SCHROETER et al. 1971) since IgM, C_3C, C_3D, C_5 are often observed in normal skin (NIEBOER 1981). The biopsy from a single individual is only of value if its exact timing relevant to the initiation of the pathology is known. There is evidence that immunoglobulins and C_3 are early signs that may be cleared by later cellular activity (CREAM et al. 1971). Adrenalin and histamine can be inoculated and biopsies taken at a set interval, may indicate deposition rather than clearance. Studies using electron microscopy (COPEMAN 1975; RUITER and MOLENAAR 1970; SOTER et al. 1976; PERROT et al. 1971) have mainly confirmed mechanisms such as gaps in vessel walls causing leakage and deposition of complexes and are of little additional value for diagnosis in skin disease. Sampling is always a problem. Apart from IgA_2 in Henoch Schonlein purpura, sub-classifying is of little value. Not many studies have been based on more than a single biopsy which need not be a representation of all lesions at all times. The findings of specific viral material confirms the involvement of, for instance, hepatitis B antigen (ALMEIDA and WATERSON 1969; NEUMANN et al. 1981).

3.2.3 Fibrinoid Necrosis

Fibrinoid necrosis is an important histological finding which has been observed by histologists for more than a century, and has been emphasised as a diagnostic feature of vasculitis. There are perivascular and intramural deposits of not only fibrin, but also its precursors and metabolites (fibrinogen and fibrinopeptides), as well as immunoglobulins, complement, platelets, plasma proteins and lipids.

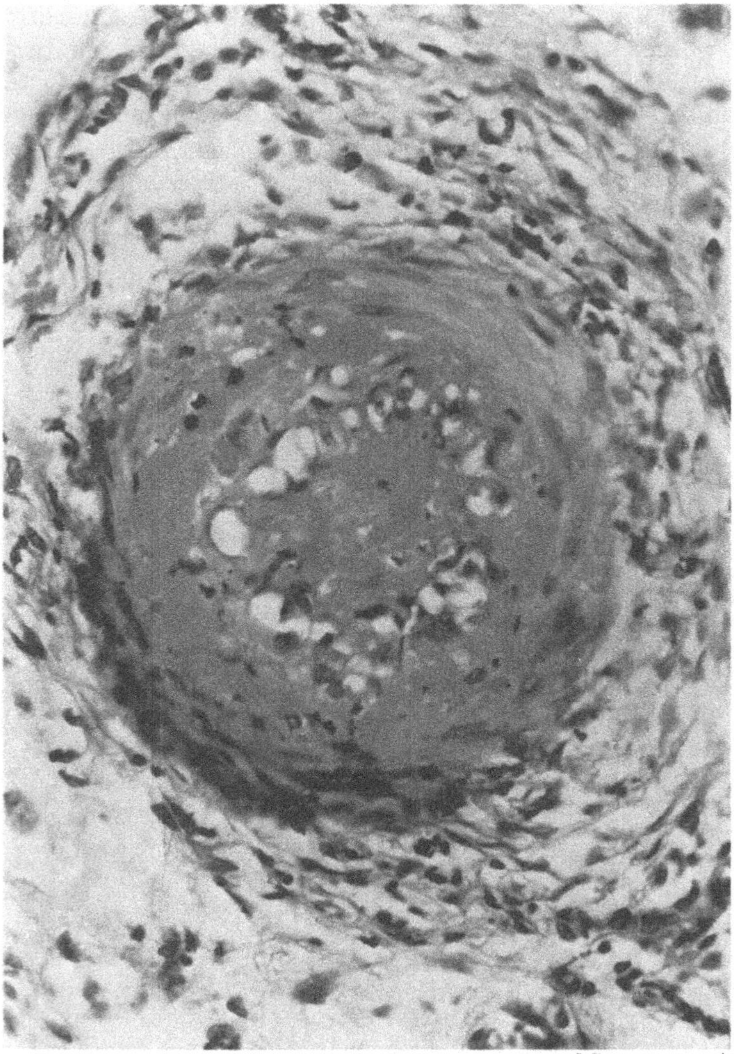

Fig. 10. Extensive fibrinoid degeneration of a small vessel. There are deposits of eosinophilic homogenous material both around and within the vessel wall, but few accompanying inflammatory cells. It is a sign of severe vessel wall disruption and may occur due to ischaemia caused by vasospasm, embolisation, coagulation or inadequate perfusion of the surrounding tissue because of acute inflammation in that tissue. HE ×430

It is not always accompanied by many inflammatory cells (Fig. 10), and the term necrosis too may be omitted if vessel wall destruction is not obvious but fibrinoid material is considerable (PHANUPHAK et al. 1980).

Intravascular debris observed in biopsy material includes normal red cells, fibrin, white cells in varying degrees of disintegration and platelet aggregates. Vessels may be occluded by cryoglobulins (Fig. 11) or emboli, e.g. bacterial endocarditis, atheroma. Platelet emboli and cholesterol emboli (DYMOCK 1981; ROZANSKY 1982) (Fig. 12) are distinctive in a HE section. A gram stain may

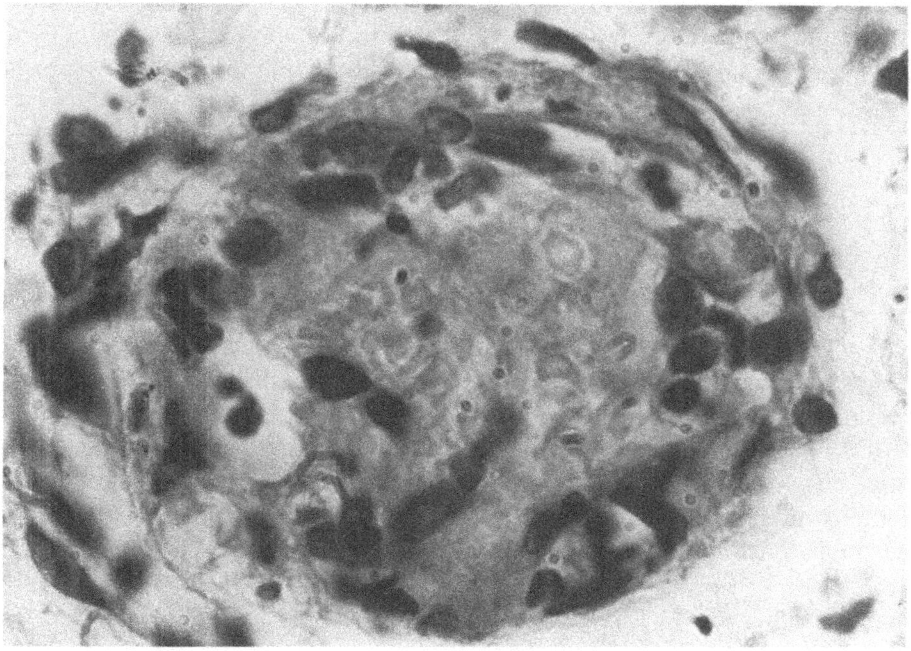

Fig. 11. A small dermal vessel completely occluded by amorphous eosinophilic material in a patient with cryoglobulinaemia. HE ×1,470

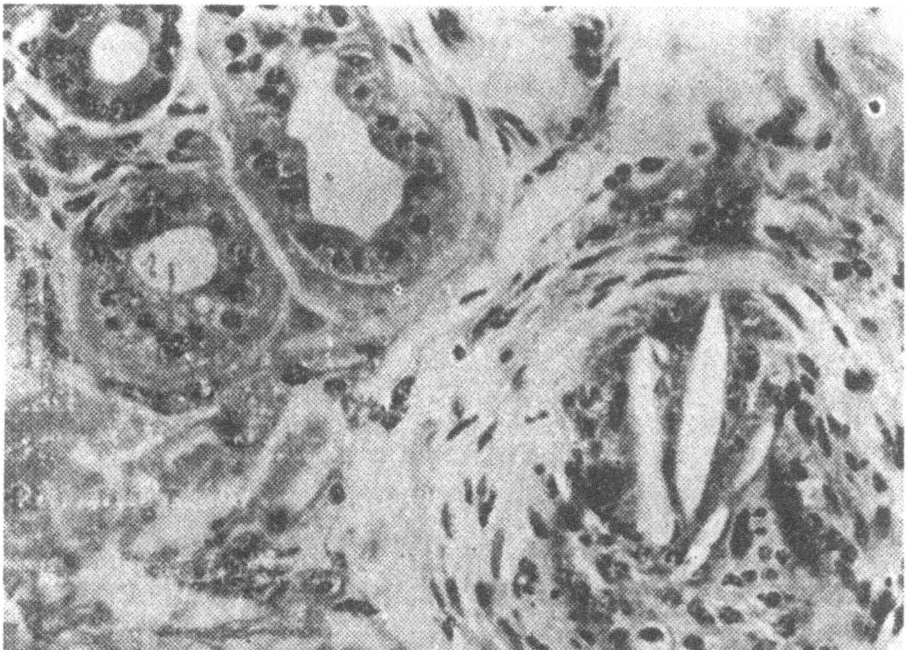

Fig. 12. Cutaneous cholesterol embolism: needle-shaped cholesterol clefts within the lumen of a dermal arteriole, one of the few diagnostic features of arteriolar pathology dueto proximal atheroma. (Published with permission of Australian J. of Dermatology R. Dymock, 1981). HE ×800

be of value in septic sources. Leucoembolisation is an important cause of tissue damage and has perhaps been under-estimated in vasculitis (JACOB 1980). The next move is to take into account the clinical history and the site of the biopsy and with this information begins the interpretation.

3.2.4 Age of the Lesion

Experimental induction of vasculitis suggests that there may be several hours between the moment of initiation and the first clinical sign of a lesion even in the most superficial of lesions. Subcutaneous lesions may take several days before they become clinically manifest. Injury to the skin by the inoculation of histamine (BRAVERMAN and YEN 1975) adrenalin (SCHROETER and WINKELMANN 1971) or the application of pressure, ice or nicotinate (JUHLIN and MICHAELSSON 1971) to localise immune complexes permits exact timing of the initiation of the lesion and a biopsy may be taken 4–6 h later. Most often neutrophils predominate in early lesions while mononuclear cells appear later (RYAN et al. 1976) (see below). The clinician does not always know the time of vascular injury and because in some cases neutrophils persist for many days or lymphocytes are found very early (ANDREWS et al. 1979), the pathologist too may have difficulty in deciding the age of the lesion.

3.2.5 Site and Depth

Biopsies should include the subcutis, because the site of maximal injury is often in the vessels of the dermal subcutaneous junction or underlying fat. Punch biopsies are on the whole less likely to pick up such tissue than a properly executed excision with a scalpel. Some causes of vessel injury, such as cholesterol emboli (Fig. 12), primarily involve deeper and larger vessels (FISCHER and KISTNER 1971; DYMOCK 1981).

While the pathologist first has to state whether there is evidence of vascular injury, he should also clearly recognise where such injury has taken place. Thus dermal inflammation may be secondary to pathology in the epidermis or fat, e.g. the epidermal irritation of scabies may be associated with a vasculitis (FERNANDEZ et al. 1977; ACKERMAN 1978; VAN NESTE and SALMON 1978) and fat injury may have associated dermal changes in nodular vasculitis. The pathologist should indicate whether the vascular pattern is scarred or altered in any way by a previous injury. The vessels in the lower leg may be elongated and tortuous due to chronic gravitational stasis or venous hypertension (Fig. 13), while arterial hypertension may have caused arteriolar hypertrophy (KULWIN and HINES 1950; WALKER et al. 1973; WILLIAMSON et al. 1971).

Increased permeability, red cell extravasation and lumen obliteration are a succession of events that characterise the response to injury. A minor injury may do no more than increase permeability while a severe injury may destroy the vessel and its lumen. This severe injury may be the consequence of cumulative minor insults resulting in exhaustion of the capacity to repair. This may be

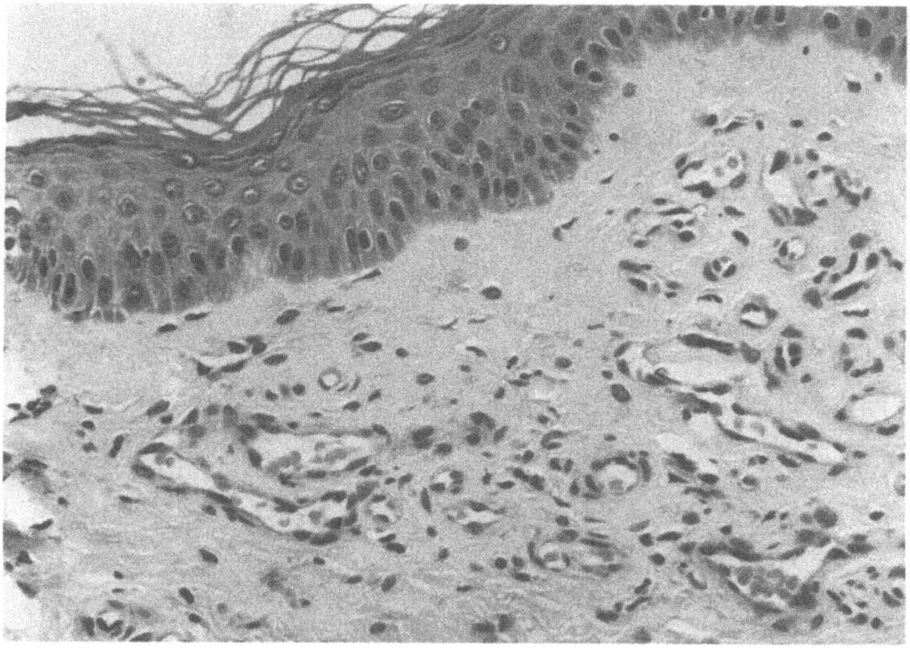

Fig. 13. Elongated and tortuous superficial dermal vessels in the lower leg. Chronic gravitational stasis or venous hypertension will induce these changes and predispose the vessels to localise haematogenous irritants such as immune complexes. Such vessels may bleed or thrombose in response to external trauma of the surface of the skin. HE ×380

no more than failure to remove fibrin or platelet aggregates. A vessel that has been previously injured and is depleted of fibrinolytic activity or prostacylin is more vulnerable than a vessel showing no signs of previous injury (RYAN 1976).

3.2.6 The Diagnosis of Histopathologic Pattern

ACKERMAN (1978) had delineated certain patterns of inflammatory skin disease and includes superficial perivascular dermatitis; superficial and deep perivascular dermatitis; and vasculitis as his first three sub-groups. He separates vasculitis from perivascular dermatitis by recognising fibrin, degeneration of collagen and necrosis; emphasising that the changes which distinguish vasculitis are in the vessel walls rather than around them. The pathology of perivascular dermatitis does not disrupt the vessel wall, blood supply to the overlying tissue is maintained, and there is neither purpura nor infarction.

The immunological processes that are believed to characterise vasculitis are detectable in perivascular inflammatory disorders, but the latter are distinguished by the absence of necrosis, indicating that blood supply is maintained.

If one takes this definition seriously, then urticarial allergic eruptions, rocky mountain spotty fever, erythema multiforme, acute febrile neutrophilic dermato-

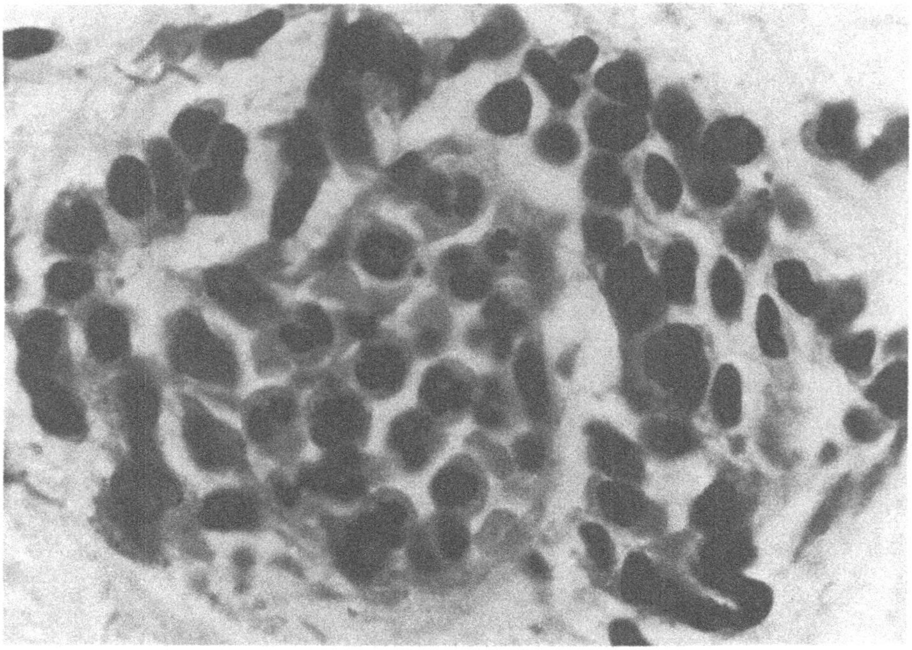

Fig. 14. An insect bite reaction: A dermal capillary filled with neutrophils and surrounded by lymphocytes. The vessel wall is preserved; there is no fibrinoid degeneration and no leukocytoclasis. Depending on the definition of vasculitis, this may be or may not be regarded as a sign of vessel injury. HE ×1,470

sis, pityriasis lichenoides et varoliformis acuta, fixed drug eruption, pigmented purpuric eruption and secondary syphilis should be mostly excluded from the vasculitides (ACKERMAN 1978). However, although we recognise the value of distinguishing disruption of the vessel wall whenever possible, we include many of these entities within our broad definition of vasculitis as microvascular injury, whereas ACKERMAN (1978) would merely describe evidence of a superimposed vasculitis in the rare cases in which he admits overlap might explain skin necrosis.

Dermatitis artefacta (HARPER and COPEMAN 1983) and *insect bites* are sometimes mistaken by the clinician for vasculitis. The late stages of injuries to the surface of the skin often have the appearance of infarcts as trauma may interfere with microcirculation and hence obstruct the flow through supplying arterioles. It is always necessary to examine early lesions for evidence of excoriation, burns or inoculation of noxious agents. Insect bites are characterised by a perivascular dermatitis often with eosinophils, plasma cells, and depending on the stage and type of insect, almost any other inflammatory cell (Fig. 14). A lymphocytic vasculitis occasionally occurs after insect bites or scabies (ACKERMAN 1978).

3.2.7 Arteritis

One must decide whether to take the line of a purist and reserve the term arteritis for primary arterial injury; or to accept a rather looser definition,

Table 2. Obliterative endovasculitis. List of diseases in which it has been observed from RYAN (1976)

Pigmented purpuric eruptions	Scleroderma	Anterior poliomyelitis
Gravitational stasis	Lupus erythematosus	Sjogren's syndrome
Thrombophlebitis	Dermatomyositis	Capillary naevi
Thrombo-angiitis obliterans	Rheumatoid arthritis	Drug eruptions
Polyarteritis nodosa	Hashimoto's disease	Trauma
Diabetes mellitus	Sickle cell anaemia	Carcinoma

as the clinician so often does when he uses the term polyarteritis nodosa, including much that primarily affects smaller vessels and which only subsequently causes injury to large vessels which may be either arteries or veins. Arteries are damaged by hypertension, platelet aggregation and coagulation; ischaemia may occur solely as a consequence of outflow obstruction. In each case it is, in our view, more appropriate to use a diagnostic label other than polyarteritis. Inflamed vessels lose their identity: small inflamed vessels look larger, and venules may resemble damaged arterioles. The pathologist must be aware of these pitfalls so that damaged capillaries or veins are recognised. The pathogenesis of arterial disease is different from capillary and venular disease. Primary venous or capillary disease must be excluded from the definition of arteritis.

Obliterative endovasculitis is a feature of a number of diseases listed in Table 2. The end result is a white porcelin-like scar, often with dilated capillaries surrounding it. Degos' malignant atrophic papulosis (SOTER et al. 1982) has its dire reputation because of the common intestinal complication of perforation but other more benign processes can give rise to a similar histological picture in the skin. Thus atrophie blanche, which is of similar appearance is frequently associated solely with gravitational disturbances of the lower leg. Confluent lesions may be spotted by enormously dilated and tortuous capillary venules (RYAN and WILKINSON 1985). The essential feature that distinguishes obliterative endovasculitis is a slow, acellular obliteration of an arteriole and consequent death and fibrosis of the dermis and epidermis supplied by the vessel (Fig. 15a) (BARD and WINKELMANN 1967). The porcelin white scar may be a single round lesion of 2 mm (Fig. 15b) or several grouped together like the petals of a flower due to several branches of a single vessel being involved. This reaction pattern is rarely pure, so that some biopsies may show more acute areas of leucocytoclastic angiitis or perivascular lymphocytes. There is usually thrombosis and obliteration of the vessel from within, but no damage whatsoever to the media and adventitia. The pink oedematous ring surrounding the lesion described by Degos is initially a hyperaemia, but may become a frank telangiectasia as in atrophie blanche. Special stains for fibrin may reveal the thrombotic process or fibrinoid in any of such lesions. The scarring of the dermis is often preceded by an accumulation of mucin. The endothelial cell obliteration in Degos' disease and in atrophie blanche is associated with absence of functions such as fibrinolysis and with intracytoplasmic tubular aggregates which may be seen in ultrastructural studies of injured vessels in this disease as well as in other collagen diseases and in experimental wounds.

Polyarteritis nodosa is a carelessly and commonly made diagnosis. In our

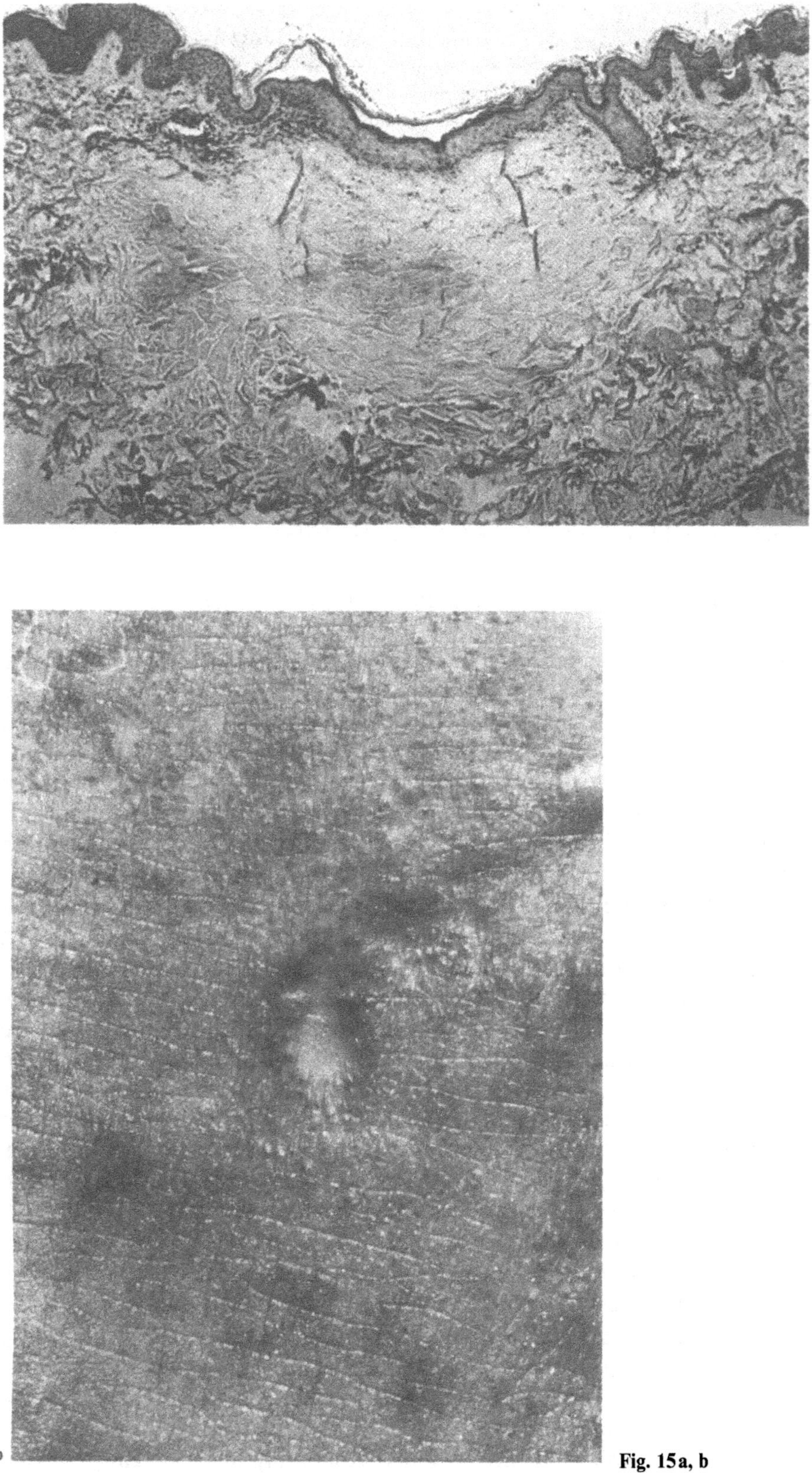

Fig. 15a, b

view it should not supercede diagnoses that both explain the pathology and are better understood such as malignant hypertension, platelet embolisation, rheumatoid vasculitis or intravascular coagulation. ZEEK (1952) excluded malignant hypertension 40 years ago but even now a diagnosis of polyarteritis nodosa is made in persons known to have severely elevated blood pressure, or it is made on the basis of biopsies from nerve or muscle taken from the lower leg of persons with chronic ischaemia, liposclerosis or lymphoedema in which interpretation is especially difficult. Endothelial proliferation and thrombotic occlusion are features seen in the skin of patients with essential hypertension (FARBER et al. 1947). Superimpose an immune complex disease such as may occur in rheumatoid arthritis and the pathology of a necrotising arteritis is to be expected.

Platelet embolisation is recognised as playing a part in the aetiology of aneurysms in small arteries in the kidney in thrombotic thrombocytopaenic purpura (UMLAS and KAISER 1979) Aneurysms are also found in microangiopathic haemolytic anaemia (KLEIN et al. 1972). Thus such aneurysms are not specific for polyarteritis nodosa. The polyarteritis nodosa of children in which the coronary arteries are affected, is probably synonomous with the mucocutaneous lymph node syndrome (KAWASAKI's disease) (SASAGURI and KATO 1982) and this is now better understood as platelet behaviour is further analysed (HIDAKA et al. 1983). In this decade in which platelet endothelial interaction is becoming so much better understood, the common denominator in many of these arterial diseases should not be obscured by morphologists. A presentation of urticaria and erythema which some authors loosely describe in chapters on polyarteritis nodosa is an example of a reaction pattern which could have something to do with platelets, coagulation or the secretions of the endothelial cell and may be associated with but could not be caused by inflammation in the wall of an artery.

Cutaneous polyarteritis nodosa was identified as a large vessel vasculitis of the deep dermis and subcutis with a benign prognosis (BORRIE 1972). We would argue that there is no advantage in separating this from what would otherwise be called nodular vasculitis which, except for local persistence or recurrent lesions, is well recognised to have a good prognosis. The evidence that it is a primary arteritis is tenuous to say the least. It is always confined to the lower leg in which gravitational factors act especially on veins, and biopsies are frequently taken late in its pathogenesis so vessels are not always easy to identify and, even when clearly arterial, the pathogenesis includes prior inflammation in the tissues supplied as well as localised lymphoedema. The clinical pattern of lesions which heal without any scarring in spite of recurrences over many years, is particularly unlikely to be due to arterial disease.

Fig. 15. a Degos' disease. A wedge-shaped ischaemic infarct in the dermis and epidermis secondary to obliterative endovasculitis of an arteriole. The dermal collagen is swollen with an homogenous smudged appearance. The picture suggests a primary arteriolar injury and a failure of distal perfusion. HE ×60 (Courtesy of M.M. BLACK). **b** The porcelin white scar is a feature of atrophie blanche, Degos' disease and lichen sclerosis atrophicus. It is secondary to obliterative endovasculitis of arterioles predominently in the superficial dermis. This does not rule out a failure of perfusion due to earlier and more distal capillary engorgement and injury

Table 3. Diseases affecting the skin which the clinician expects the histopathologist to diagnose

Erythema nodosum	
Nodular vasculitis	
Leukocytoclastic vasculitis	
Granulomatous vasculitis	Wegeners, Churg-Strauss lymphomatoid granulomatosis
Giant cell arteritis	
Septic vasculitis	
Cryoglobulinaemia	
Diffuse intravascular coagulation	
Erythema multiforme	
Sweet's disease (acute febrile neutrophilic dermatosis)	
Pyoderma gangrenosum	
Granuloma faciale	
Erythema elevatum diutinum	
Obliterative endovasculitis	

Lividoid vasculitis with its morphologically reticulate pattern of vascular origin, is a vasculitis in the broad sense of microvascular injury, but it is, in our view, no more so than atrophie blanche. The microvasculature of the lower leg is protected from hypertension by arteriolar vasoconstriction (LEVICK and MICHEL 1978) and hence the arterioles are always predisposed to spasm and block, and this is likely to be exaggerated where there is venous hypertension. As Levick and Michel have pointed out, the protective arteriolar vasoconstriction of the dependent leg is prevented by a rise in temperature. Livedo with summer ulceration is a clinical entity in which vasculitis is enhanced by warm weather. Normal, protective mechanisms are blocked and there is vasodilatation, causing capillary hypertension. The suggestion that such reticulate patterns are primarily immunologically induced is not well founded but the vessels involved are permeable or sieve-like and therefore will localise any immune complexes that are circulating.

3.2.8 Fitting the Pathology to the Clinical Picture

Up to this point we have concentrated on the essentials of vessel injury and the difficulties inherent in the concept of vasculitis. Table 3 lists the disease entities that the clinician may expect to diagnose and hence would seek confirmation by, or occasionally the initiation of such diagnoses by the pathologist.

3.2.9 Erythema Nodosum, Nodular Vasculitis and Panniculitis

There is overlap in the histological appearance of these disorders Erythema nodosum is primarily septal inflammation which may extend into the fat and deeper dermis. The vascular element is at the most a capillaritis or venulitis. Large vessels, arteries or veins, are not involved and there is little or no ischaemic

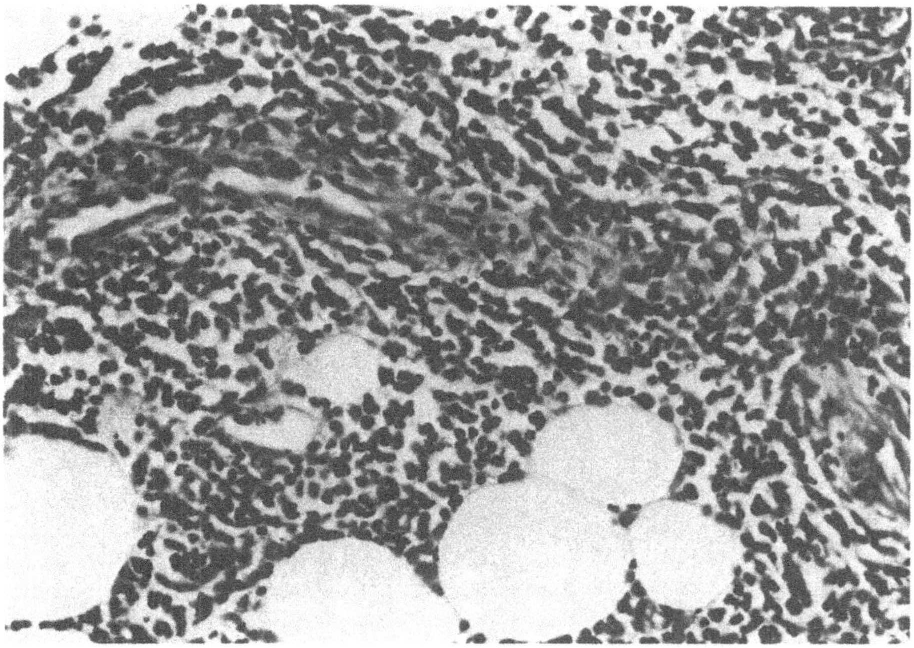
a

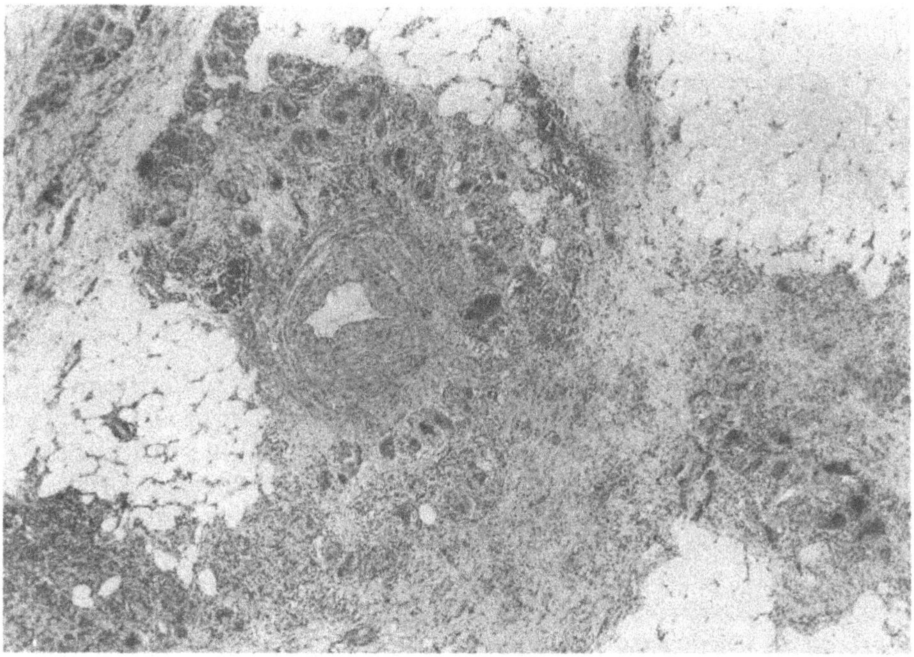
b

Fig. 16. a Erythema nodosum. In the late stages after at least one week the septal infiltrate consists primarily of lymphocytes and histiocytes with some spillover into adjacent fat. There may be patchy involvement of small and medium vessels but minimal fat necrosis. Earlier lesions often show greater neutrophil accumulation but are unlikely to be biopsied. HE ×380. **b** Chronic 'migratory' erythema nodosum. Long-standing lesions show an infiltrate of lymphocytes, histiocytes and many giant cells. Non-caseating granulomas may form; possibly a response to damaged fat and to protein accumulation. HE ×60

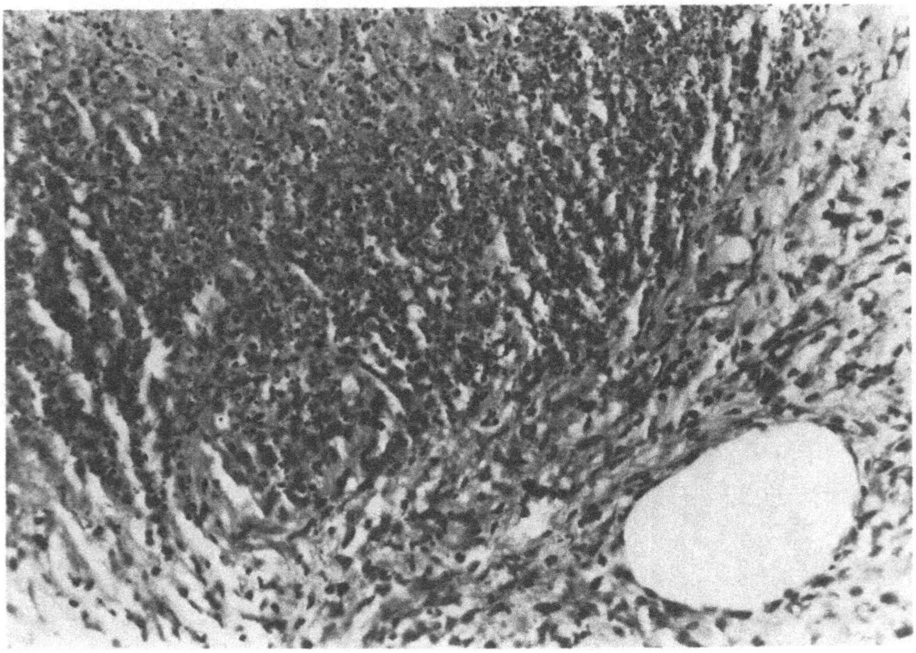

Fig. 17. Acute nodular vasculitis. A large septal vessel is completely destroyed by a necrotising vasculitis. Multiple sections may be required to demonstrate an affected vessel. Poor perfusion and damage of the vessel by intermittent hypoxia, secondary to prior more distal inflammation, may play a role in the aetiology. HE ×605

necrosis (Fig. 16a, b). It is a deep urticarial vasculitis, which heals without scarring. It may initially be neutrophilic but a lymphohistiocytic infiltrate usually predominates. If any fat cells die a mild granulomatous picture may be observed. Many fat cells remain entirely unaffected. There are less acute migratory forms which show a more mixed infiltrate with more pronounced granuloma formation (Fig. 16b) and some overlap with thrombophlebitis (RYAN and WILKINSON 1985).

On the other hand, in acute nodular vasculitis there is a severe necrotising vasculitis of a large septal vessel (Fig. 17) leading to ischaemia and extensive fat necrosis, so that the predominate picture is a patchy, lobular panniculitis. Numerous foamy and multinucleated histiocytes are present in the necrotic fat. Chronic and recurrent forms occur in cold dependant areas, e.g. "erythema induratum" affecting the calves of the scrofulus washer woman who stood all day in cold outhouses. The reaction pattern is also seen in the buttocks and thighs of cold female horse riders wearing tight jodhpurs, and is partly a consequence of ischaemia (BEACHAM et al. 1980). There is gradual thickening of the septa by oedema, granulation tissue and macrophages. Healing procedes by fibrosis of all or part of the fat lobule. In suspected cases of nodular vasculitis, multiple sections should be taken through the tissue block until large vessel vasculitis can be demonstrated.

The aetiology of nodular vasculitis is not fully understood but it has long been believed that both cold and a low grade thrombophlebitis, aggravated

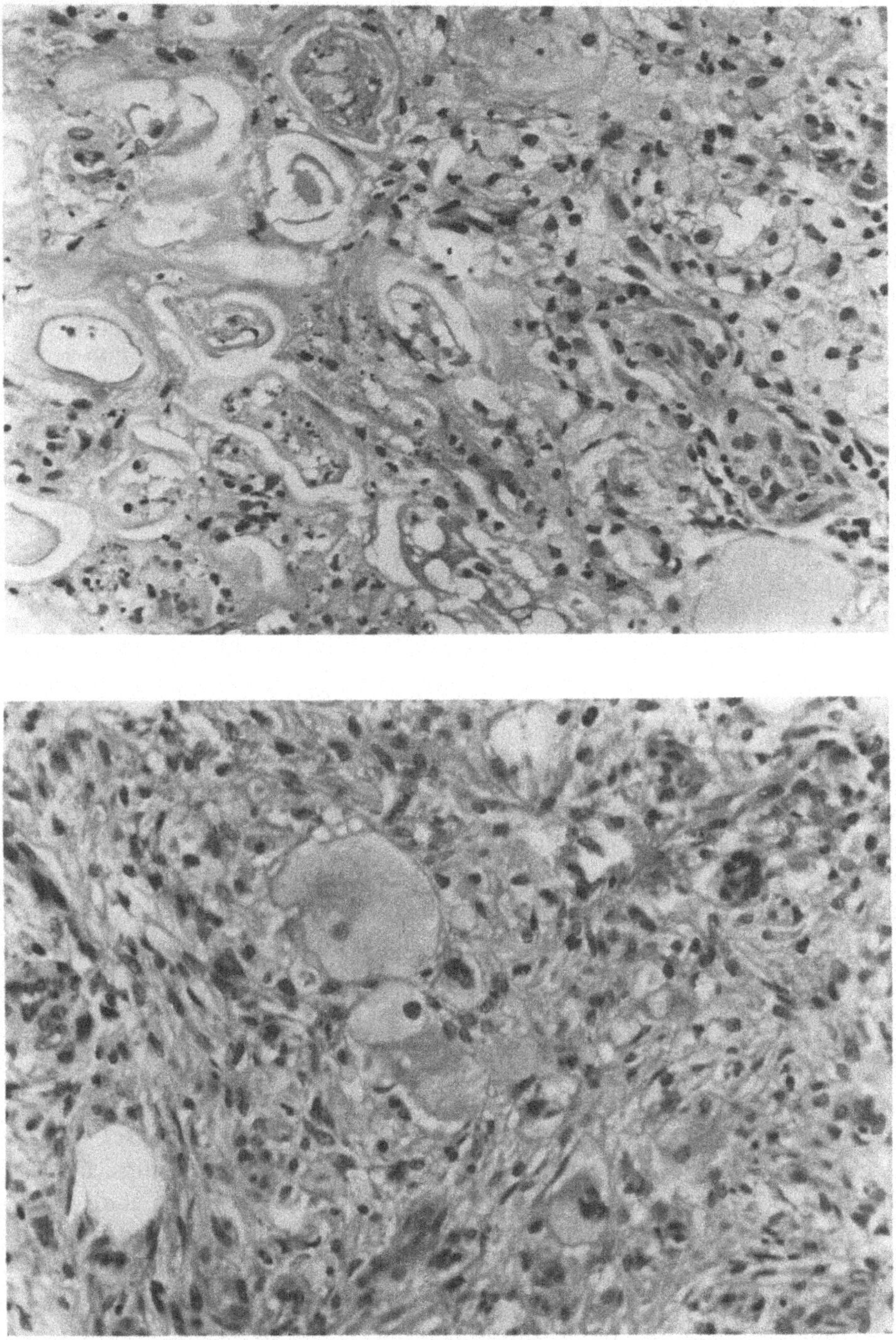

a

b

Fig. 18. a Subcutaneous nodular fat necrosis secondary to pancreatitis. There are many areas of fat necrosis with 'ghost-like' fat cells and basophilic deposits of calcium within and around fat cells. HE ×380. **b** A mixed infiltrate of neutrophils, lymphocytes, histiocytes and foam cells surrounds the foci of fat necrosis. HE ×380 by venous hypertension, play some part (WILKINSON 1954). To this may be added immune complex deposition, platelet embolisation and ischaemia. It is often a chronic recurring process confined to the lower leg and damage is cummulative. It is possible that bacterial antigens, immune complexes or platelet aggregates are deposited at sites of previous vascular damage, where there is an altered vascular pattern and inhomogeneity of flow in the fat lobule.

A lobular panniculitis without vasculitis affecting all the cells in an inflamed lobule has many associations, e.g. lupus erythematosus profundus, pancreatitis (Fig. 12a, b) factitial. There is disproportionate fat cell death compared with the surrounding septal inflammation and the fat is more uniformly damaged than in nodular vasculitis.

Pathologists should not themselves give support to the clinical morphologist seeking a difference between nodular vasculitis, erythema induratum, sub-acute nodular migratory panniculitis and erythema nodosum migrans. The problem of overlap is inevitable; larger vessels are likely to become involved even if only due to impairment of flow through them. Fat necrosis inducing a granuloma or followed by liquefaction and suppuration is a likely consequence of inflammation or ischaemia. As a consequence, there are variants of varied intensity and chronicity, that are given a number of names which should now be obsolete, e.g. Weber Christian disease, Rothman and Makai disease and migratory erythema nodosum (BAVERSTED 1968).

3.2.10 The Granulomatous Diseases

Purely arterial diseases tend to spare the lungs. However, pulmonary hypertension may develop in chronic respiratory disease, gradually destroying the normal vascular pattern and predisposing to secondary arterial disease. There is a spectrum from benign exudative and eosinophilic pulmonary disease to the malignant obstructive phase of necrosis described by WEGENER 1939. In the skin, these diseases have similar exudative to obstructive phases of vascular pathology. Clinically, such lesions range from space-occupying hyperaemia or granulomata to infarction and ulceration with rapid total destruction of the vessel and surrounding tissue. The pathologist should avoid ridiculous sub-classification. Classifications including Loffler, Choffler, Churg, Chegener and Wegener were well described, as the "Choffler Train" (BURTON and BURTON 1972).

These diseases are usually chronic with intermittent acute phases. Much depends whether an acute, chronic or acute on chronic lesion is biopsied. Wegener's granulomatosis (HU et al. 1977; FAUCI et al. 1983; RONCO et al. 1983) allergic granulomatosis (CHURG and STRAUSS 1951) and lymphomatoid granulomatosis have to be distinguished. Biopsies of acute lesions in Wegener's granulomatosis show leucocytoclastic vasculitis and any size of vessel may be affected. A granuloma is seen around a central core of degenerate basophilic collagen, apparently outside the vessel and associated with masses of polymorphonuclear cells and leucocyte debris. Around this is a sleeve of lymphocytes and palisading histiocytes. We will argue that this granuloma is not necessarily initially extravascular but it is a histiocytic response around a venule totally destroyed by

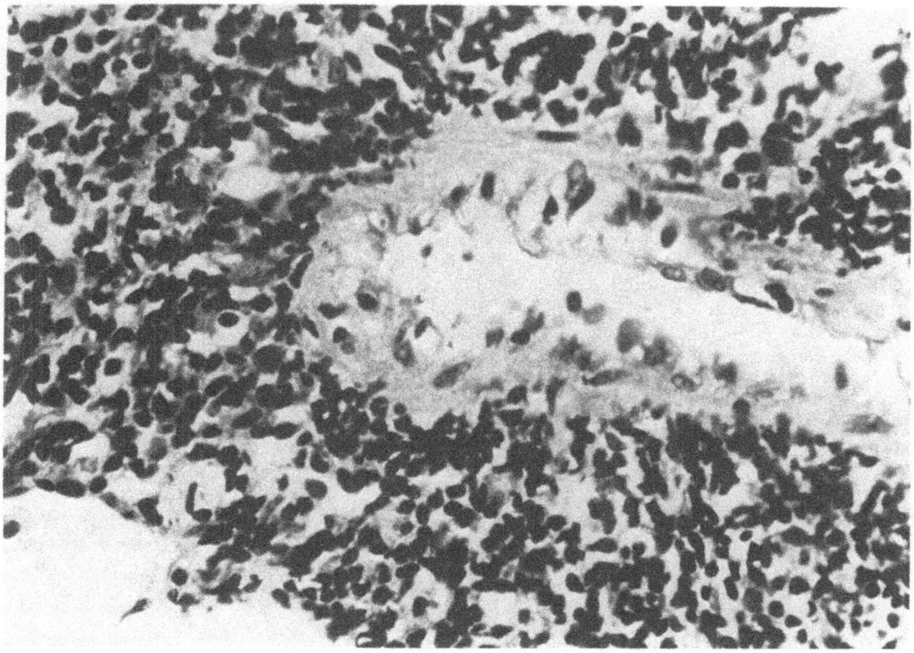

Fig. 19. Lymphomatoid granulomatosis in a non-ulcerated area; the lymphocytic infiltrate surrounds but does not disrupt a large vessel so that blood supply is maintained. Infarction is not a feature unlike the aggressive injury in some sites of Wegener's granulomatosis. HE ×605

prior vasculitis. The larger parent vessel may rarely be the centre of a granuloma. A dense angiocentric, necrotising, fibrinoid reaction may obliterate the large vessel and this is surrounded by epithelioid and giant cells. This is a much larger lesion extending through the entire dermis and contributing to its total destruction. There is sometimes an ischaemic infarct of the tissues because the supplying vessel has its outflow obstructed within the granuloma. Eosinophils and neutrophils have a relatively short life and are supplied only from the blood stream. Their presence is therefore an indication of continuing blood supply. The late obstructive phase of vasculitis shows few neutrophils and a prominent histiocyte response. When this process incites a T- or B-cell response there will be evidence of some blast cell formation and mitotic figures giving rise to the picture known as lymphomatoid granulomatosis (LIEBOW et al. 1972; LIEBOW 1973; MURPHY et al. 1981; JAMES et al. 1981). The lesions in this condition usually preserve their blood supply so that clinically ulceration is rare and histologically the vessels of non-ulcerated lesions are preserved in the centre of the lesion (Fig. 19), but there may be angio-destruction and necrosis in ulcerated areas. Allergic granulomatosis is associated with the same spectrum of changes but eosinophils are more prominently involved and the clinical picture is more acute and fulminant.

Lymphomatoid papulosis (BLACK 1982; WILLEMZE et al. 1982) is included in this chapter because there is a phase in its evolution in which vascular damage is prominant. Mostly, however, the papules show no vasculitis but the evolution

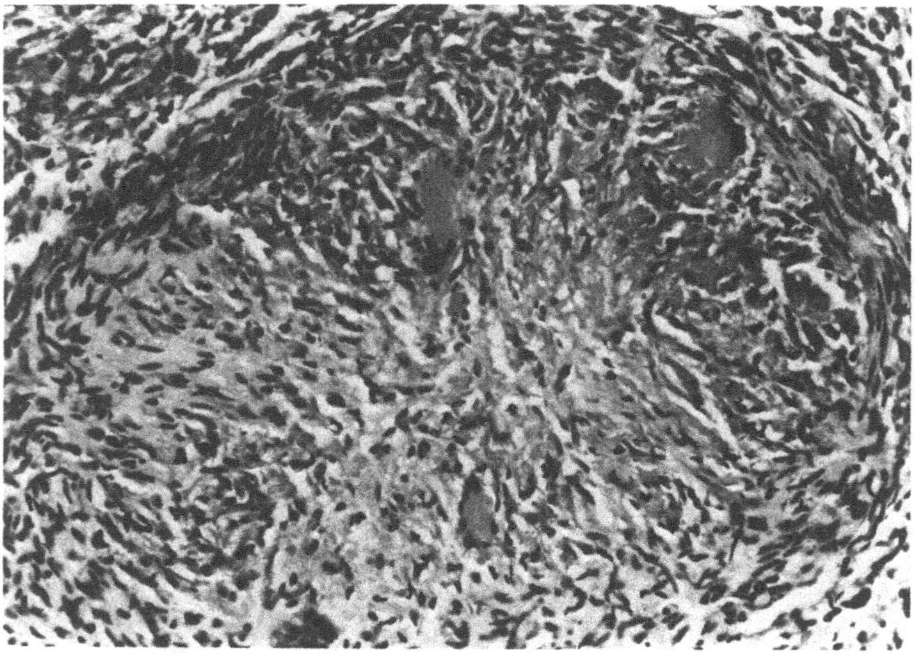

Fig. 20. Temporal (giant cell) arteritis. The wall of the artery has degenerated and there is an intramural infiltrate of mononuclear cells, plasma cells and multinucleated giant cells. HE ×380

of the papules over a number of days evokes an increasingly heavy perivascular infiltrate that eventually may progress to vessel obliteration and central necrosis. The clinician has a choice of numerous papular lesions, some with epidermal spongiosis and lymphocyte infiltration underlying a parakeratotic scale and some with dilated capillaries surrounded by lymphocytes. A biopsy of a lesion showing incipient necrosis will inevitably show the heaviest infiltrate with some large and bizarre mononuclear cells, some the identity of T-cells and others, Langerhans cells (WILLEMZE et al. 1982).

3.3 Cranial (Giant Cell) Arteritis

Occasionally, temporal arteritis presents with scalp ulcerations. There is a patchy panarteritis involving large and medium-sized temporal or other cranial arteries. The trigger appears to be degeneration of the elastic lamina and this stimulates a macrophage response. Many of the macrophages evolve into multinucleated giant cells (Fig. 20). There is an infiltrate of mononuclear cells and plasma cells, fibrinoid degeneration and eventually fibrosis of the vessel wall.

3.4 Leucocytoclastic Angiitis (Fig. 21)

The diseases recognised by clinicians that have this pathology in common are listed in Table 4. There is a variable superficial, neutrophil versus lymphocyte

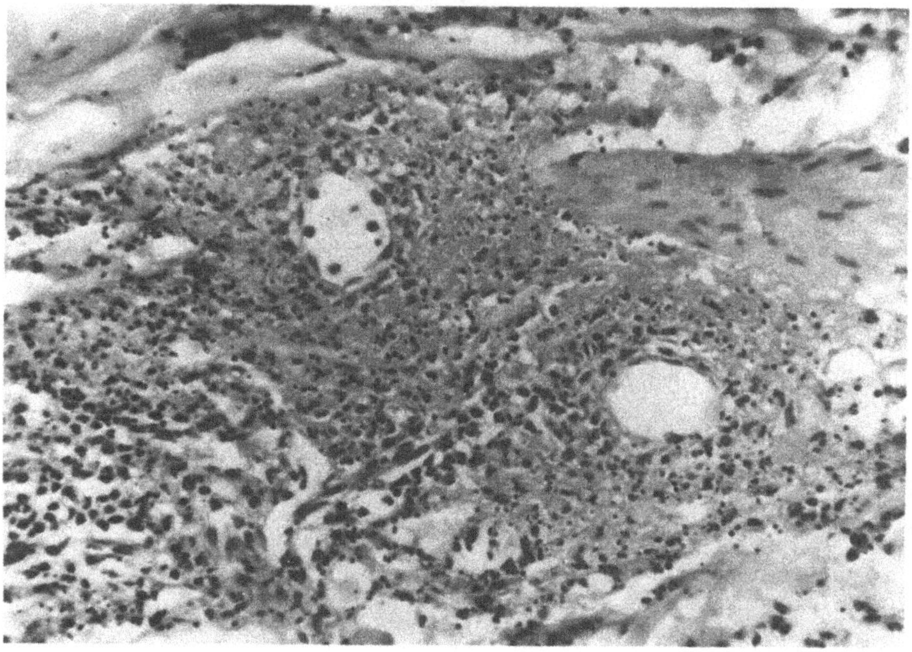

Fig. 21. Leukocytoclastic vasculitis of dermal capillaries. There is endothelial swelling, fibrinoid degeneration and neutrophils around and within the vessel walls, associated with abundant nuclear fragments. Up to this stage perfusion has been maintained and neutrophils continue to accumulate. HE ×380

Table 4. Disorders associated with a cutaneous leukocytoclastic vasculitis

Henoch-Schönlein disease urticarial vasculitis erythema elevatum diutinum connective tissue disorders	rheumatoid arthritis systemic lupus erythematosus dermatomyositis
Chronic infections	subacute bacterial endocarditis chronic gonococcaemia erythema nodosum leprosum hepatitis B herpes simplex
Ulcerative colitis lymphoproliferative diseases	Hodgkins' disease lymphosarcoma
Malignancies mixed cryoglobulinaemia granulomatous vasculitis	allergic granulomatosis Wegener's granulomatosis
Drug sensitivities	sulphonamides, thiazides, penicillin
Food allergies	benzoates, tartrazine
Trauma	cold, tick bites

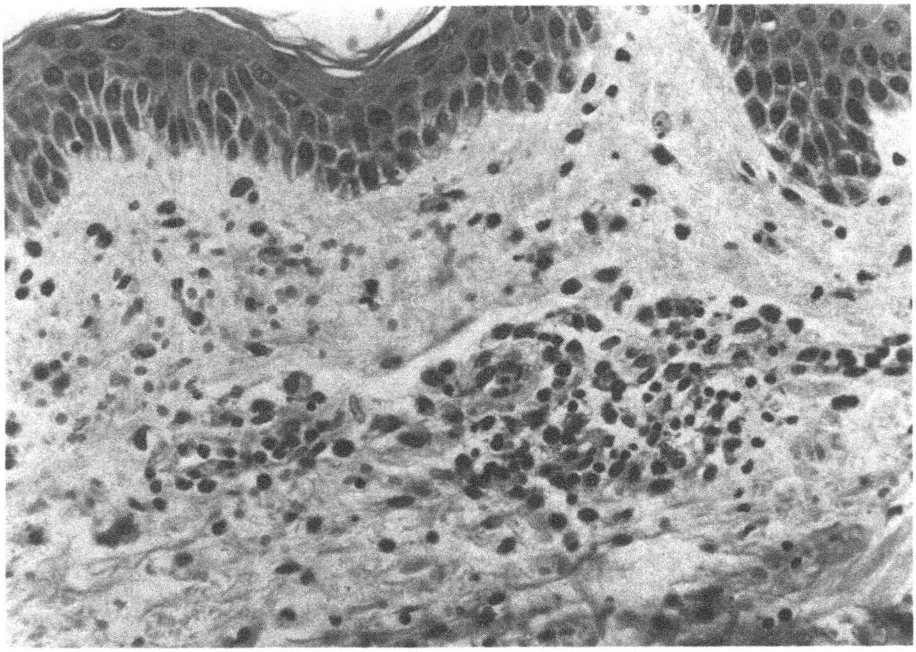

Fig. 22. A predominantly lymphocytic vasculitis in a patient with palpable purpuric vasculitic lesions. There is extensive extravasation of red blood cells and lymphocytes around and within the vessel walls. HE ×380

response which depends on the age of the lesion and the mechanism. The early acute lesion, associated with complement consumption, will have a heavy neutrophilic component and severe ischaemia and necrosis may develop. Urticarial vasculitis does not develop necrosis but is, however, associated with hypocomplementaemia and a predominantly neutrophilic response. Hypocomplementaemia and urticaria or ischaemia and necrosis occur at polar ends of the spectrum (Fig. 7) (RUSSELL JONES et al. 1983).

The infiltrate involves and disrupts the vessel wall. There is evidence of endothelial swelling, vacuolisation or shrinkage. The neutrophils are disrupted releasing abundant nuclear fragments(dust). Fibrin and plasma protein deposition (fibrinoid) occurring within and around the vessel walls and extending between collagen bundles are a classic, but not inevitable feature since fibrinoid is not seen in early more urticarial lesions. Extravasation of red cells is less obvious in chronic lesions in which cells are replaced by haemosiderin and in which fibrosis tends to be a feature. Acute ischaemia due to obliteration of the microvasculature may lead to ischaemic necrosis of the wall of the supplying arterioles and infarction of the centre of an inflammatory lesion.

Fig. 23. a Chronic gonococcal sepsis: A superficial pustule has formed within the dermal papilla and epidermis. Papillary vessels show vascular dilatation and congestion with fibrinoid material HE ×380. **b** Microthrombi are common in small vessels in gonococcal sepsis. Central infarction and necrosis of the lesion forming a haemorrhagic pustule is the clinical consequence. HE ×1,470

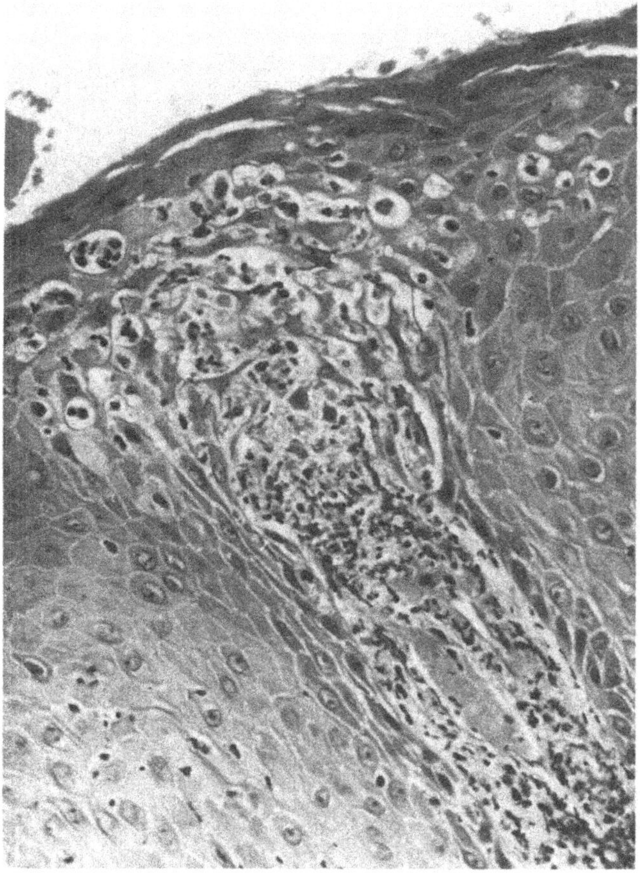

a

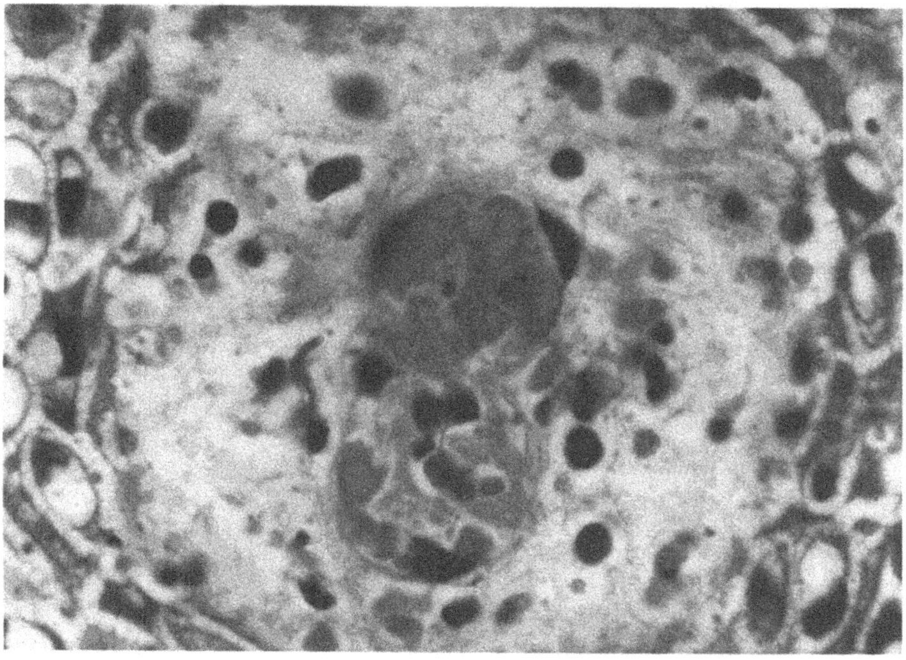

b

Fig. 23a, b

a

b

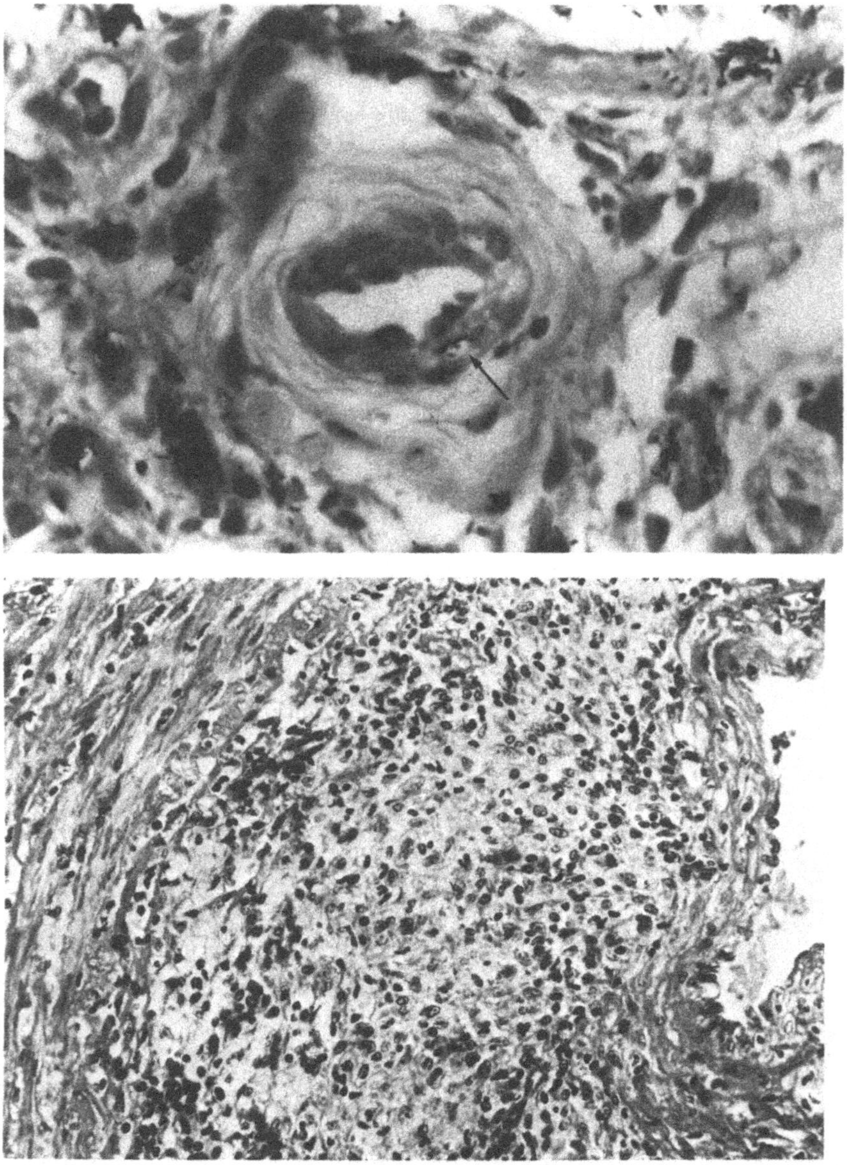

Fig. 24. a Lepromatous leprosy: solid staining bacilli (*arrowed*) in the media and endothelium of an arteriole in the lower dermis. Numerous bacilli and macrophages are present in the surrounding tissues. Fite-Faraco stain (RIDLEY 1977). ×960 (Courtesy of CORUH and McDOUGALL 1979). **b** Granulomatous inflammation around a subcutaneous vein in lepromatous leprosy. HE ×300. (Courtesy of MUKHERJEE et al. 1983)

4. Mixed Vasculitis

Vasculitis is rarely monocellular and some degree of neutrophil and lymphocyte mixing is usual (Fig. 22). SOTER et al. (1976) emphasised the distinctiveness of neutrophilic versus lymphocytic infiltration. There is a trend to equate neutro-

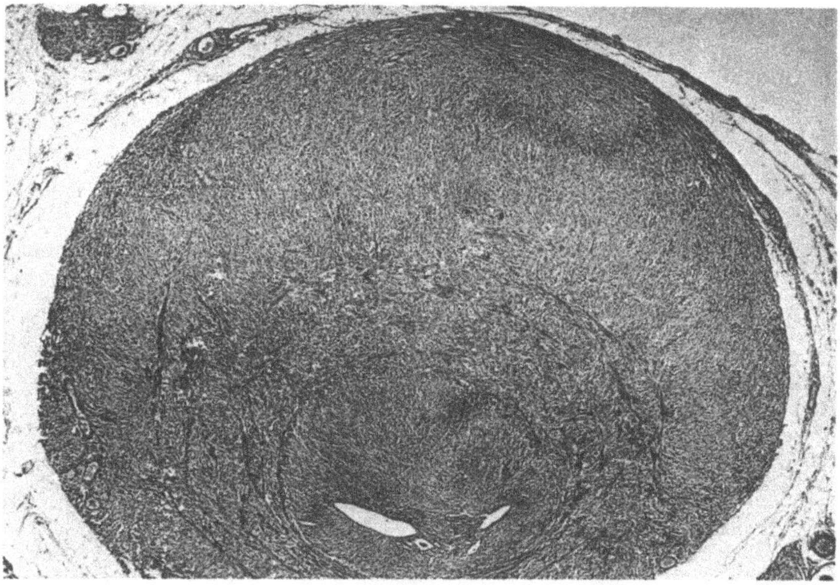

Fig. 24. c Subcutaneous vein with a diffuse lepromatous granulomata replacing the whole intima and causing nearly total occlusion of the lumen. HE ×50. (Courtesy of MUKHERJEE et al. 1983)

phils with complement activation and lymphocytes with cell mediated immunity. Clinically identical lesions can have predominence of either cell type, but the infiltrate in drug eruptions or connective tissue diseases such as lupus erythematosus tends to be more lymphocytic. Even when there are circulating immune complexes, there is an overall lack of correlation between the pathological picture and the identification of the complexes (ANDREWS et al. 1979). Thus, while a neutrophilic response may be more common in early lesions, even in the same subject a lymphocytic response may be observed in some lesions earlier or later (MITCHELL SAMS 1980).

The proponents of arguments that timing is important can produce evidence that neutrophils (RYAN 1976) or mononuclear cells (GOWER et al. 1977) appear first but chronicity and repair is usually equated with mononuclear cells. However, ANDREWS (1979) found timing of biopsy did not determine the predominant cell type. There are few opportunities for studies using serial biopsies, but where more than one biopsy is done they serve mostly to emphasise variability and mixed pictures (PHANUPHAK et al. 1980; CREAM et al. 1971).

4.1 Septic Vasculitis

Septic embolisation and vasculitis due to bacteria antigens (REA and RIDLEY 1979; ACKERMAN et al. 1965; SHAPIRO et al. 1973) or bacteria themselves (HURWITZ et al. 1984), encourage pus formation. Masses of neutrophils form abscesses well beyond the vessel and often within the epidermis. In chronic gonococcaemia, a superficial pustule is often formed surrounded by intense vascular dilatation and congestion (Fig. 23a). Fibrinoid material and microthrombi are com-

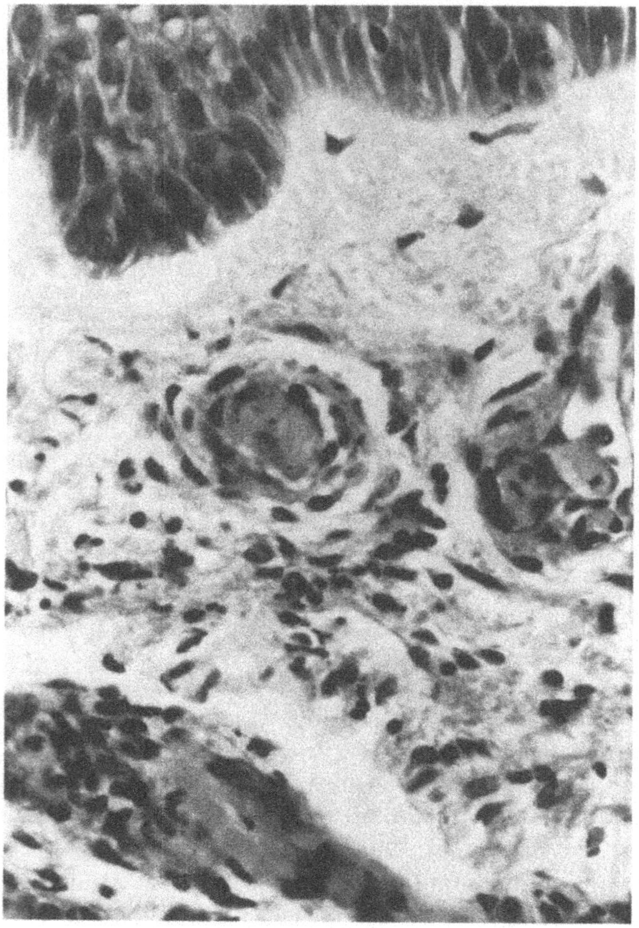

Fig. 25. Mixed cryoglobulinaemia: Dermal vessels are occluded by amorphous eosinophilic material and there is a vasculitis. The infiltrate is predominently mononuclear and there are some nuclear fragments in the surrounding tissue. HE ×605

mon in capillaries,venules and small arteries (Fig. 23b). Leukocytoclasis is often present.

In lepromatous leprosy large numbers of bacilli may invade cutaneous and subcutaneous vessel walls (Fig. 24a) (CORUH and McDOUGALL 1979). If large veins are involved there may be a granulomatous phlebitis (Fig. 24b) with eventual occlusion of the lumen (Fig. 24c) (MUKHERJEE et al. 1983).

Purpura Fulminans (HJORT et al. 1964; SPICER and RAU 1976); *Coumarin necrosis* (NALBANDIAN 1965; RUSSELL JONES and CUNNINGHAM 1979) and *Disseminated Intravascular Coagulation* (ROBBOY et al. 1973) are disorders with features of intravascular coagulation and consumption of clotting factors. There is loss of vessel wall integrity and bleeding into the tissues. Thus the fibrin clot, mainly in venular capillaries is a prominent feature associated with extensive red cell extravasation. The rate of development probably determines the

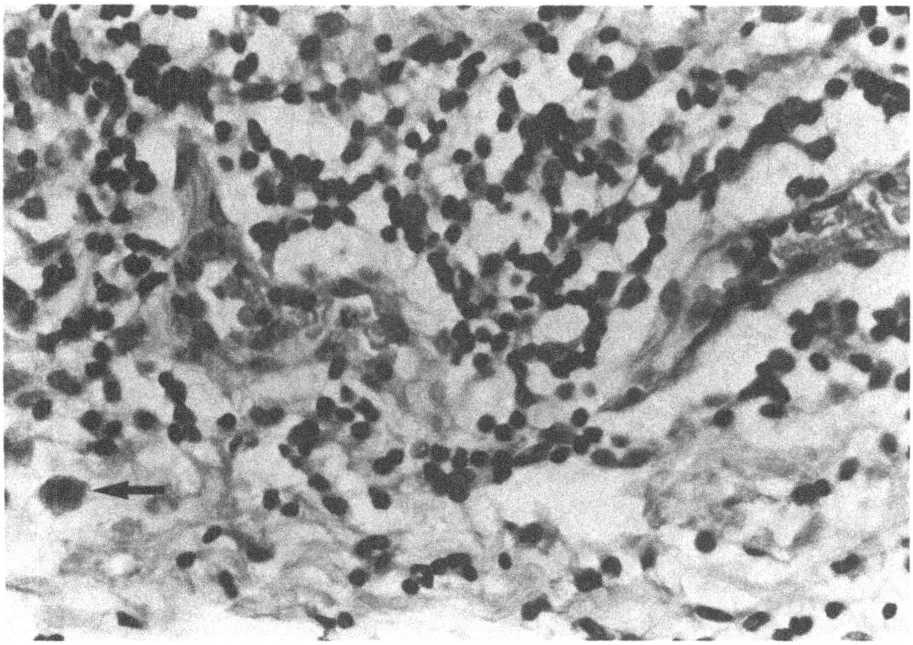

Fig. 26. Pigmented purpura: Elongated tortuous vessels are surrounded by mononuclear cells. In long-standing cases, extravasated red blood cells may be difficult to find, but there is haemosiderin within macrophages (*arrowed*). HE ×605

cellular response, which may include either neutrophils or lymphocytes, but complete absence of inflammation is common. The endothelial cell damage could be a sign of either a toxic injury or ischaemia.

In *Thrombotic Thrombocytopenic Purpura*, widespread hyaline thrombi may be recognised containing platelets, red blood cells and leucocytes. The consequence is ischaemic necrosis of the vessel wall in this case, usually an arteriole (FELDMAN et al. 1966; BONE et al. 1978; NEAME et al. 1973; ORBISON 1952). Thus, as mentioned above, this is one of the few causes of arterial versus venular injury.

4.2 Cryoglobulinaemia

Cryoglobulins may be monoclonal or mixed. Monoclonal cryoglobulins, usually IgM or IgG, are associated with immuno-proliferative disorders such as myeloma, Waldenstrom's macroglobulinaemia or lymphoma. In areas of cooling or stasis, the cryoglobulins are precipitated, occluding and damaging small vessels and frequently causing extensive red cell extravasation. The vessels, usually dermal capillaries or venules, are filled with an amorphous eosinophilic substance (Fig. 11). There may be a mild perivascular lymphocytic infiltrate, but leukocytoclasis and fibrinoid deposition are not a feature.

Mixed cryoglobulins are circulating immune complexes. They are found in

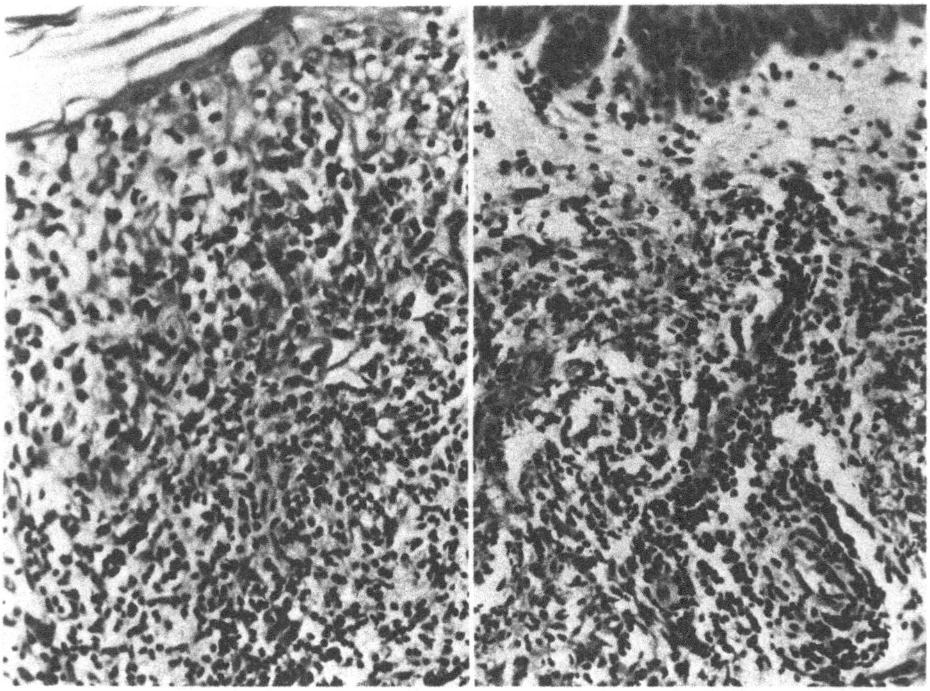

Fig. 27. a Erythema multiforme – epidermal type: The epidermal changes are pronounced with basal cell vacuolar degeneration and necrotic keratinocytes throughout the epidermis. The mononuclear cell infiltrate is relatively mild. HE ×270. **b** Erythema multiforme – dermal type: There is a pronounced infiltrate of mononuclear cells within the superficial dermis, but very little epidermal involvement. There are some extravasated red cells but no leukocytoclasis or fibrinoid necrosis. HE ×270

auto-immune disorders such as systemic lupus erythematosus and rheumatoid arthritis, or diseases associated with hyperglobulinaemia. The cryoglobulin complex activates complement and induces a leukocytoclastic vasculitis (Fig. 25).

Pigmented purpuric eruptions are characterised by upper dermal capillary elongation and tortuosity (DAVIS and LAWLER 1958) and extravasation of red cells (Fig. 26). The inflammatory response consists mainly of mononuclear cells. There is often an excess of haemosiderin or iron with melanin in the macrophages, and mild fibrosis. The pathology is usually confined to the lower legs (RYAN and WILKINSON 1985) emphasising a gravitational factor.

Erythema multiforme, Sweet's disease and Pyoderma gangrenosum are inflammatory processes which show overlap in aetiology and histopathology. A vascular component is common especially in later stages in which the damage to the vessel wall may be a consequence of heavy white cell infiltrates, clotting or ischaemia.

The changes in erythema multiforme may be predominently dermal or epidermal (LEVER and SCHAUMBERG LEVER 1983). Classic erythema multiforme presents with intense upper dermal oedema, papillary vessel dilatation evidence of epidermal basal cell damage, or more extensive keratinocyte necrosis

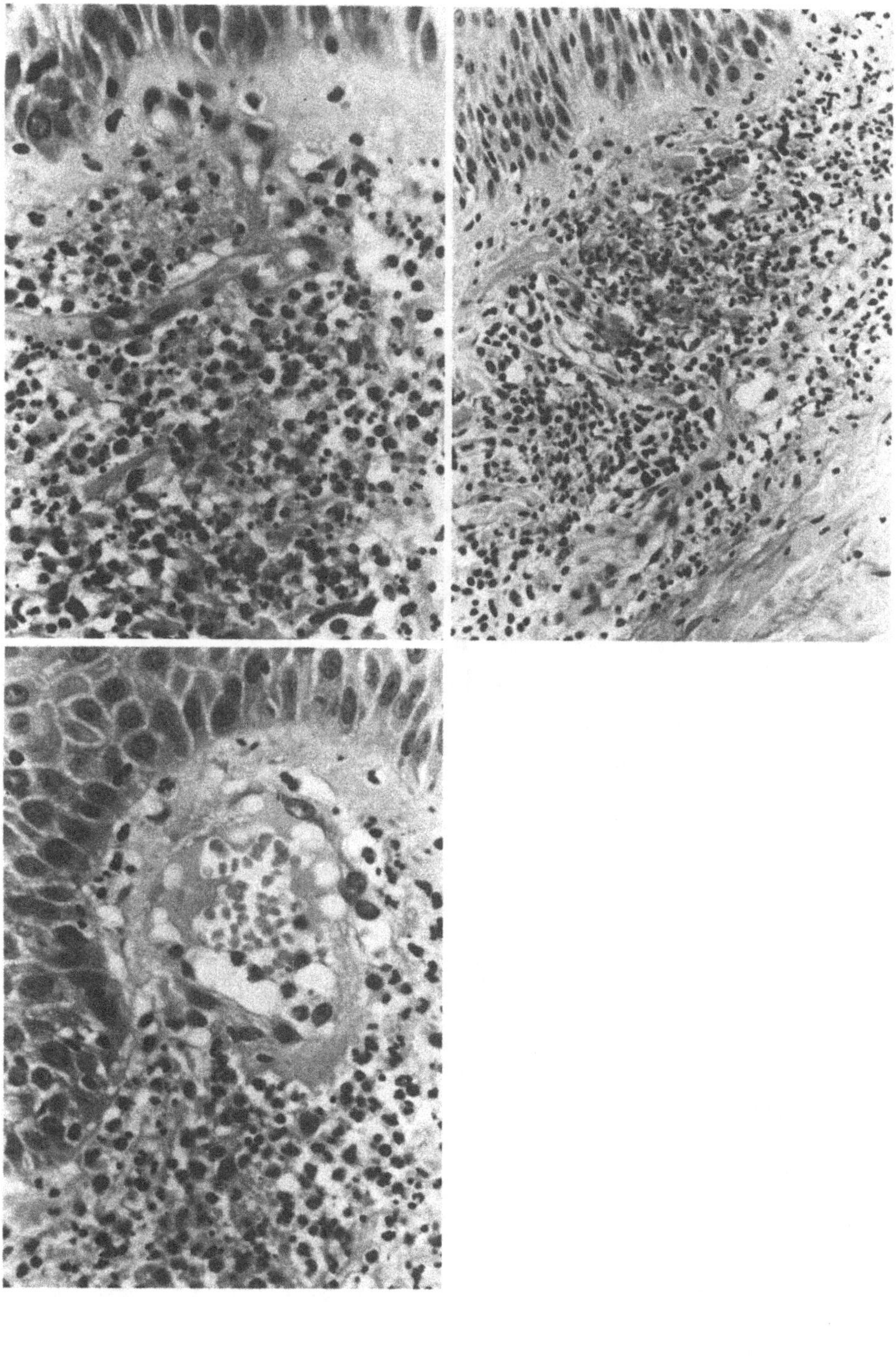

Fig. 28a–c. Sweet's disease (acute neutrophilic dermatosis). **a** There is a dense infiltrate, mainly of neutrophils, within the dermis, separated from the epidermis by a zone of oedema. HE ×432,5. **b** In some areas lymphocytes predominate and there is an overlap with the dermal form of erythema multiforme. HE ×270. **c** Many of the neutrophils show leukocytoclasia but blood vessels are well preserved. HE ×432,5

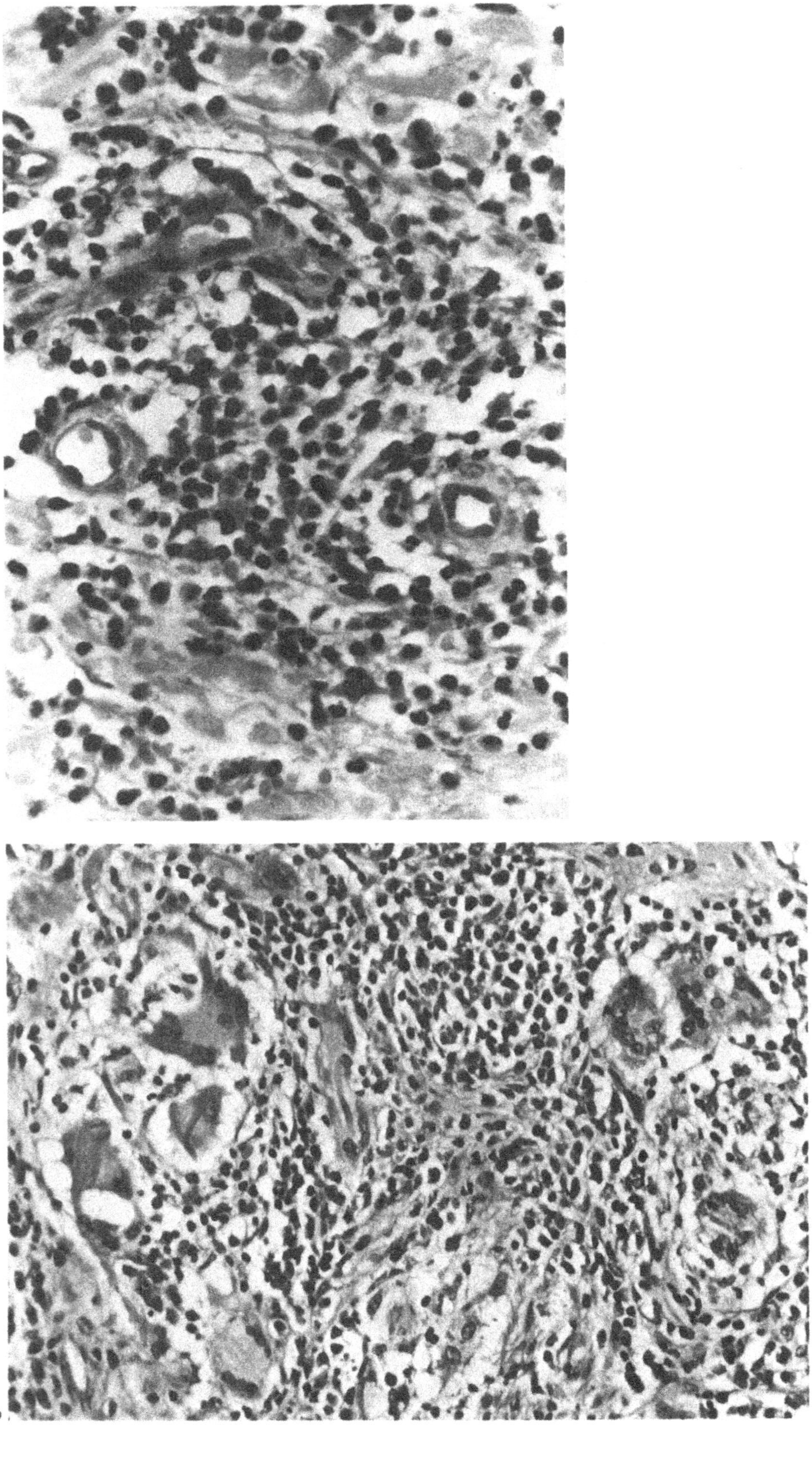

a

b

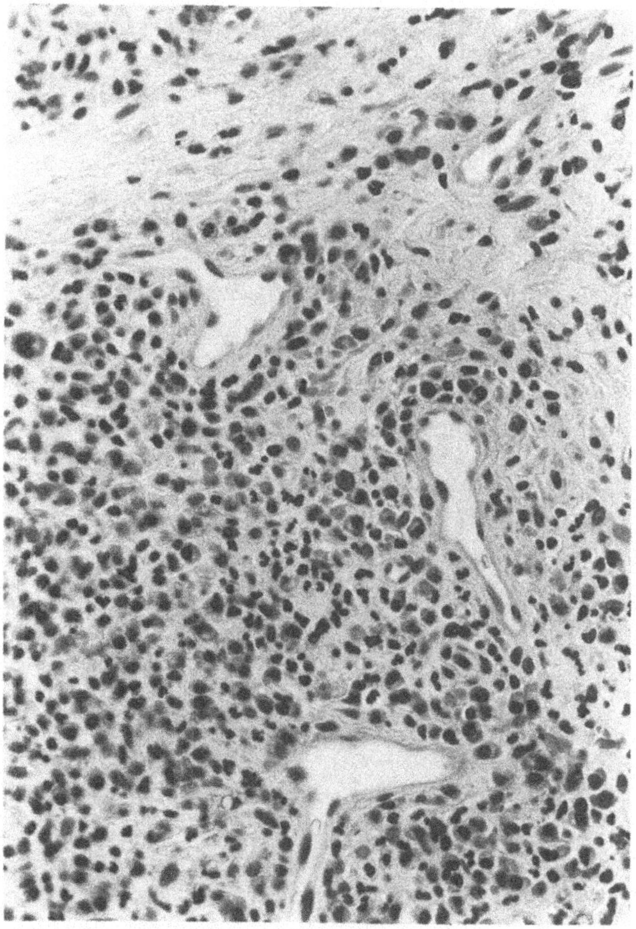

Fig. 30. Granuloma faciale: The upper dermis contains a dense polymorphic infiltrate which characteristically leaves a zone of normal collagen adjacent to the epidermis. Neutrophils and eosinophils predominate and frequently nuclear dust is formed. In some areas there may be evidence of vasculitis. HE ×380

(Fig. 27a). Once the epithelium and upper dermis have been disrupted, upper vessels are inevitably injured with extravasation of erythrocytes. The type of cell wall infiltrate depends on the timing and intensity of the reaction, but it is usually lymphocytic rather than neutrophilic and "nuclear dust" is not found. Macular and many papular lesions show predominently dermal changes (Fig. 27b), while in some target lesions epidermal changes are pronounced (Fig. 27a).

Fig. 29. a Pyoderma gangrenosum: A variable neutrophil, eosinophil or mononuclear response may be seen. Vessel walls are usually normal in the early lesion unless impaired perfusion and ischaemic infarction supervenes. HE ×605. **b** Pyoderma gangrenosum: The infiltrate is lymphocytic frequently with a granulomatous component in deeper dermis or fat. Poorly perfused tissues are attempting to clear debris and to repair. HE ×380

Sweet's disease (SWEET 1964) known as acute febrile neutrophilic dermatosis has some similar clinical and histological features to erythema multiforme. However, the heavy, focal dermal infiltrate is usually largely neutrophilic with some leucocytoclasis but, many lesions show a neutrophilic infiltrate mixed with lymphocytes and even eosinophils (Fig. 28a, b, c). The degree of oedematous reaction in the overlying dermis is variable and rarely there are intradermal vesicles. The vessel walls may show some endothelial swelling but there is no perivascular fibrinoid material or extravasation of red blood cells and necrosis is rare since blood supply remains good through patent vessels.

Pyoderma gangrenosum may show a similar superficial neutrophil response associated with epidermal ulceration (Fig. 29a). Granulation tissue and pseudo-epitheliomatous hyperplasia are features of more persistent incompletely resolving lesions. There may be micro-abscess formation either superficial or deep. The infiltrate tends to be mononuclear in the deeper dermis with a granulomatous component in fat or around damaged adnexa (Fig. 29b). The congestion and clotting within within the venules is greater than in Sweet's disease, but vessel walls are usually normal (Fig. 29a). Clinically and pathologically, anything from a superficial pustule to a deep erythema nodosum-like lesions can be seen. The diagnosis rests with the clinician.

Erythema elevatum diutinum is a chronic recurrent leucocytoclastic (neutrophilic) vasculitis in which ischaemic necrosis is rare but fibrosis is usual. Characteristically, large amounts of fibrinoid surround the upper dermal vessels without vessel obliteration. Cholesterol (lipid) deposition known as extracellular cholesterosis (URBACH et al. 1932) is seen in some cases and probably does not justify separate classification (RYAN and WILKINSON 1985).

Granuloma faciale (COBANE et al. 1950). This rare chronic disorder is of unknown cause. Clinically it seems hardly to justify the term vasculitis, but pathologically there is evidence of vasculitis with fibrinoid deposition within and around capillary walls, red cell extravasation and leukocytoclasia. The upper dermis contains a dense mixed infiltrate predominently of neutrophils and eosinophils, which may extend into subcutaneous fat. The epidermis is characteristically spared and there is a narrow 'grenz' zone of normal papillary dermis (Fig. 30).

Granuloma faciale is distinguished from erythema elevatum diutinum by the presence of eosinophils and the zone of normal collagen beneath the epidermis.

Acknowledgement: The authors wish to thank Richard L. Jones for technical assistance.

References

Ackerman AB (1978) Histologic Diagnosis of Inflammatory Diseases. Lea & Febger, Philadelphia

Ackerman AB, Miller RCA, Shapiro L (1965) Gonococcaemia and its cutaneous manifestations. Arch Dermatol 91:227–232

Alarcon-Segovia D (ed) (1980) Clinics in Rheumatic Diseases. Vol. 6/No. 2: The Necrotising Vasculitides. W.B. Saunders, London

Almeida JD, Waterson AP (1969) Immune complexes in hepatitis. Lancet 2:983–986

Altorfer J, Hedinger C, Clodius L (1977) Light and electron microscopic investigation of extremities of dogs with experimental chronic lymphostasis. Folia Angiologica 25:140–155

Andrews BS, Cains G, McIntosh J, Petts V, Perry R (1979) Circulating and tissue immune complexes in cutaneous vasculitis. J Clin Lab Immunol 1:311–320
Baferstedt B (1968) Erythema nodosum migrans. Acta Dermato-Vener 48:381–384
Bard J, Winkelmann RK (1967) Livedo vasculitis: segmental hyalinizing vasculitis of the dermis. Arch Dermatol 96:489–499
Beacham BE, Cooper PH, Buchanan S, Weary PE (1980) Equestrian cold panniculitis in women. Arch Dermatol 116:1025–1027
Black MM (1982) Lymphomatoid papulosis. Br J Dermatol 106:717–721
Bone RC, Henry JE, Petterson J, Amare M (1978) Respiratory dysfunction in thrombotic thrombocytopaenic purpura. Am J Med 65:262–269
Borrie P (1972) Cutaneous polyarteritis nodosa. Br J Dermatol 87:87–95
Borrie P, Stansfeld A (1966) Cutaneous vasculitis. In: Mckenna RMB (ed) Modern Trends in Dermatology. Vol 3. Butterworths, London, 167–195
Braverman IM (1981) The Angiitides. In: Braverman IM (ed) Skin Signs of Systemic Disease. 2nd Edn. W.M. Saunders, Philadelphia, 378–444
Braverman IM, Keh-Yen A (1984) Ultrastructure of the human microcirculation in valve containing collecting veins at the dermal-subcutaneous junction. J Invest Dermatol 81:438–442
Braverman IM, Yen A (1975) Demonstration of immune complexes in spontaneous and histamine induced lesions in normal skin of patients with leukocytoclastic angiitis. J Invest Dermatol 64:105–112
Braverman IM, Yen A (1977) Ultrastructure of the human dermal microcirculation: II the capillary loops of the dermal papillae. J Invest Dermatol 68:44–52
Burton JL, Burton PA (1972) Pulmonary eosinophilia associated with vasculitis and extravascular granulomata. Br J Dermatol 87:412–419
Casley-Smith JR, Gaffney RM (1981) Excess plasma proteins as a cause of chronic inflammation and lymphoedema. Aust J Pathol 133:243–272
Caulin-Glaser T, Gallo GR, Lamm ME (1983) Non-dissociating cationic immune complexes can deposit in glomerular basement membrane. J Exp Med 158:1561–1572
Cherry GW, Ryan TJ (1976) The effect of ischaemia and reperfusion on tissue survival. In: Ryan TJ (ed) Microvascular Injury (Vol 7 Major Problems in Dermatology). Lloyd Luke Medical, London, 93–115
Churg J, Strauss L (1951) Allergic granulomatosis, allergic angiitis and periarteritis nodosa. Am J Pathol 27:277–301
Cobane JH, Straith CL, Pinkus H (1950) Facial granulomas with eosinophilia. Their relation to other eosinophilic granulomas of the skin and to reticulo granuloma. Arch Dermatol 61:442–454
Copeman PWM (1975) Cutaneous angiitis. J R Coll Physicians Lond 9:103–119
Copeman PWM (1983) Cutaneous angiitis: more than immune complex venulitis. In: Saunders KB (ed) Advances in Medicine. Pitman Medical Publishers, London, 165–183
Copeman PWM, Ryan TJ (1970) The problems of cutaneous angiitis with reference to histopathology and pathogenesis. Br J Dermatol 82:2–14
Coruh G, McDougall AC (1979) Untreated lepromatous leprosy: histopathological findings in cutaneous blood vessels. Int J Lep 47:500–511
Cream JJ, Bryceson ADM, Ryder G (1971) Disappearance of immunoglobulin and complement from the Arthus reaction and its relevance to studies of vasculitis in man. Br J Dermatol 84:106–109
Cupps TR, Fauci AS (1981) The Vasculitides (Major Problems in Internal Medicine, Vol. 21). W.B. Saunders, Philadelphia
Davis MJ, Lawler JC (1958) Capillary alterations in pigmented purpuric disease of the skin. Arch Dermatol 78:723–731
DeBono D (1983) White blood cells and the vessel wall. In: Woolf N (ed) Biology and Pathology of the Vessel Wall. Praeger Publishers, New York, 101–118
Dodman B, Cunliffe WJ, Roberts BE (1973) Observations on tissue fibrinolytic activity in patients with cutaneous vasculitis. Br J Dermatol 88:229–235
Dymock RB (1981) Cutaneous atheromatous embolism. Aust J Derm 22:30–32
Eady RAJ, Wilson Jones E (1977) Pseudopyogenic granuloma: Enzyme histochemical and ultrastructural study. Hum Pathol 8:653–668
Farber EM, Hines EA, Montgomery H, Craig W (1947) Arterioles of skin in essential hypertension. J Invest Dermatol 9:285–298

Fauci AS, Haynes BF, Katz P, Wolff SM (1983) Wegener's granulomatosis: prospective clinical and therapeutic experience in 85 patients for 21 years. Ann Intern Med 98:76–85

Feldman JD, Mardiney MR, Unanue ER, Cutting H (1966) The vascular pathology of thrombotic thrombocytopaenic purpura. Lab Invest 15:927–946

Fernandez N, Torres A, Ackerman AB (1977) Pathologic findings in human scabies. Arch Dermatol 113:320–324

Fischer DA, Kistner RL (1971) Athero thrombotic emboli in the lower extremities. Arch Dermatol 104:533–537

Fishman AP (1982) Endothelium. Ann NY Acad Sci 401:1–274

Foldi M, Casley Smith JR (1983) Lymphangiology. F.K. Schattauer Verlag, Stuttgart

Freemont AJ (1982) The small blood vessels in areas of lymphocytic infiltration around malignant neoplasms. Br J Cancer 46:283–288

Gowans JL, Knight EJ (1964) The route of recirculation of lymphocytes in the rat. Proc R Soc Lond [Biol] 159:257–282

Gower RG, Sams WM, Thorne EG, Kohler PF, Claman HN (1977) Leukocytoclastic vasculitis: sequential appearance of immunoreactants and cellular changes in serial biopsies. J Invest Dermatol 69:477–484

Graham RC, Shannon SL (1972) Peroxidase arthritis II lymphoid cell – endothelial interactions during a developing immunologic inflammatory response. Am J Pathol 69:7–24

Granstein RD, Soter NA, Haynes HA (1983) Necrotising vasculitis within cutaneous lesions of mycosis fungoides. J Am Acad Derm 9:128–133

Hammersen F (1972) The fine structure of different types of experimental oedemas for testing the effect of vasoactive drugs demonstrated with a flavonoid. Angiologica 9:326–354

Harper JI, Copeman PWM (1983) Dermatitis artefacta presenting as a Vasculitis. J R Soc Med 76:970–971

Hidaka T, Nakano M, Ueta T, Komatsu Y, Yamamoto M (1983) Increased synthesis of thromboxane A2 by platelets from patients from Kawasaki disease. J Pediatr 102:94–96

Higgins JC, Eady RAJ (1981) Human dermal microvasculature I its segmental differentiation. Light and electron microscopic study. Br J Dermatol 104:116–130

Hjort PF, Rapaport SI, Jorgensen L (1964) Purpura fulminans: report of a case successfully treated with heparin and hydrocortisone. Review of 50 cases from the literature. Scand J Haematol 1:169–192

Hu C, O'Loughlin S, Winkelmann RK (1977) Cutaneous manifestations of Wegener's granulomatosis. Arch Dermatol 113:175–182

Hurwitz RM, Leaming RD, Horine RK (1984) Necrotic cellulitis: A localised form of septic vasculitis. Arch Dermatol 120:87–92

Jacob HS (1980) Complement induced vascular leukostasis: its role in tissue injury. Arch Pathol Lab Med 104:617–620

James WD, Odom RB, Katzenstein AA (1981) Cutaneous manifestations of lymphomatoid granulomatosis. Arch Dermatol 117:196–202

Juhlin L, Michaelsson G (1971) Abnormal cutaneous reactions to a nicotinic acid ester. Acta Dermato-Vener 51:448–452

Klein PJ, Schaefer HE, Feaux de Lacroix W, Fischer R (1972) Morphological findings in microangiopathic hemolytic anaemia. Hemostasis 1:304–314

Kulwin MH, Hines EA (1950) Blood vessels of the skin in chronic venous insufficiency: Clinical and pathological study. Arch Dermatol Syph 62:293–304

Lever WF, Schaumber-Lever G (1983) Histopathology of the Skin. J.B. Lipincott Co, Philadelphia

Levick JR, Michel CC (1978) The effect of position and skin temperature on the capillary pressures in the fingers and toes. J Physiol 274:97–109

Levinsky RJ (1981) Role of circulating immune complexes in renal diseases. J Clin Pathol 34:1214–1222

Liebow AA (1973) Pulmonary angiitis and granulomatosis. Am Rev Resp Dis 108:1–18

Liebow AA, Carrington CRB, Friedman PJ (1972) Lymphomatoid granulomatosis. Hum Pathol 3:457–558

Mitchell Sams W (1980) Models of necrotising vasculitis. In: Wolff K, Winkelmann RK (eds) Vasculitis (Major Problems in Dermatology, Vol. 10). Lloyd Luke, London, 108–116

Moretti G (1968) Blood vessels of the skin. In: Jadassohn J (ed) Handbuch der Haut und Geschlechtskrankheiten. Springer-Verlag, Berlin, 491–623

Mortimer PS, Cherry GW, Jones RL, Barnhill RL, Ryan TJ (1983) The importance of elastic fibres in skin lymphatics. Br J Dermatol 108:561–566
Mukherjee A, Girdhar BK, Malviya GN, Ramu G, Desikan KV (1983) Involvement of subcutaneous veins in lepromatous leprosy. Int J Lep 51:1–6
Murphy GF, Harrist TJ, Sato S, Mihm MC (1981) Microvascular Injury in lymphatoid granulomatosis involving the skin. Arch Dermatol 117:804–808
Nalbandian RM, Mader IJ, Barrett JL, Pearce JF, Rupp EC (1965) Petechiae, ecchymoses and necrosis of skin induced by coumarin congeners. JAMA 192:603–608
Neame PM, Lechago J, Ling ET, Koval A (1973) Thrombotic thrombocytopenic purpura: report of a case with disseminated intravascular platelet aggregation. Blood 42:805–814
Neumann HAM, Berretty PJM, Reinders-Folmer SCC, Cormane RH (1981) Hepatitis B surface antigen deposition in the blood vessel walls of urticarial lesions in acute hepatitis B. Br J Dermatol 104:383–387
Nieboer C (1981) Immunofluorescence patterns in sun-exposed and non-sun-exposed skin of healthy individuals. Acta Dermato-Vener 61:471–479
Orbison JL (1952) Morphology of thrombotic thrombocytopaenic purpura with demonstration of aneurysms. Am J Pathol 28:129–143
Perrot H, Leung TK, Leung J (1971) Etude ultrastructurale des lesions vasculaires dermiques du trisyndrome de Gougerot. Arch Dermatol Forsch 241:44–55
Phanuphak P, Kohler PF, Stanford RE, Schocket AL, Carr RI, Claman HN (1980) Vasculitis in chronic urticaria. J Allergy Clin Immunol 565:436–444
Rea TH, Ridley DS (1979) Lucio's phenomenon: A comparative histological study. Int J Lep 47:161–166
Ridley DS (1977) Skin Biopsy in Leprosy. Documenta Geigy. Ciba Geigy, Basle, Switzerland
Robboy SJ, Mihm MC, Colman RW, Minna JD (1973) The skin in disseminated intravascular coagulation. Br J Dermatol 88:221–229
Romanus M, Bagge U, Seifert F, Branemark PI (1978) Intravital microscopy of the microcirculation in man during and after experimentally controlled ischaemia. Scand J Plast Reconstr Surg 12:181–187
Ronco P, Verroust P, Mignon F, Kourilsky O, Vanhille P, Meyrier A, Mery JP, Morel-Maroger L (1983) Immunopathological studies of polyarteritis nodosa and Wegener's granulomatosis. Q J Med 206:212–223
Rozansky SJ (1982) Multiple cholesterol emboli syndrome. South Med J 75:677–680
Ruiter M, Molenaar I (1970) Ultrastructural changes in arteriolites (vasculitis) allergica cutis superficialis. Br J Dermatol 83:14–26
Russell Jones R, Bhogal B, Dash A, Schifferli J (1983) Urticaria and vasculitis: a continuum of histological and immunopathological changes. Br J Dermatol 108:695–703
Russell Jones R, Cunningham J (1979) Warfarin skin necrosis. Br J Dermatol 100:561–565
Russell Jones R, Eady RAJ (1984) Endothelial cell pathology as a marker for urticarial vasculitis in a light microscopic study. Br J Dermatol 110:139–150
Ryan TJ (ed) (1976) Microvascular Injury (Vol 7 Major Problems in Dermatology). Lloyd Luke Medical, London
Ryan TJ (1980) Anatomical features relevant to vasculitis. In: Wolff K, Winkelmann RK (eds) Vasculitis (Major Problems in Dermatology, Vol. 10). Lloyd Luke, London, 25–30
Ryan TJ (1983) Cutaneous circulation. In: Goldsmith L (ed) Biochemistry and Physiology of the Skin. Oxford University Press, Oxford, 817–877
Ryan TJ, Kanan MW, Cherry GW (1976) The pathology of ischaemia, stasis and vasculitis. In: Ryan TJ (ed) Microvascular Injury (Vol 7 Major Problems in Dermatology). Lloyd Luke Medical, London, 51–92
Ryan TJ, Wilkinson DS (1985) Vasculitis and Angiitis. In: Rook A, Wilkinson DS, Ebling R (eds) Textbook of Dermatology. 4th Edn. Blackwell Scientific Publication, Oxford, 11111
Sasaguri Y, Kato H (1982) Regression of aneurysms in Kawasaki disease; a pathological study. J Pediatr 100:225–231
Schneeberger EE (1982) Circulating proteins and macromolecular transport across continuous nonfenestrated endothelium. Ann NY Acad Sci 401:25–37
Schroeter AL, Copeman PWM, Jordan RE, Sams WM, Winkelmann RK (1971) Immunofluorescence of cutaneous vasculitis associated with systemic disease. Arch Dermatol 104:254–259

Schroeter AL, Winkelmann RK (1971) A human model to study cutaneous necrotizing angiitis using intradermal epinephrine. Clin Res 19:364

Schwartz SM (1982) Disturbance in endothelial integrity in endothelium. Ann NY Acad Sci 401:228–233

Shapiro L, Teisch JA, Brownstein MH (1973) Dermatohistopathology of chronic gonococal sepsis. Arch Dermatol 107:403–406

Simionescu M, Simionescu N, Palade GE (1982) Biochemically differentiated microdomains of the cell surface of capillary endothelium. Endothelium. Ann NY Acad Sci 401:9–24

Skalak R, Branemark PI, Ekholm R (1970) Erythrocyte adherence and diapedesis. Angiologie 21:224–239

Soter NA, Mihm MC, Gigli I, Dvorak HF, Austen KF (1976) Two distinct cellular patterns in cutaneous necrotizing angiitis. J Invest Dermatol 66:344–350

Soter NA, Murphy GF, Mihm MC (1982) Lymphocytes and necrosis of the cutaneous microvasculature in malignant atrophic papulosis: A refined light microscope study. J Am Acad Derm 7:620–630

Spicer TE, Rau JM (1976) Purpura Fulminans. Am J Med 61:566–571

Stalker AL, Brown LJ, Hall J (1969) Microcirculatory and histological observation on experimental defibrination. Bibliotheca Anatomica 10:366–373

Sweet RD (1964) An acute febrile neutrophilic dermatosis. Br J Dermatol 76:349–356

Tilton RG, Larason KB, Udell JR, Sobel BE, Williamson JR (1983) External detection of early microvascular dysfunction after no-flow ischaemia followed by reperfusion in isolated rabbit hearts. Circ Res 52:210–225

Tripathi RC, Tripathi BJ (1984) Bulk flow through vacuolar trans-endothelial channels. Int J Microcirc Clin Exp. In press

Umlas J, Kaiser J (1970) Thrombohaemolytic thrombocytopaenic purpura (TTP): A disease or syndrome? Am J Med 49:723

Urbach E, Epstein E, Lorenz K (1932) Extrazellulare cholesterinose. Arch Dermatol Syph (Berlin) 166:243–272

Van Neste D, Salmon J (1978) Circulating antigen and antibody complexes in scabies. Dermatologica 157:221–224

Walker F, Dhal DP, Walker MG, Mavor GL (1973) The normal and arterialised saphenous vein (7th European Conference on Microcirculation, Aberdeen, 1972). Bibliotheca Anatomica 11:495–498

Wegener F (1939) Ueber eine eigenartige rhinogene granulomatose mit besonderer beteiligung des arteriensystems und der nieren. Beitr Pathol Anat Allge Path 102:36–68

Wilkinson DS (1954) The vascular basis of some nodular eruptions of the legs. Br J Dermatol 66:201–213

Willemze R, Meyer CJ, Van Vloten WA, Scheffer E (1982) The clinical and histological spectrum of lymphomatoid papulosis. Br J Dermatol 107:131–144

Williamson JR, Vogler NJ, Kilo C (1971) Regional variation in the wall of the basement membrane of muscle capillaries in man and giraffe. Am J Pathol 63:359–370

Wilms-Kretchmer K, Majno G (1969) Ischaemia of the skin. Am J Pathol 54:327–343

Winkelmann RK (1980) Classification of Vasculitis. In: Wolff K, Winkelmann RK (eds) Vasculitis (Major Problems in Dermatology, Vol. 10). Lloyd Luke, London, 1–24

Winkelmann RK, Ditto WB (1964) Cutaneous and visceral syndromes of necrotising or "allergic" angiitis: A study of 38 cases. Medicine (Baltimore) 43:59–89

Witkowski JA, Parish CP (1982) Histopathology of the decubitus ulcer. J Am Acad Derm 6:1014–1021

Wolff K, Winkelmann RK (eds) (1980) Vasculitis (Major Problems in Dermatology, Vol. 10). Lloyd Luke, London

Woolf N (ed) (1983) Biology and Pathology of the Vessel Wall. Praeger Publishers, New York

Yen A, Braverman IM (1976) Ultrastructure of the human dermal microcirculation: The horizontal plexus of the papillary dermis. J Invest Dermatol 66:131–142

Zahavi J, Wetwick J, Al-Hasani SFA (1980) Enhanced in vivo platelet release reaction, increased thromboxane synthesis and decreased prostacyclin release after tourniquet ischaemia. Lancet 2:663–667

Zeek PM (1952) Periarteritis nodosa. A critical review. Am J Clin Pathol 22:777–790

Genetic and Developmental Aspects of Pathological Pigmentation Patterns

R.B. GOUDIE, A.S. JACK, and B.M. GOUDIE*

1. Introduction

This review attempts to relate current ideas about pattern formation in normal development to the anatomical patterns formed by the lesions of certain poorly understood pigmentary disorders of the human skin. Although there is as yet little direct experimental evidence linking the two topics, the principles derived from laboratory experiments on pattern formation in other species do provide

* Some of the studies described here were supported by the Scottish Hospitals Endowments Research Trust and by the Research Support Group of the Glasgow Area Health Board

insight into the way some of the clinical conditions develop and, conversely, the diseases themselves serve as natural experiments of basic biological interest.

Abnormal skin pigmentation has several advantages for the study of pattern, being two dimensional, easily recorded by photography, persistent and relatively innocuous. The idea of using pigmentary disorders as experiments of nature applicable to general physiological processes is not new. Albinism was one of the four inborn errors of metabolism which led GARROD (1909) to postulate the relationship between genes and enzymes – an idea which was to have a profound influence on the subsequent progress of biochemistry and genetics. Because of their frequently bizarre appearance, patterned abnormalities of pigmentation have aroused much curiosity (MEIROWSKY 1942; WHIMSTER 1968, 1971) but scientific progress has been slow, owing to the great difficulty of devising experiments which are meaningful and technically feasible. Hopefully, the application of new experimental techniques in molecular biology and genetics and the use of pigmentary disorders of the skin as model developmental systems will help to solve the mystery of pattern formation, one of the most resistant problems in basic biology and one of the least explored aspects of the pathology of human disease.

2. Overview of Melanin Pigmentation of Skin and Hair

It is now firmly established in mammals and birds (RAWLES 1947, 1948) that cutaneous melanocytes are derived from cells of the neural crest, which may also give rise to numerous other structures including part of the acoustic ganglion (DEOL 1967), sensory neurones of spinal and other cranial ganglia, sympathetic and parasympathetic neurones and some of the mesenchyme of the head and trunk (LE DOUARIN 1982; WESTON 1982). The melanocyte precursors migrate ventro-laterally in the dermis from which they enter the basal layer of the epidermis and hair bulbs. There they function as unicellular glands (BILLINGHAM 1948) and synthesise and secrete melanin to surrounding keratinocytes. In man recognisable melanocytes are not seen in the skin until the tenth week of gestation (ZIMMERMAN and BECKER 1959). By this time the basic anatomical pattern of the body is already formed and, provided the cells of the neural crest are normal, it is this pattern which will determine the ultimate location and function of the melanocytes and the pigment pattern of the body.

Skin and hair colour depends on numerous factors well reviewed by SEARLE (1968) and SILVERS (1979). These include the kind of melanin produced – brown or black eumelanin and yellow or red phaeomelanin; the same melanocyte can switch from one to the other at least in the hair follicles of mice with the agouti gene (SAKURAI et al. 1975). The function of epidermal and follicular melanocytes differs; thus white hair may be present with a dark epidermis or vice versa, a point which emphasises the importance of the local environment on melanocyte function. Skin colour is markedly influenced by the amount and character of melanin stored in the keratinocytes and this accounts for the difference between dark and fair skinned races rather than the population density of epidermal melanocytes.

In an excellent chapter on the biology of the melanin pigmentary system FITZPATRICK et al. (1979) have reviewed factors which affect the numbers and activity of melanocytes. Keratinocyte melanin is influenced by genetic factors, MSH or ACTH secretion and exposure to ultraviolet light. About twice as many functioning melanocytes are present on the skin of head or forearm as over the rest of the body, and the number can be increased by UV radiation which activates dormant melanocytes and stimulates mitosis. The number of active melanocytes can also be influenced by hormones: according to SNELL (1967) an enhanced effect of oestrogen and progesterone probably accounts for darkenning of nipples, areolae, genitalia and the midline of the abdomen during pregnancy. Hair follicle melanocytes are associated with the hair matrix epithelium, having the same relationship as epidermal melanocytes do with keratinocytes. During the growth (anagen) period of the hair cycle, follicular melanocytes synthesise and secrete melanin into the hair matrix cells, while in the resting (telogen) phase these functions are in abeyance and melanocytes can be found only with difficulty. In mice over 130 different mutations involving more than 50 different loci affect size, shape, number, clumping and position of melanin granules in the hair shaft to influence its colour (SILVERS 1979).

3. Pattern Formation in Embryogenesis

The following brief summary is largely based on the book by SLACK (1983) and the chapter on cellular mechanisms in development in ALBERTS et al. (1983).

As late as the eight cell stage of the developing mammalian embryo the individual cells (blastomeres) are interchangeable with each other and therefore uncommitted to any particular line of development. This explains how an embryo can split in two to form twins, an event which may occur by division of the mammalian embryo even at the gastrula stage (KAUFMAN and O'SHEA 1978). For the same reason, fusion of dissimilar embryos can take place (in mice up to the eight cell stage) resulting in a single chiameric individual which can grow to maturity (TARKOWSKY 1961), the cells of each component undergoing considerable random mixing before they become committed to form specific structures such as the mesoderm, neural crest etc. (MINTZ 1971; MCLAREN 1976).

The formation of anatomical patterns during embryogenesis (i.e. the spatial organisation of the developing embryo) is poorly understood. It is not known, for example, how such fundamental patterns as the order of head, body and tail in the cephalocaudal axis, or bilateral symmetry of skeletal structures, come about. It is now known that cells which find themselves on the surface of the preimplantation embryo give rise to the trophoblast because of their superficial position while those on the inside form the inner cell mass from which the embryo proper develops (ADAMSON and GARDNER 1979). After implantation patterns are thought to arise in areas not exceeding 100 cells (1 mm) in diameter, the prospective developmental fate of the various cells in these areas apparently depending on their position within the group. The mechanism is not clear but various theoretical models have been proposed including cellular interactions which involve dose-related responses of cells to gradients of diffusible substances ("morphogens") produced by neighbouring cells (WOLPERT 1978, 1981).

Intercellular adhesion is obviously important in maintaining existing patterns while changes in adhesiveness will permit cell migration and the formation of new patterns, thus allowing new cellular interactions to take place. Our understanding of the molecular basis of intercellular adhesion has been advanced by the use of antibody probes which have facilitated the identification and isolation of cell adhesion molecules (CAMs). It seems probable that from the earliest stages of development a relatively small repertoire of CAMs markedly influences pattern formation as a result of modulation of the amount expressed on the surface of individual cells at appropriate times (EDELMAN 1983). In neural crest cells, for example, N (nerve) – CAM appears early, disappears during migration of the cells, and reappears at sites where ganglia are formed (THIERY et al. 1982).

The general picture of mammalian development which emerges is one of adhesion and induction of neighbouring cells which become determined to follow particular developmental pathways and then proliferate to form clones, some of which may be modified later by further induction. The opportunity for a cell to receive a particular inductive signal depends on its being in the right place at the right time, and its competence to respond to that signal depends on its existing state of determination. Accordingly, there is a hierarchy of developmental events which may lead to further determination, commitment to make a specific anatomical structure (e.g. arm rather than leg), migration by a given pathway, or differentiation to form a particular type of cell.

It must be emphasised that during embryogenesis cells may be determined to certain lines of development some time before there is morphological evidence of the structures they are committed to form, for example the prospective muscle cells which are morphologically indistinguishable from the remainder of the mesenchymal cells of the developing limb bud (CHEVALLIER et al. 1977). Determination is a heritable state handed down from cell generation to cell generation. Little is known of its molecular basis. Nuclear transplantation experiments suggest that early in development cytoplasmic determinants are more important than those in the nucleus. Later in development changes in DNA are thought to play a part. Among the few clear-cut examples are methylation of cytosine (RAZIN and RIGGS 1980) and chromosomal re-arrangements and somatic mutations at the site of the immunoglobulin genes in B lymphocytes and plasma cells (LEDER 1982).

4. Clonal Origin of Pigment Patterns in Mice

The word "clone" is used in various ways in different branches of biology. In effect a clone is a family of somatic cells which inherit their behaviour from a common ancestor from which they are all descended – the founder cell of the clone. Here the definition by MINTZ and SANYAL (1970) is followed – "the mitotic progeny of one cell in which a specific constellation of gene loci first becomes active or derepressed and has remained active as a cell heredity". A considerable amount is known about the clonal basis of development, and much of this has been derived from study of skin and hair pigmentation. It is hoped to show in sections 5, 6 and 7 that clonal mechanisms provide an explanation for some curious pigment patterns in man and give interesting insight on the probable arrangement of cell populations at a very early stage of human development.

The recognition of clones is difficult in most normal individuals since there is usually no marker to allow distinction or demarcation between clones which have originated in a number of identical founder cells. Important information has been obtained from melanocyte clones in chimaeric mice. These animals are made by fusing morulae of two different strains, reimplanting the composite embryo in the uterus of a pseudopregnant "foster mother" mouse and allowing development to continue till term. If the embryos of different coloured strains are fused, the offspring have a variegated appearance often taking the form of transverse bands of alternating pigment type round the body. The bands vary in width and terminate sharply at the dorsal and ventral midlines (Fig. 1). MINTZ (1971) has analysed the findings in considerable numbers of chimaeric mice and concludes from the width of the narrowest bands that there are 17 melanocyte clones on either side of the body, each derived from a separate founder cell. She has shown that the clones are randomly arranged with respect to genotype and the pattern of stripes on one side of the body is independent of that on the other. This latter finding is attributed to the migration of the melanocyte clones before fusion of the neural folds in the mid dorsal line.

The same phenomenon as that seen in the somewhat artificial chimaeric animal is observed in normal female mice heterozygous for X-linked coat colour genes (LYON 1961). In these animals, random inactivation of one or other X chromosome in all somatic cells and their clonal progeny leads to a characteristic variegated pattern composed of bands of normal and mutant hair. As in the chimaeras described above the bands do not cross the midline.

A third situation in which melanocyte clones are sometimes visible arises by somatic mutation in a melanocyte precursor leading to altered pigmentation in the mutant clone. Excellent examples are seen in mice homozygous for the unstable recessive gene p^{un} (pink-eyed unstable). In these animals a back mutation often occurs during a cell division early in embryonic life, and this leads to a clone of revertant darkly pigmented p^{un} + cells ("+" referring to to the normal dominant wild type gene which produces dark melanin). The revertant clones are readily seen against the pale homozygous fur (Fig. 2). (It is of interest that the white spotting gene piebald (*s*) can alter the size and discreteness of individual bands of the variegated animal by diminishing the amount of mixing of cells between neighbouring clones (SEARLE 1978).

All the clones discussed above are composed of melanocytes and are made visible by the products of cell-autonomous genes which influence melanin. In agouti mice the situation is different (see SILVERS 1979). Agouti refers to a special form of hair pigmentation in which the bulb and tip have dark eumelanin separated by a wide zone of pale phaeomelanin in the intervening hair shaft.

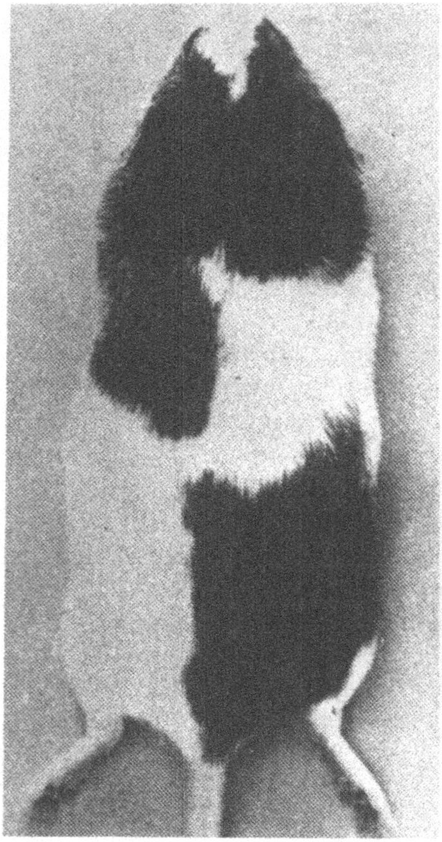

1

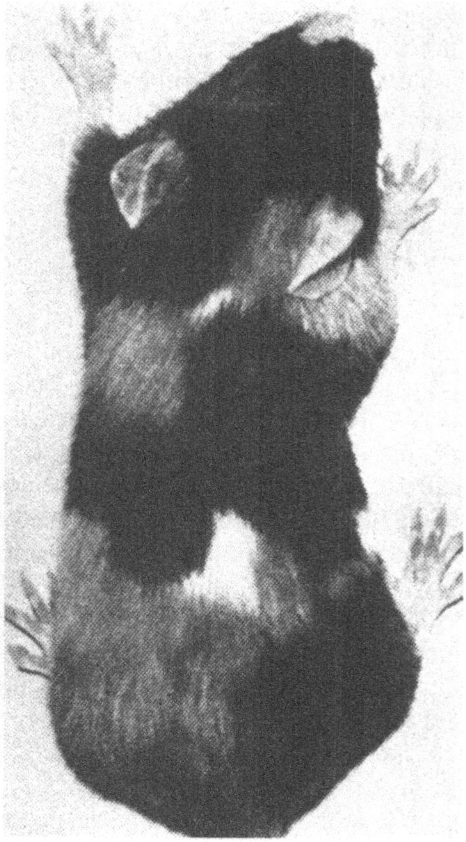

2

Fig. 1. Chimaeric mouse. The dark and white melanocyte clones terminate sharply at the midline and form independent patterns on the two sides of the body. Reproduced from Whitten (1978) with permission of Plenum Press

Fig. 2. Coat colour mosaicism in mouse homozygous for pinkeyed unstable (p^{un}/p^{un}). Clones of p^{un}/p^{un} cells (grey) and revertant $p^{un}/+$ (black) melanocytes, sharply separated at the midline, are randomly arranged on the two sides of the body. The white spots are due to homozygosity for piebald (*s*/*s*). Reproduced from Searle (1978) with permission of the author and Plenum Press

The kind of melanin produced by the melanocytes of the hair follicles in these animals is not controlled by an autonomous gene in the melanocyte, but by the activity of the agouti gene in dermal hair follicle cells. The agouti locus is strikingly responsive to positional information as exemplified by a^t (black-and-tan). In mice of this genotype hair follicles of identical genotype may produce yellow hairs on the belly, agouti on the sides and black the middle of the back. Recombination experiments of a^t/a^t dorsal and ventral dermis with ventral and dorsal epidermis show clearly that the pigmentation of the hair in this strain is determined by the dermis (Poole and Silvers 1976). Though agouti does not occur in man, it serves to illustrate the importance of external regulatory signals in melanocyte behaviour and the possible influence of clones of cells of another type (mesodermal) on the cells of melanocyte clones.

In black (*aa*) ↔ agouti (*AA*) chimaeric mice light and dark transverse bands are seen around the body, but these are much narrower than those of melanocyte clones (Fig. 3) and correspond in number (75–100) to the somites, a pattern attributed by MINTZ (1971) to mesodermal clones. Whereas the allocation of uncommitted cells to become founders of melanocyte clones is generally agreed to be random and to occur independently on the two sides of the body, MCLAREN (1976) considers that there is less evidence that this is so in the case of "dermal" clones in which the agouti gene is expressed. Thus in the C3H ↔ C56BL combination there is regularly a non-agouti area between the ears (Fig. 3). One possible explanation for this could be that the non-agouti cells are the first to become competent to respond to the cephalocaudal inductive signal which determines the formation of the somites.

One example of a black-and-tan (a^t/a) ↔ black (*aa*) chimaera has been described (PETERS and MARKERT 1979). Fairly large coherent irregular ventral patches of tan pigmentation were present, a different pattern from that commonly observed on the dorsum of agouti ↔ non-agouti chimaeras. A possible explanation is that the ventral dermis originates from the somatopleural mesoderm unlike that of the dorsum which arises from somites. Interestingly, none of the ventral patches showed a midline cut-off. Further studies of such chimaeras is clearly indicated.

Bicoloured patterns resembling those produced by hair follicle clones in chimaeras are seen in some mice homozygous for certain autosomally inherited alleles at the agouti locus e.g. viable yellow (A^{vy}) and mottled agouti (a^m). These, and comparable effects produced by particular alleles at other loci, are briefly reviewed by SILVERS (1979). Unlike p^{un} the genes concerned are stable, and they are of course not subject to X-inactivation. Their tendency to produce variations in pigmentation among genetically identical litter mates and mottled patches within an individual animal is unexplained and perhaps due to non-genetic factors.

In the mouse, many pigmentation patterns result from patches of white fur devoid of recognisable hair follicle melanocytes. These are due to "white spotting" genes at various loci including piebald (*s*), dominant spotting (*W*), microphthalmia (*Mi*) and belted (*bt*) all of which are discussed in detail by SILVERS (1979). There is some evidence that white spotting results from programmed cell death of clones of melanocytes at certain anatomical positions. Providing this occurs sufficiently late in embryonic life it is presumed that the loss is not made good by the tendency of melanocytes from adjacent viable clones to occupy the empty spaces, especially at anatomical sites such as the peri-umbilical area and forehead which are last to be colonised by melanocytes during normal development. Consistent with this view is the finding that white spotted – wild type chimaeras either resemble white spotted or wild type animals and do not present the banded appearance of chimaeras with alternating clones of melanocytes of different colours (e.g. following fusion of albino and black embryos).

To summarise, in chimaeric and mosaic mice of carefully selected genotype it is possible to recognise patterns due to clones of genetically different melanocytes or of dermal cells which control melanocyte function. The patterns consist

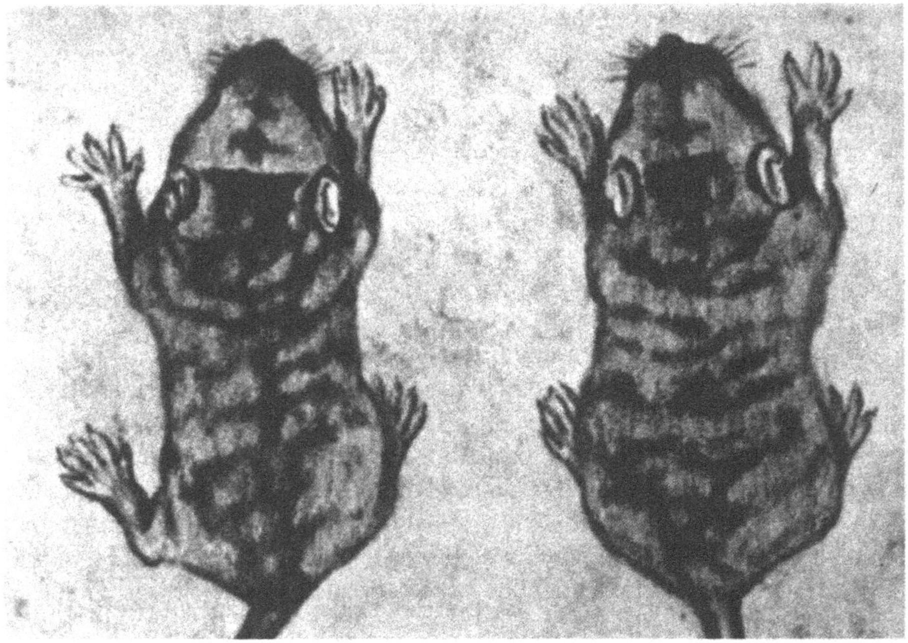

Fig. 3. Black (aa) – agouti (AA) chimaeras. The "dermal" clones are much narrower than those of melanocyte clones. Note the regular (non random) presence of dark non-agouti fur between the ears. Reproduced from McLAREN (1976) with permission of the author and Cambridge University Press

essentially of a series of bands which terminate abruptly at the dorsal and ventral midlines and are randomly arranged on each side of the body. Melanocyte clones form broader bands than dermal clones but the differences may be obscured if there is extensive mixing of cells from adjacent clones or if the genetic consitution of the animals is unsuitable.

5. Skin Pigmentation in Human Chimaeras

Human beings who have two cell lines differing from one another in several genetically determined features must have been derived from more than one zygote i.e. they are spontaneous chimaeras. If one of the cell lines is found only in the blood, transfusion of blood cells from the mother or a twin may have caused the chimaerism, but if both lines are present in the solid tissues it is assumed that the individual has arisen from fusion of two non-identical zygotes at a very early stage of development with production of a primary chimaera. McLAREN (1976) has described various mechanisms to explain this and considers that fusion of egg and second polar body following fertilisation by two separate spermatozoa is biologically the most plausible. The study of proven examples of human chimaerism associated with pigmentary anomalies

Table 1. Published human chimaeras with abnormal skin pigmentation

Case No.	Evidence of chimaerism	Cell line markers	Number of contributions demonstrated		Skin biopsy Histol.	Reference
			Maternal	Paternal		
1	Blood and skin	XX/XY, ABO, S, Jr, Sickling	2	2	–	ZUELZER et al. (1964)
2	Skin, hermaphroditism	XX/XY, ABO, Lu, Fy. Haptoglobin, Phosphoglucomatase	2	2	–	COREY et al. (1967)
3	Blood and skin	ABO, S, Ra, Fy, HLA, acid phosphatase etc.	1	2	–	MOORES (1973), FINDLAY and MOORES (1980)
4	Skin, hermaphroditism	XX/XY	1	2	No melanocytes seen in basal layer of unpigmented specimen	FITZGERALD et al. (1979)
5	Skin, blood	ABO, acid phosphatase, peptidase A			Melanocytes normal	FINDLAY and MOORES (1980)

of the skin is of interest in view of the clonal origin of the abnormal patterns observed, and the insight they might be expected to provide as models of the likely effects of mitotic errors (mutation etc.) in somatic cells concerned with human skin pigmentation.

Human chimaeras have been reviewed by RACE and SANGER (1975), MCLAREN (1976) and TIPPETT (1983). Table 1 lists the cases showing abnormalities of skin pigmentation which form the basis of the present discussion. In general the patterns resemble those seen in chimaeric mice but because of our ignorance of the genetic backgrounds in the human patients it is not possible to distinguish melanocyte from dermal clones.

A striking feature is the marked variation in pattern observed from patient to patient and even in different parts of the skin of the same patient. In case 5 for example, the appearance ranged from a spray-like pigmentation with a fine granularity of 1 mm or less, through larger solid rounded patches of varying darkness resembling the café-au-lait spots in neurofibromatosis, to confluent darker areas. The edges of many of the larger lesions are frequently ill defined and very irregular with fine stippling indicative of mixing of dissimilar cell lines. In general, sizeable clonal patches which abut on the dorsal or ventral midline tend to be limited to their own side of the body though the line of demarcation is as a rule neither sharp not straight. It therefore seems likely that a minority of cells from clones involved in skin pigmentation on one side of the body do cross the midline, and that the latter does not form the boundary of a permanent anatomical compartment like that which restricts the mixing of polyclones during insect development (CRICK and LAWRENCE 1975).

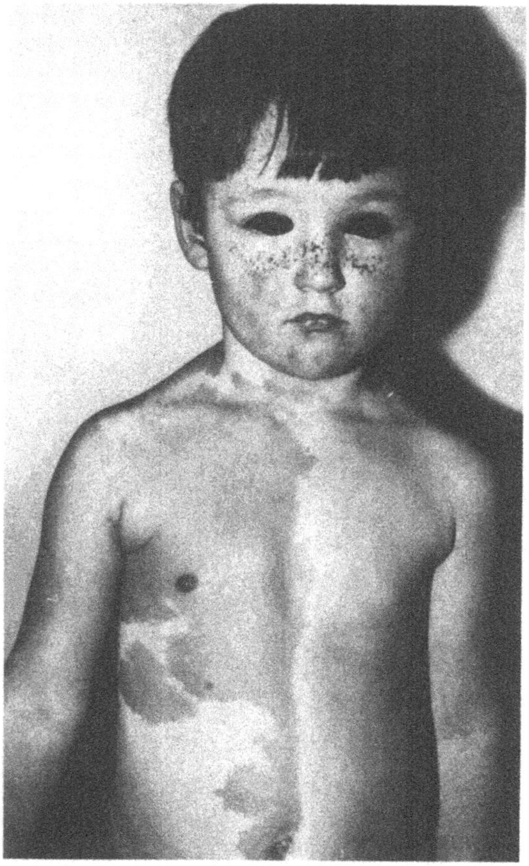

Fig. 4. Skin pigmentation in a human chimaera. The irregular interface between dark and pale skin and the occasional small macules result from mixing of cells of adjacent clones. Midline demarcation is rather imprecise and apparently absent over the larynx. Note the differences in pigmentation of the eyebrows. The dark macules across the centre of the face are freckles

The larger clonal patches on the trunk have a tendency to form transverse bands or wedges extending in a lateral direction. In case 3 the darker areas of skin were arranged in striae resembling the so-called lines of Blaschko (BLASCHKO 1901; JACKSON 1976). The largest blocks (case 5) had horizontal upper and lower limits and so tended to meet in the midline at right angles giving a square cut outline. In cases 1, 2, 3 and 5 the patches on the two sides of the body were dissimilar and asymmetrical and clearly had developed independently of each other in keeping with observations on pigment patterns in chimaeric mice.

The pattern in case 4, which unfortunately is poorly illustrated, appeared exceptional. At least two bands passed straight across the anterior abdomen, the left upper and right lower parts lacking in pigment so that a curious harlequin-like appearance was produced. According to the authors no melanocytes were seen in the basal layer in a biopsy of the unpigmented skin but they

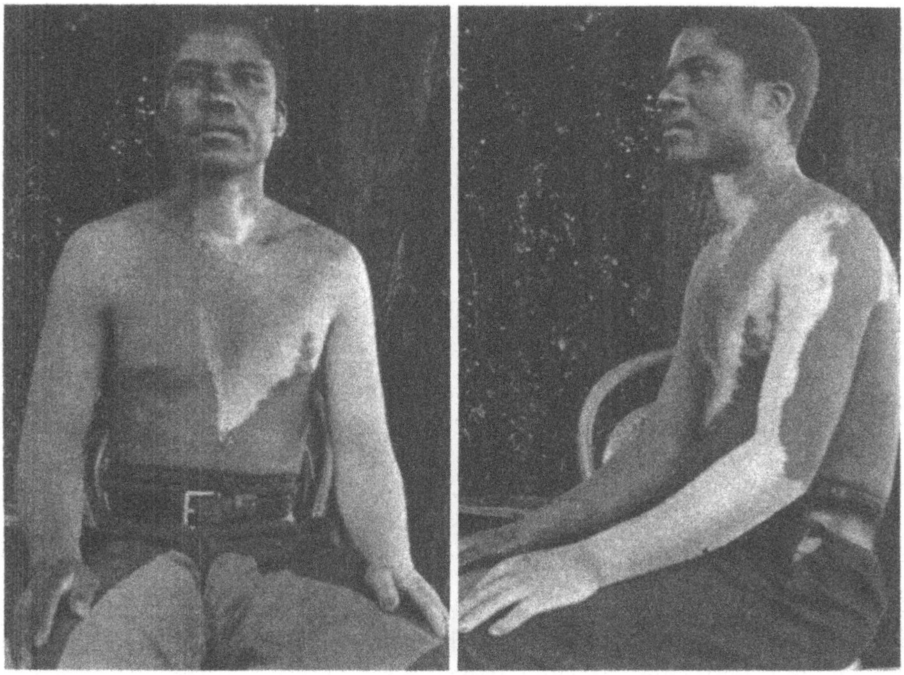

Fig. 5. Presumed example of mosaicism showing distribution of clone of revertant albino melanocytes. The midline demarcation is rather imprecise and apparently absent over the larynx. From PEARSON et al. (1911a)

were present in a pigmented area. The anatomical distribution of the unpigmented skin in case 4 is quite unlike that encountered in other conditions in which epidermal melanocytes are lacking e.g. piebaldism and vitiligo. It is possible that the absence of melanocytes in this case may be the result of chimaerism and reflect defective regulatory interactions between melanocytes and other cells (epidermal or mesodermal) of different genotype.

Figure 4 illustrates the appearance of a hitherto unpublished four year old chimaera recently seen by us. His blood contained two populations of red cells of different rhesus groups. The midline phenomenon is well seen in addition to the very irregular outline of the hyperpigmented areas. The darkly pigmented skin mainly forms large blocks, but there are occasional small macules indicative of mixing of light and dark cells. The left eyebrow was brown and much darker than the red right eyebrow and the hair on the scalp was variegated. The skin on the left side of forehead was dark. The presence of a dark patch extending across the midline on the front of the neck is of interest since a similar phenomenon is also seen in the patient illustrated in Fig. 5.

There is a major difference between the human chimaeras discussed above and the presumed human mosaics to be described in later sections; all the chimaeras have light and dark pigmentation on both sides of the body whereas this is quite exceptional in the mosaics (see section 7.3 for discussion).

While the chimaeric patterns described above all reflect the clonal behaviour of human skin cells, multiple factors must contribute to the details of the pattern observed in each individual case. These include the nature and amount of pigment which the different melanocyte clones produce and secrete, and the tendency of the melanocytes to adhere to others of the same genotype and so produce coherent patches. Similar considerations will apply to clones of dermal cells which regulate melanocyte function. Furthermore, each type of melanocyte may be associated with and respond differently to each type of dermal cell. As a rule, it is not possible to interpret the patterns in detail because, in contrast to the mouse chimaeras, much less is known about the genetic constitution of the human embryos which have fused.

Attempts have been made to relate which line of fibroblast underlies each type of skin pigmentation in cases 1, 2 and 4, each of which was an XX ↔ XY chimaera. Differences were noted in cases 1 and 2, but the number of samples tested was too small to be statistically significant.

6. Skin Pigmentation in Presumed Human Mosaics

The term "mosaic" is used to describe a genetically composite individual derived from a single zygote that is formed by the union of one egg with one sperm. By definition the different cell populations in a mosaic arise during development by a process such as somatic mutation or chromosal non-disjunction. In practice it is often difficult to establish how a spontaneously composite individual has been formed and the distinction between chimaeras and mosaics is often presumptive. The following paragraphs describe the skin pigmentation patterns in three probable human mosaics, two with trisomy of chromosome 18.

Figure 5 shows the appearance of a negro with 15 complete albinos in four generations of his family (PEARSON et al. 1911a). He is one of three siblings whose skin appears to express the albino mutation in a patchy fashion. This remarkable occurrence probably results from each sibling being homozygous for albinism with one of the mutant albino genes unstable and prone to revert to a pigmented phenotype in the manner of the p^{un} allele in mice. This case is of special interest since the albino locus is primarily expressed in melanocytes and the pattern observed almost certainly reflects the cutaneous distribution of melanocyte clones in man. A notable feature is again the somewhat imperfect midline phenomenon with apparent spread of albino melanocytes across the front of the larynx as in the human chimaera illustrated in Fig. 4. The reason for this is quite obscure.

Two possible examples of human mosaicism with abnormal skin pigmentation have been described in males with mental retardation, facial and body asymmetry and trisomy 18 in some of their fibroblasts and peripheral blood lymphocytes. The cytogenetic abnormality may have resulted either from chromatid non-disjunction in a euploid cell or chromatid loss during mitosis of an aneuploid cell. In the case reported by CHEMKE et al. (1983), the trunk and upper and lower extremeties showed linear hyperpigmented areas with precise limitation at the midline. Unfortunately, the description and illustrations of the hyperpigmented areas are lacking in detail, the abnormality being described as anaevus unius lateralis. It is unknown whether the clones responsible for the appearance are epidermal, dermal or melanocytic. Dermal fibroblast cultures from the hyperpigmented area showed pure trisomy 18 while the karyotype of the unaffected side was normal. The patient's right side showed several unilateral developmental abnormalities known to be associated with trisomy 18 – hypoplasia of eye and external ear, flattening of the chest and other skeletal abnormalities. However, there were also bilateral congenital defects, notably narrow ear canals and conductive hearing loss, and syndactyly of the fingers, features suggesting the presence of abnormal cells on both sides of the body at least in some tissues. In the case described by SASAKI et al. (1972), the right side of the body was hypoplastic and (except for the face) more deeply pigmented than the left; the karyotype of fibroblasts from the left side was normal but 25% of those from the right showed trisomy 18.

These presumed mosaics differ from all the human chimaeras described above in that light and dark pigmentation is present only on one side of the body, with the exception of some albino skin over both sides of the larynx. The findings indicate a lesser degree of cell mixing and movement in human mosaics than in human chimaeras.

In the next section, further examples of possible human mosaicism are described under a separate heading, the reason being that their genetic backgrounds are even less clear than those described above.

7. Syndromes Associated with Lentigines

A lentigo is a flat, round, oval or irregular pigmented spot up to 5 mm in diameter, characterised by a marked increase of the melanin within the keratinocytes and often by slight melanocytic and epidermal cell hyperplasia with elongation of the rete pegs (MOSHER et al. 1979). The melanocytes lie singly in the epidermis and do not form aggregates or "theques" which are typical of pigmented naevi. The intensity of pigmentation may vary in different lentigines in the same patient and even in different parts of the same lentigo. Lentigines usually develop during childhood and differ from freckles in being unrelated to sun exposure. The focal nature of the lesions is unexplained and it is not known whether the defect is primarily in the melanocytes or in neighbouring cells.

Lentigines are relevant to the present subject partly because there are certain inherited disorders in which they are present in large numbers and form distinctive patterns. Of greater interest is the partial involvement of the skin with large lentiginous patches which probably results from mosaicism and reflects movements of cells adjacent to the midline in the early embryo. Finally, it can be speculated that each individual lentiginous macule may be the result of the release from a point source of a diffusible substance which initiates proliferation and pigment production in adjacent melanocytes, a possible example of pattern induction during postnatal life. Lentigines do not appear to have been recognised or studied in species other than man.

7.1 Moynahan's Syndrome

This condition is well described by GORLIN et al. (1969) and POLANI and MOYNAHAN (1972). It is inherited as a Mendelian dominant with incomplete penetrance. It is characterised by multiple lentigines "from scalp to feet". These are more numerous over the upper part of the trunk and neck thus forming a characteristic anatomical pattern. Sometimes there are also several larger café-au-lait spots. The mutation is pleiotropic and it exhibits variable expression – all the abnormalities not being present in individual cases. The pleiotropic effects include hypertrophic cardiomyopathy with conduction defects, ocular hypertelorism, prognathos, sensineural deafness, retardation of physical and mental development, skeletal abnormalities such as pectus carinatum or excavatum or kyphosis, gonadal hypoplasia and hypospadias.

The syndrome has been attributed either to a systemic (hormonal) effect of the lentigines on the development of the other tissues, or, perhaps more likely, to a defect in the neural crest leading to abnormal behaviour of cells derived from it – melanocytes, autonomic innervation of the heart etc. The latter explanation does not readily account for the skeletal defects and it is conceivable that all the abnormalities could be due to a primary fault in mesoderm causing widespread induction of change in neural crest behaviour. There are single reports (NORLUND et al. 1973; WEISS and ZELICKSON 1977) of ultrastructural abnormalities of melanosomes but these do not appear to be constant and cannot be taken to indicate a primary defect in melanocytes.

7.2 Peutz-Jeghers Syndrome

(Perioral lentiginosis)

This syndrome, inherited as an autosomal dominant, is characterised by two main features, the presence of multiple pigmented spots predominantly on the oral mucosa and skin around the mouth, nose, hands and feet, and the occurrence of polyps in the gastrointestinal tract (JEGHERS et al. 1949). The lentigines usually appear in early childhood and are irregularly distributed in the affected areas. The lesions themselves are round, oval or irregular in outline and tend to be smaller on the skin (1 mm) than in the oral mucosa (up to 12 mm). The histology of the pigmented lesions has not been adequately studied (ZEGARELLI et al. 1956). The cutaneous lesions tend to regress after puberty, suggesting that a continuing stimulus is required to maintain them. The intestinal polyps are usually multiple and mainly affect the jejunum, though examples can be found at any site from stomach to rectum (BARTHOLOMEW et al. 1962). Their histological appearance and clinical behaviour suggest they are hamartomatous rather than true tumours but malignant change, possibly fortuitous, occasionally supervenes. Intestinal haemangiomatosis has also been described (BANDLER 1960), and further evidence of the pleiotropic nature of the mutation is the occurrence of peculiar ovarian tumours in a small proportion of affected females (SCULLY 1970).

Table 2. Partial unilateral lentiginosis

Author	Anatomical distribution	Side	Biopsy	Associated conditions
McKelway (1904)	Roots of hair to knee	L	–	Mental retardation
Adamson (1911)	Nipple to inguinal fold	L	–	Supernumerary nipple on opposite side
MacLeod (1913)	Axilla to buttock	L		Capillary naevus R wrist and hand
Shumate (1941)	Forehead, entire nose, cheek, lips, chin and anterior neck	R	–	
Cappon (1948)	Clavicle and occipital hairline to ankle. Affected skin uneven	R	–	Mental retardation
Pickering (1973)	Above clavicle to line convex upward from umbilicus	L	+	Epilepsy. Left cerebral telangiectasia and cutaneous vascular naevi in distribution of left maxillary nerve
	6th – 9th thoracic dermatomes anterior only	L	–	Nil
Thomson and Diehl (1980)	Umbilicus to ankle (café au lait spots present)	R	–	Familial goitre
Hughes et al. (1983)	4th cervical to 5th thoracic dermatomes (café au lait spots present)	L	+	Sickle cell anaemia

7.3 Partial Unilateral Lentiginosis

A number of cases have been described in which there are multiple lentigines confined to part of one side of the body (Table 2) – partial unilateral lentiginosis. In none of these cases is there a family history of multiple lentigines and the anatomical distribution of the lesions does not correspond to that seen in the inherited syndromes. Two of the eight patients with partial unilateral lentigines were, however, mentally retarded, a feature of Moynahan's syndrome.

The nature of partial unilateral lentiginosis has not been established, but the pattern is very much in keeping with a clone of abnormal cells which has arisen early in development and occupied a considerable area of the body surface. Unfortunately, samples of normal and abnormal skin from such cases have not been examined for karyotypic or biochemical evidence of mosaicism and this clearly needs to be done in future cases.

If partial unilateral lentiginosis actually does result from a genetic abnormality such as mutation, recombination or non-disjunction in a somatic cell during development, then it is of great interest that the abnormal clone, despite its considerable size does not cross the midline or form alternating bands with normal clones of the same type. There are three possible explanations. (1) There may as already suggested, be much less cell mixing in human mosaics than in chimaeras. (2) The abnormal cells may be unusually adherent to each other and much less likely than their normal counterparts to migrate and mix with neighbouring clones. (3) Cohesive growth may be a normal property of the kind of cell which primarily gives rise to the lentigo pattern. Until the nature of this cell is discovered, the problem will not be solved.

7.4 Multiple Lentigines with a Harlequin Pattern

In 1964 DAVIS and SHAW reported an example of multiple lentigines which had developed in a negress at the age of three years. The pattern of the lesions is shown diagramatically in Fig. 6. In the lighter area, the skin was medium tan. There were scattered ovoid lentiginous macules in the darker areas, with the long axes of the lesions apparently orientated along lines of dermatomal development. In each half of the head, neck and trunk the light and dark areas alternated so that corresponding areas of the two sides of the body had mirror image boundaries and were reciprocally light and dark with sharp demar-

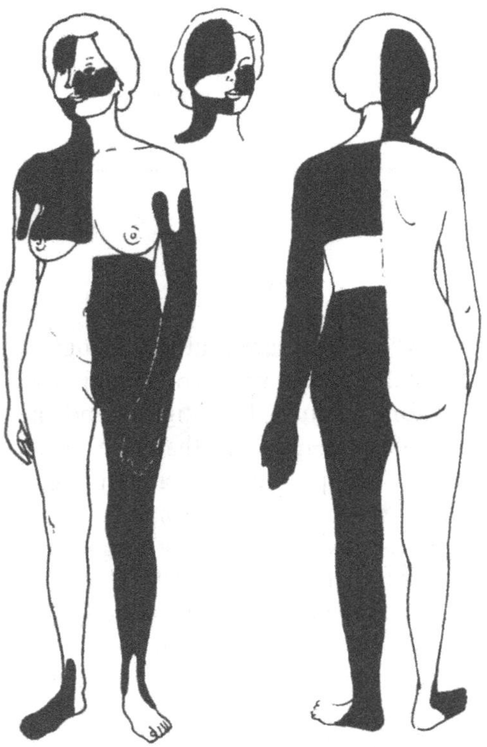

Fig. 6. Diagram of lentiginous (black) and nonlentiginous (white) skin in presumed human mosaic. Apart from a lentigo-free girdle round the upper abdomen there is a reciprocal "harlequin" pattern of affected and unaffected skin at corresponding positions on each side of the midline. Reproduced from DAVIS and SHAW (1964) with permission of the New England Journal of Medicine

cation from one another at the dorsal and ventral midlines. The mirror image boundaries and reciprocal arrangement of normal and lentiginous skin on the two sides of the body (which will be referred to as a "harlequin" pattern) also involved the limbs, but there was a light coloured girdle round the upper abdomen unaffected by lentigines. The patient was otherwise well. There was no objective evidence of chimaerism or mosaicism from the karyotype of lymphocytes and fibroblasts or from blood grouping at eight loci. Histological examination of skin showed an apparent increase in melanin in the clinically lentiginous specimen and prominent rete pegs in both the normal and abnormal skin.

Despite lack of positive in vitro evidence of the presence of two genetically different cell lines, it seems almost certain that the patient is a mosaic. The distribution of the lentiginous areas cannot be attributed to any known adult anatomical structures and its band-like arrangement with limitation at the midline resembles that of melanocyte or hair follicle clones in chimaeric mice (see Fig. 1). Furthermore, family studies of the Moynahan and Peutz-Jeghers syndromes show that multiple lentigines may be the result of mutation. The following discussion is based on the assumption that the harlequin pattern is due to a genetic event which took place in a somatic cell very early in embryonic development.

If indeed the harlequin pattern is composed of two genetically distinct clones, their behaviour is remarkable in that apart from the lentigo-free girdle round the upper abdomen, the position of the clonal boundaries corresponds exactly on the two sides of the body and the reciprocal arrangement of lentiginous and non-lentiginous skin across the midline is so regular. It will be recalled that in chimaeric and mosaic mice the cephalocaudal sequence of melanocyte clones is random, the pattern on each side being independent of the other. The same is true of the arrangement of human clonal pigmentation in all but one of the chimaeras already described in section 5, the exception being case 4 of Table 1 in which the abdominal skin had a flag-like or harlequin pattern. The only other published example of a harlequin pattern of which the authors are aware (Pearson et al. 1911b) affected the face (Fig. 7) as in Davis and Shaw's case – perhaps a phenomenon of some developmental significance in view of the rarity of unilateral involvement of facial pigmentation in presumed human mosaics.

A simple explanation for the Davis and Shaw harlequin is that the mutant clone originally lay along one side of the midline as in the cases of partial unilateral lentiginosis already described, and that mutant and non-mutant cells subsequently exchanged mirror image positions on either side of the cephalocaudal axis. This would suggest that the cephalocaudal and mediolateral positions these cells were to occupy were already determined before they exchanged places but there was no commitment at the time to one particular side of the body. The lentigo free band round the upper abdomen of Davis and Shaw's case would represent regulatory repair following loss of some mutant cells. The pattern having been formed in this way at a very early stage of development the clonal descendents must have retained their relative positions to one another during subsequent growth and migration from the neighbourhood of the mid-

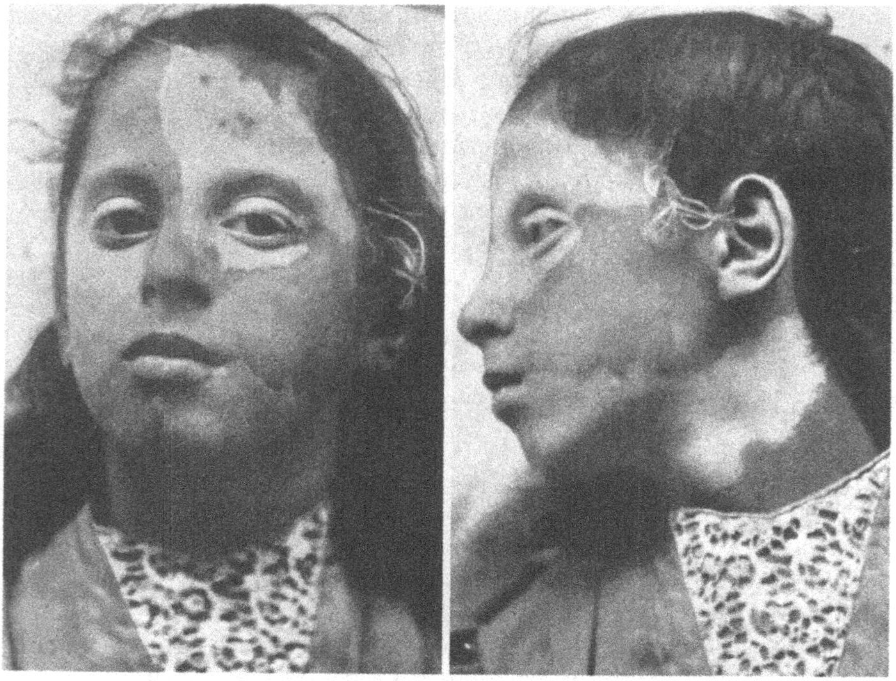

Fig. 7. Harlequin depigmentation pattern of head and neck. The body was unaffected. From PEARSON et al. (1911 b)

line. This seems the most plausible scenario and it provides a unique glimpse of the alignment and morphogenetic movements of a small group of cells near the midline of the early human embryo.

Unfortunately, it is by no means clear what kind of cells originally formed the harlequin pre-pattern. Proximity to the midline would be in keeping with neuroectodermal precursors of the neural crest or with cells of the mesoderm. In a previous analysis of Davis and Shaw's case by GOUDIE et al. (1980), the possibility of a neuroectodermal origin was rejected because the regularity of the harlequin pattern seemed inconsistent with the random distribution of melanocyte clones encountered in chimaeric and mosaic mice. It was therefore concluded that the pattern probably originated in a set of mesodermal cells which developed after the phase of extensive cell mixing thought to characterise the blastocyst stage. Vascular endothelium was considered a possibility in view of its time of development, distribution through the superficial dermis in close proximity to melanocytes and its anatomical continuity. For these reasons it was postulated that endothelial cells are arranged in monoclonal zones, each of which occupies an accurately predetermined site in the cardiovascular system, and that the clones impose detailed developmental patterns on the vascular tree itself, providing positional information relevant to the morphogenesis of surrounding tissues including patterns of skin pigmentation. This mechanism would fit with the association between partial unilateral lentiginosis and the vascular abnormality of skin and brain in the case described by PICKERING

(1973). It would also provide an explanation for the curious case described by SANDERSON (1960) in which multiple vascular lesions (telangiectases) developed and rapidly transformed into telangiectatic cellular pigmented naevi. Unfortunately, it has not been possible to test the vascular clone hypothesis in chimaeric mice because of lack of suitable markers of endothelial genotype.

If the harlequin pattern is due to endothelial clones it is rather surprising that in Moynahan's syndrome there is an association between multiple lentigines and other disorders affecting the nervous system and various derivatives of the neural crest. It is in fact possible to reconcile the harlequin pattern with melanocyte clones if it is assumed as in partial lentiginosis that there is very much less cell mixing in the prospective neuroectoderm during normal gastrulation than occurs in chimaeric or mosaic mice or in human chimaerism. The studies by JACOBSON (1978) and JACOBSON and HIROSE (1978) on the fate of labelled blastomeres in the Xenopus embryo show that there is remarkably little random exchange of cells across the midline of the developing neural plate though programmed reciprocal interchange of cells does occur between corresponding positions on opposite sides, for example in the development of the primordial retinae. By analogy a harlequin pattern of melanocyte precursors could well be derived from a neural plate composed of normal cells on one side of the midline and mutant cells on the other.

8. Piebaldism

Piebaldism refers to a group of rare congenital pigmentary disorders of skin and hair usually inherited as a Mendelian dominant (MOSHER et al. 1979). As shown in Fig. 8 there is a white forelock and forehead accompanied often with hypomelanosis of chin, anterior abdomen and chest, the elbow and knee regions, and sometimes parts of the hands and feet. The lesions are roughly symmetrical, but not exactly so, a feature common to most inherited pigmentary disorders. A second characteristic of piebaldism is the presence of irregularly distributed pigmented macules which are of course most obvious in the areas otherwise lacking in pigmentation. Although the anatomical distribution of hypomelanosis differs in detail from case to case even in members of the same family (SUNDFOR 1939), it is much more predictable than that of the pigmented macules.

It is generally assumed that the primary defect lies in the melanocytes themselves or in their precursors (COMINGS and ODLANDS 1966; SELMANOWITZ 1979). Certainly, in the pale areas, recognisable melanocytes were greatly reduced in number while even in the pigmented skin various ultrastructural abnormalities were found in the melanosomes of the one case studied by electron microscopy (BREATHNACH et al. 1965) and this again points to disordered melanocyte function. The neural crest – melanocyte theory is supported by the occurrence of defects in other neural crest derivatives – heterochromia of the iris in some cases and rarely of megacolon (MAHAKRISHNAN and SRINIVASAN 1980), the result of defective colonic autonomic innervation derived from the neural crest, and, in certain families, cerebellar ataxia (TELFER et al. 1971). Furthermore, there

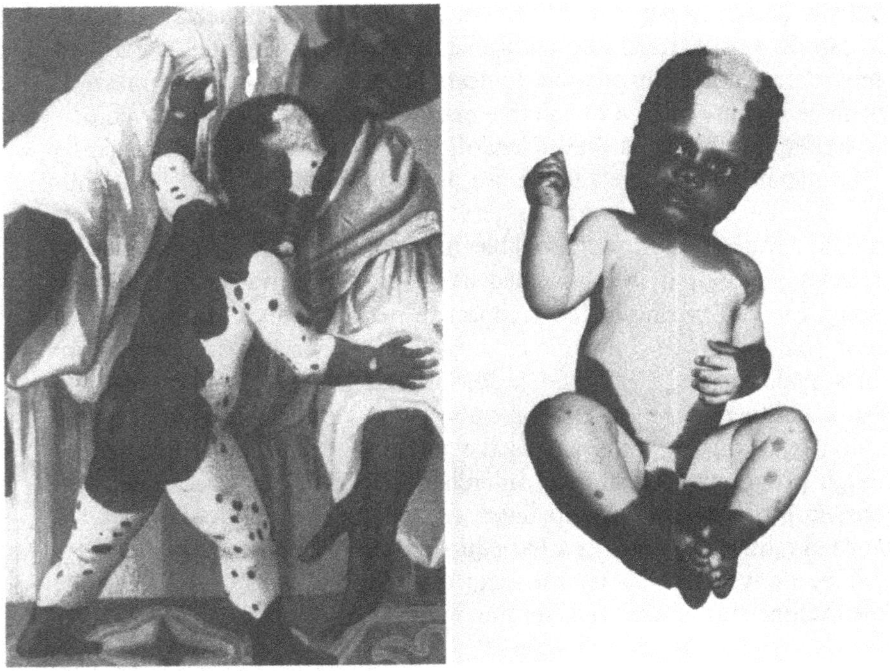

Fig. 8. Two cases of piebaldism showing characteristic pattern of amelanosis which is almost symmetrical and affects forelock, forehead, ventral aspect of trunk, and areas around elbows and knees. Randomly distributed pigmented macules are also a feature. Left, from painting by Le Mausurier 1782; right, photograph provided by Professor J.H. Edwards of Oxford

is similar patterned depigmentation in Waardenburg's syndrome (McKUSICK 1983) which is almost certainly attributable to a neural crest abnormality judging from the other common pleiotropic effects of the mutation – nerve deafness, heterochromia iridis, lateral displacement of the inner canthus, cleft palate and/or lip.

From our knowledge of pigment patterns in human chimaeras and mosaics it seems most unlikely that the pattern of hypomelanosis in piebaldism has to do with the clonal behaviour of melanocytes. The selective and roughly symmetrical involvement and non-involvement of neighbouring patches of skin of the hands and wrists illustrated in Fig. 8 point to a fault in local regulation of melanocyte behaviour. In our view the most likely explanation for the piebald pattern is a defect in melanocytes of cell surface receptors which are involved in local tissue interactions at certain anatomical sites during normal melanocyte migration or development. The defect appears to be quantitative and unstable, hence the occurrence of numerous random pigmented macules, the occasional darkening of hypomelanotic skin after exposure to sunlight (SELMANOWITZ 1979) and the spontaneous expansion or contraction of the unpigmented areas in some cases (DAVIS and VERDOL 1976).

Piebald syndromes have been associated with karyotypic abnormalities of chromosome 4. In one patient (FUNDERBURK and CRANDALL 1974) there was

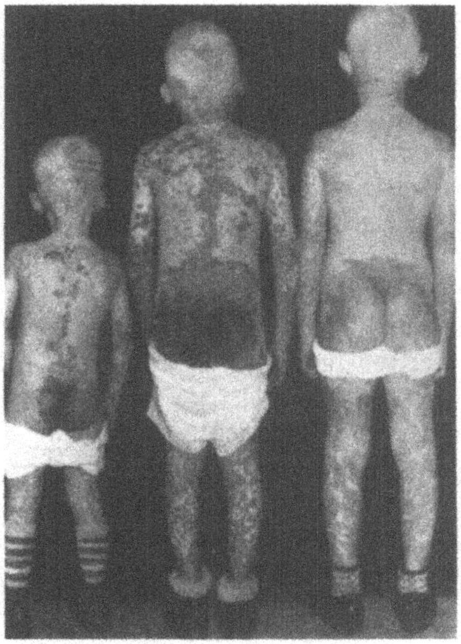

Fig. 9. X-linked partial albinism in two brothers and a cousin. The pattern is slightly asymmetrical and similar but not identical in each case. Reproduced from ZIPRKOWSKI et al. (1962) with permission of Archives of Dermatology

a reciprocal translocation and intercalary deletion in one of the chromosomes, while in a second case (LACASSIE et al. 1977) there was an interstitial deletion of the long arm adjacent to centromeric heterochromatin raising the possibility of a position effect – i.e. a change of action of a gene due to its repositioning in the genome. It is uncertain how many different mutations can result in human piebaldism. Some of the loci causing white spotting in mice, probably an analogous condition, have already been mentioned in section 4.

9. Partial Albinism with Deafness

ZIPRKOWSKI et al. (1962) described 14 members of three generations of a Jewish Sephardi family with X-linked deafness, vestibular hypofunction and partial albinism. At birth there was pigmentation affecting the gluteal and scrotal regions but otherwise the skin was albinotic. Later, sharply delineated roughly symmetrical hyperpigmented macules reminiscent of leopard skin developed mainly on the midline of the back and on the extremities (Fig. 9). Histologically epidermal melanocytes were present in normal numbers, hyperpigmentation and hypopigmentation being associated respectively with strong and weak reactions for tyrosinase. The phenotype of female carriers was normal although there must have been clonal patches in which the normal X-chromosome was inactivated (section 4). Apparently the defect is not cell autonomous and can be corrected by cellular interactions with normal cells.

Woolf et al. (1965) encountered two deaf partially albinotic brothers in a Hopi Indian family. The mode of inheritance and histopathology of the disorder was unknown. The pattern of pigment variegation was very similar in both, most of the face, upper chest and arms being albinotic with randomly scattered pigmented macules. In one of the brothers there was marked asymmetry of forearm pigmentation.

These families provide further examples of abnormalities due to different mutant genes which are almost certainly primarily expressed in the neural crest or cells derived from it. As in piebaldism there is some variation in pattern within each family and in individual cases the pattern sometimes shows significant lateral asymmetry.

Pattern asymmetry in patients with various genetic disorders of the neural crest raises several interesting questions. Are the abnormal patterns initially laid down in a symmetrical manner but subsequently distorted by cell mixing during lateral migration? Are the mutant genes particularly unstable or is the control of their expression unusually lax? It would also be interesting to know whether asymmetry is peculiar to abnormal melanocyte patterns or if it is a general feature of mutations affecting pattern formation in other tissues.

10. Vitiligo

By definition vitiligo is characterised by acquired (post-natal) depigmentation of the skin due to loss of epidermal melanocytes. As a patterened pigmentary disorder, it has several important peculiarities. (1) Since the lesions appear in post-natal life, their origin and spread can be observed with the naked eye. (2) The anatomical distribution of the lesions varies greatly from case to case, thus providing an opportunity to identify factors responsible for the localisation of the disease. Some lesions coincide with well recognised anatomical structures (Fig. 10), others seem to correspond to intrinsic cutaneous prepatterns whose existence is not apparent until they are mapped out by pigmented loss, while yet others appear to have no normal counterpart but to result de novo from pathological events. (3) Vitiligo occurs in about 1% of the population and so allows ample opportunity for clinical research on pattern formation.

Several forms of vitiligo are recognised, the most common appearing as white macules which are often roughly symmetrical and are accompanied in about 80% of cases by autoantibody formation against a 75,000 Dalton protein present on the surface of normal human melanocytes (Naughton et al. 1983). The common form of vitiligo is also closely associated with other organ-specific autoantibodies e.g. antithyroglobulin, antigastric parietal cells (Brostoff et al. 1969) and autoimmune diseases affecting thyroid (Cunliffe et al. 1968) and/or gastric mucosa (Grunnet et al. 1970). Other forms of vitiligo which include halo naevus and segmental vitiligo are encountered less frequently and their relationship to melanocyte autoimmunity is not yet known. The following discussion deals with the common form of vitiligo except where stated, and is largely based on reviews by Lerner (1959, 1971), Mosher et al. (1979) and El Mofty and El Mofty (1980).

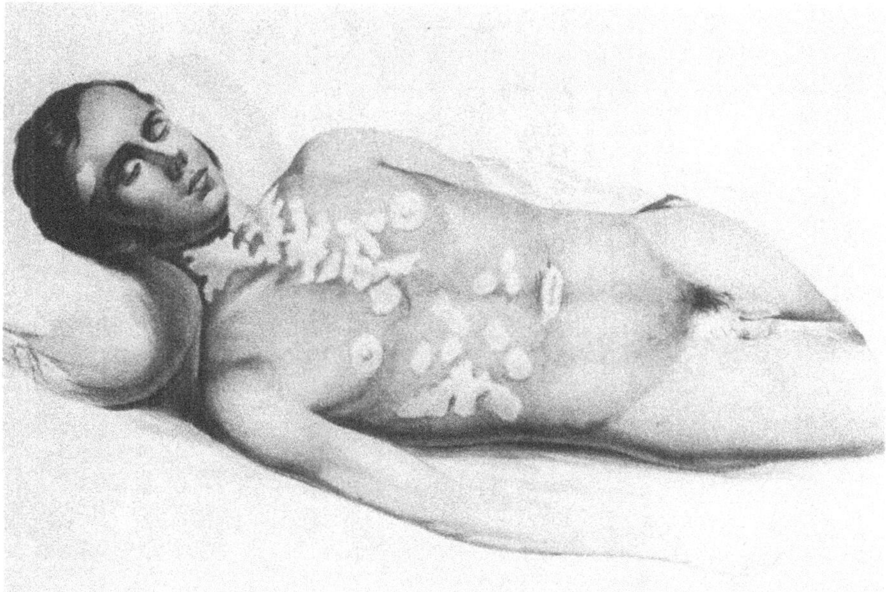

Fig. 10. Vitiligo complicating chronic adrenal insufficiency. Apart from the symmetrical involvement of nipples and areolae the anatomical basis of the pattern is obscure. Reproduced from ADDISON (1855)

In some cases only a few macules are present. These may remain unchanged for long periods but the disease tends to progress by centrifugal enlargement of the lesions and the formation of new macules. This may occur slowly or rapidly and occasionally it may lead to amelanosis of the whole skin. Initially, the pigment loss may develop round a pre-existing naevus (halo naevus), over an old or recent injury or burn, or at the site of contact with certain chemicals, notably phenols, hydroquinones and their derivatives. Neither melanocytes (as identified by tyrosinase or melanosomes) nor melanin can be found in fully developed lesions and surviving melanocytes in the adjacent epidermis are abnormally large. In keeping with the presumed autoimmune aetiology there is lymphocytic infiltration of the dermis at the expanding edge of some lesions and increased numbers of epidermal Langerhans cells (BIRBECK et al. 1961; NORLUND et al. 1978), bone-marrow derived antigen-binding mononuclears which can stimulate sensitised T lymphocytes (KATZ et al. 1979). A third of lesions are said to regress spontaneously by repopulation of the epidermis with melanocytes from the hair follicles or from unaffected epidermis at the edge of the lesion. In the interesting "trichrome" vitiligo some lesions of intermediate colour show reduction in numbers rather than complete absence of functional melanocytes.

10.1 Inheritance

Approximately a quarter of vitiligo patients have an affected relative. HAVEZ et al. (1983) have conducted the first well planned study of the mode of inheri-

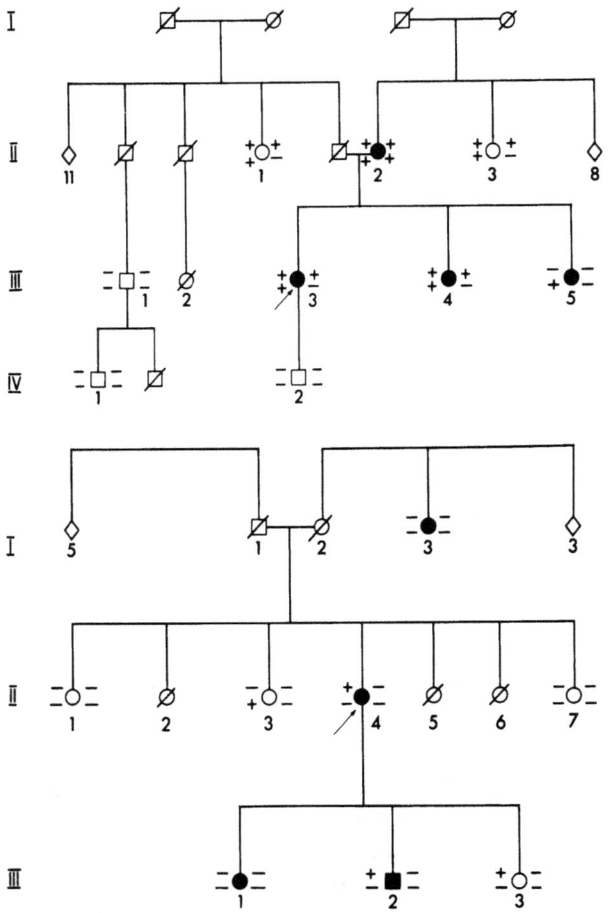

Fig. 11. Organ specific autoimmunity in two families with multiple cases of vitiligo. Index case *arrowed*. Vitiligo, solid symbols. Antibodies (+ or −): *top left*, thyroid microsomes; *top right*, thyroglobulin; *bottom left*, gastric parietal cell; *bottom right*, islet cell. *Upper pedigree*: II2 primary hypothyroidism, pernicious anaemia; III2 thyrotoxicosis; III3 thyrotoxicosis, alopecia areata; III4 primary hypothyroidism; III5 diabetes mellitus; IV1 diabetes mellitus. *Lower pedigree*: I1 diabetes mellitus; II2 thyrotoxicosis; II4 thyrotoxicosis, alopecia areata. After GOUDIE et al. (1983a)

tance in 150 families and conclude that the disease is polygenic and does not demonstrate simple mendelian ratios. Its "heritability" is calculated to be 70%. Among the genetic factors predisposing to vitiligo those determining the development of organ specific autoimmunity are probably very important. Fig. 11 illustrates the association between vitiligo and other organ-specific autoimmune diseases in two families studies by the authors (GOUDIE et al. 1983a) and indicate the need to consider the whole spectrum of organ-specific autoimmunity in pedigrees rather than vitiligo alone. It should be noted that alopecia areata is known to occur with undue frequency in patients with vitiligo and autoimmune thyroid disease (MULLER and WINKELMANN 1963) though it has not yet been associated with organ-specific autoantibody reacting with cells of the hair follicles.

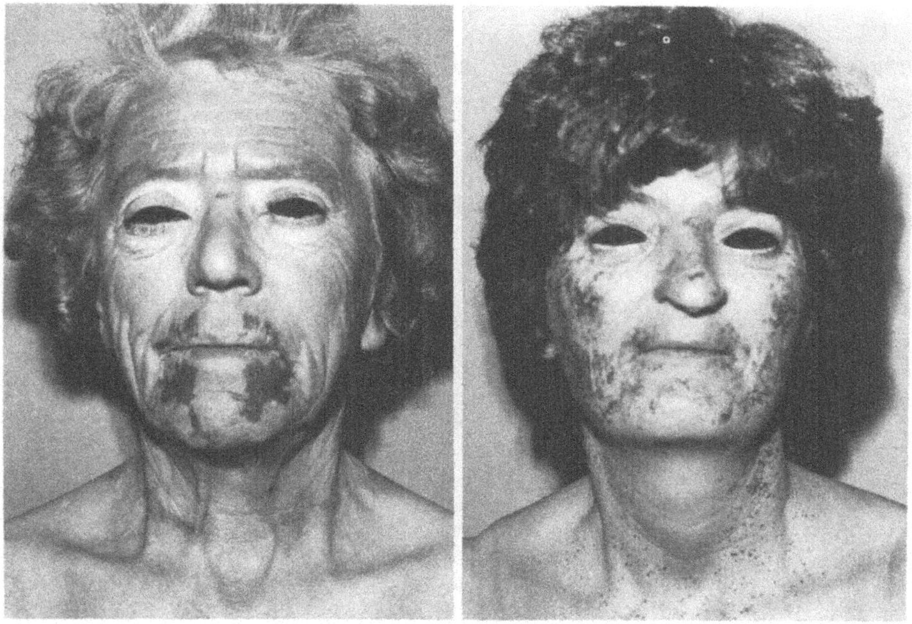

Fig. 12. Advanced vitiligo. Note the symmetry of the depigmentation and the differences in texture of the lesions in the two patients. Reproduced from GOUDIE et al. (1983b) with permission of the Scottish Medical Journal

Preliminary evidence suggestive of an association between vitiligo and HLA DR4 has been reported by FOLEY et al. (1983), and this is in keeping with the known tendency to linkage disequilibrium between DR antigens and other organ specific autoimmune diseases.

10.2 Pattern of Lesions in Vitiligo

10.2.1 Symmetry

A striking feature of the lesions of vitiligo is their occurrence at roughly corresponding sites on opposite sides of the midline (Figs. 12, 15, 16, 17 and 18). The crude bilateral symmetry persists to the late stages of the disease when most of the skin is white and only small residual areas of pigmentation remain (Fig. 12).

10.2.2 Texture

In some cases there are block-like areas of depigmentation while in others the lesions tend to have a mottled appearance. These differences also may persist until a late stage (Fig. 12). The variation in texture of vitiligo is reminiscent

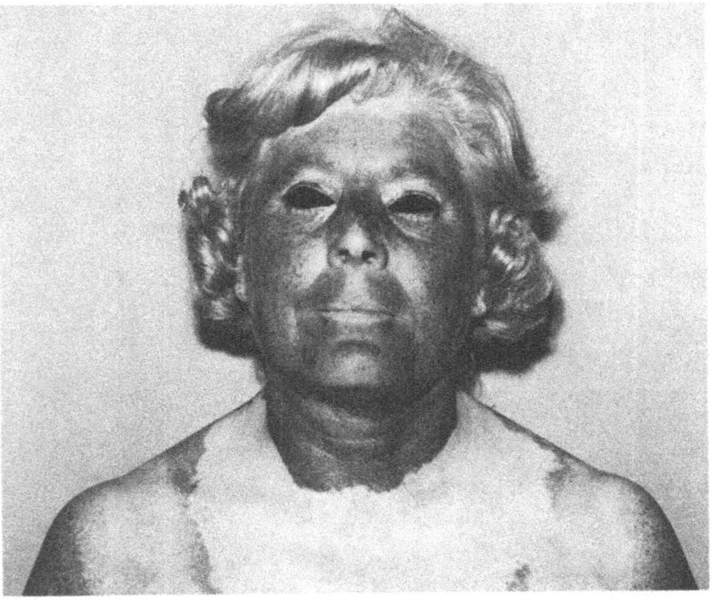

Fig. 13. Vitiligo pattern influenced by clothing. There is marked depigmentation of the area bounded by the neckline and shoulder straps possibly due to chemical damage from a high-necked garment or unaccustomed exposure to sunlight (III3 upper pedigree, Fig. 11). Reproduced from GOUDIE et al. (1983a) with permission of Scottish Medical Journal

of the range of appearances attributed to differences in extent of clonal mixing in the skin of human and animal chimaeras (sections 4 and 5).

10.2.3 Site

Some lesions of vitiligo correspond in position to well defined anatomical structures such as in the case illustrated by ADDISON (1855) in which the nipples and areolae were involved (Fig. 10). Several characteristic distribution patterns have been described including parts of the body which are normally most deeply pigmented, extensor bony surfaces, periorificial areas, axillae and low back. Depigmentation of distal digits and the lips produces the "lip-tip" syndrome.

10.3 Role of Local Tissue Injury (Köbner Phenomenon)

In patients already suffering from vitiligo, further lesions may be produced by various types of injury such as surgical incision, pressure from clothes and burns of various kinds (LERNER 1959). Such lesions are easily recognised by their anatomical distribution for they correspond exactly to the site of injury (e.g. corresponding to a garment (EL MOFTY and EL MOFTY (1980) and Fig. 13) and tend not to spread. In one notable case (SWEET 1978) in which the word "Mandy" had been scraped on the skin of the forearm four months previously

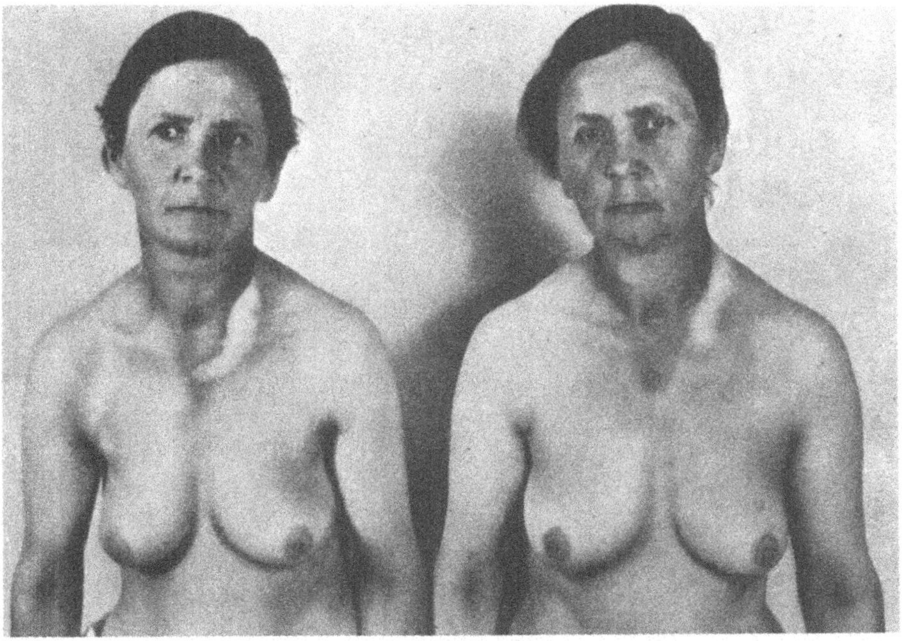

Fig. 14. Segmental vitiligo in monozygotic twins. The lesion in each is similar but not identical in position. Reproduced from LUCHSINGER and HANHART (1949) with permission of Archiv für Genetik

with a pointed piece of metal, the Köbner phenomenon became apparent only when the characteristic lesions of vitiligo developed elsewhere in the body – an intriguing example of cellular memory and prepattern formation! The development of vitiliginous lesions at the site of an injury points to the importance of local factors in the pathogenesis of melanocyte loss. In the majority of lesions these factors appear to be intrinsic and not, as in the Köbner phenomenon, the result of damage from the external environment.

10.4 Anatomical Basis of Vitiligo Patterns

The majority of lesions in vitiligo do not correspond to known anatomical structures nor do they demonstrate (except in "segmental" cases, Fig. 14) the markedly asymmetrical behaviour or midline phenomena associated with melanocyte or mesodermal clones. Often there is a discrepancy between melanocyte loss in epidermis and adjacent hair follicles (pigmented hair protruding from amelanotic skin or vice versa) reflecting non equivalent micro-environments and/or responses of epidermal and follicular melanocytes. The occurrence of reciprocal patterns (Fig. 15) suggests that the lesions of vitiligo map out otherwise inapparent sub-divisions of the skin based on a system of symmetrical regional specializations which must have been laid down much earlier in development. It is noteworthy that there is as yet no evidence that melanocyte antibody is specific for melanocytes at different anatomical sites, and this again points

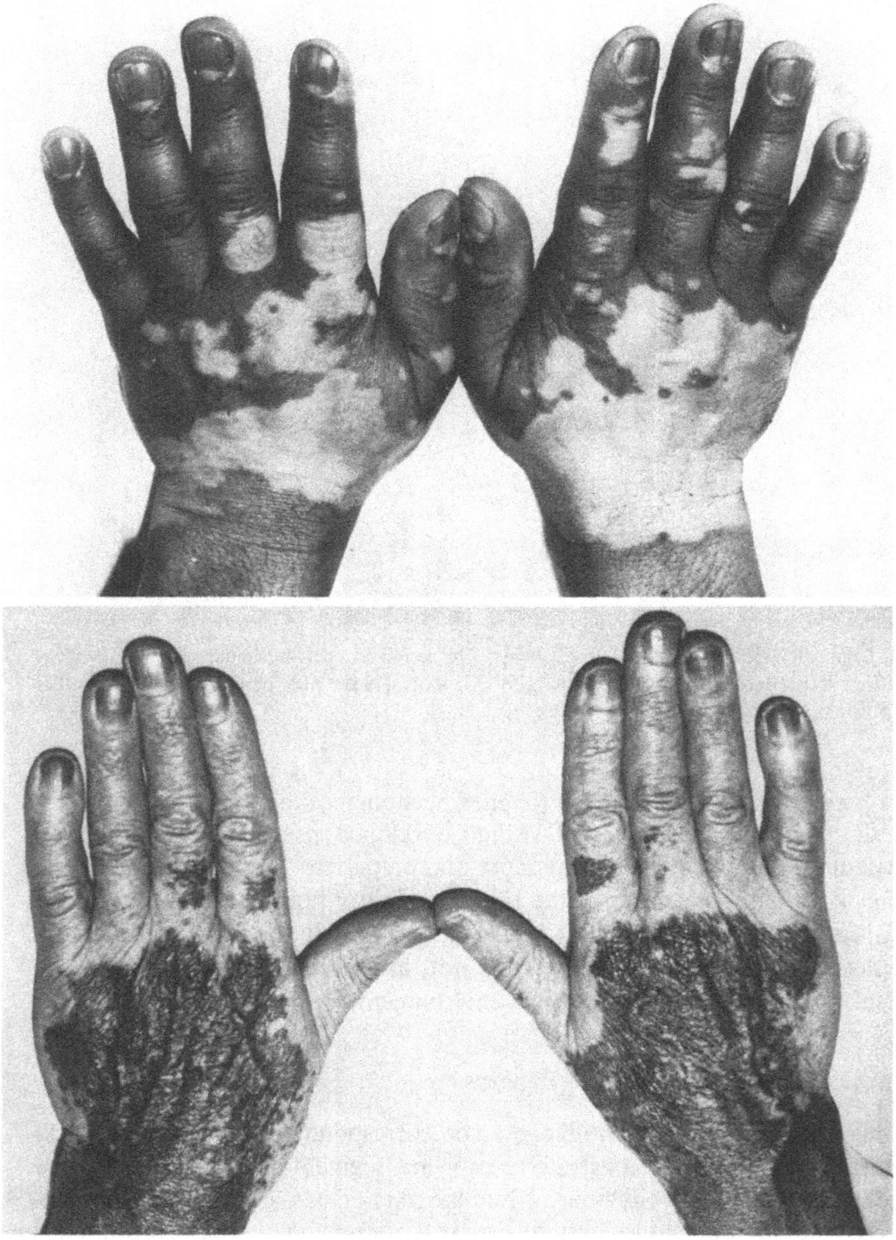

Fig. 15. Reciprocal vitiligo patterns. The predominantly distal and proximal involvement of the hands of these patients does not correspond to the distribution of known anatomical structures. Reproduced from GOUDIE et al. (1983b) with permission of the Scottish Medical Journal

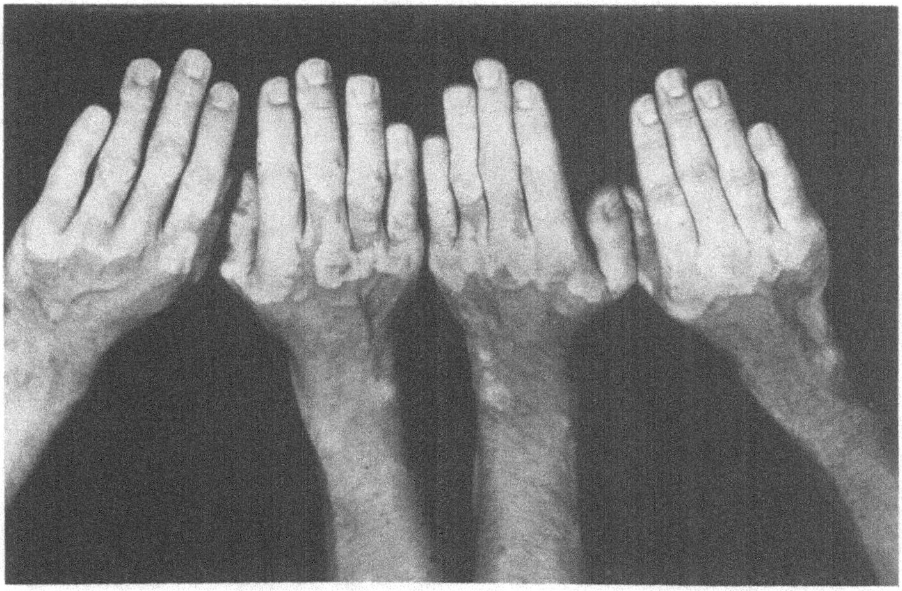

Fig. 16. Vitiligo affecting the hands of monozygotic twins. The patterns are remarkably similar in position and extent. Reproduced from v. MAYENBURG et al. (1976) with permission of Der Hautarzt and the authors

to the probable importance of local tissue factors in determining the sites at which vitiligo develops.

PINKUS (1959) has reviewed a number of transplantation experiments between normal and vitiliginous skin to elucidate whether the dermis or epidermis is the primary site of the disturbance. The results were somewhat contradictory and difficulties in interpretation of results must have arisen due to Köbner phenomena and repopulation of the epidermis of thin grafts by cells from dermal hair follicles.

10.5 Inheritance of Vitiligo Patterns

There are published photographs of 6 reputedly monozygotic twin pairs concordant for vitiligo (MOHR 1951; SIEMENS 1953; VOGEL and DORN 1964; KIMMIG and JANNER 1966; v. MAYENBURG et al. 1974 and LUCHSINGER and HANHART 1949). Members of each pair have strikingly similar patterns though with differences in detail (Figs. 14 and 16). These findings are in keeping with an hereditary basis for the location of vitiliginous lesions. It has been proposed that the differences between the patterns in such twins and even on opposite sides of the body in a single individual may be due to frequent somatic mutation at an unstable locus in the cells responsible for the localisation of melanocyte damage (GOUDIE et al. 1980). There are however, other equally satisfactory explanations. For example it is possible that an initially symmetrical pattern might be distorted by unprogrammed inequalities of subsequent cell growth or irregular cell migration from the midline.

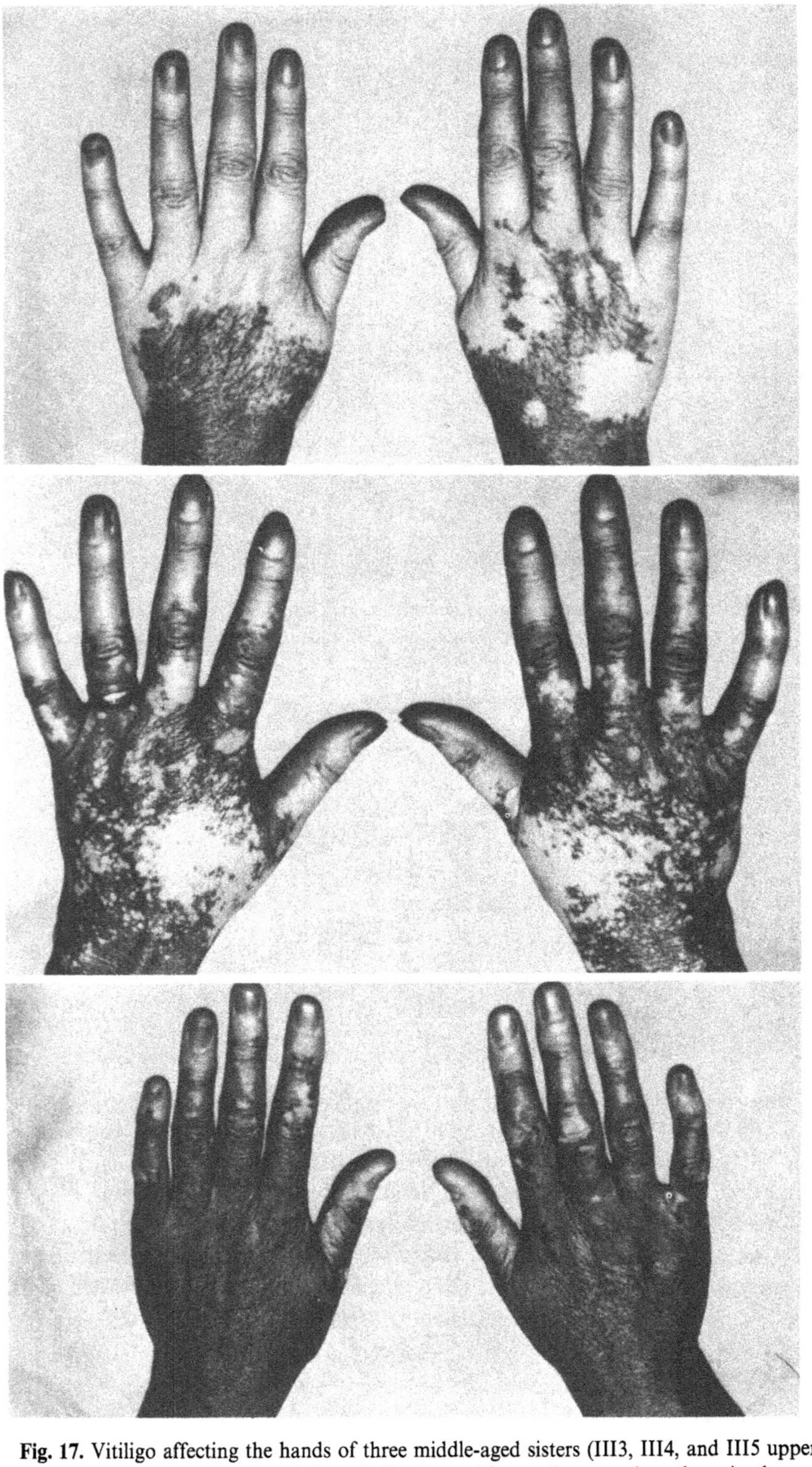

Fig. 17. Vitiligo affecting the hands of three middle-aged sisters (III3, III4, and III5 upper pedigree, Fig. 11). The patterns are much less similar in position and extent than those in the monozygotic twins illustrated in Fig. 16. Reproduced from GOUDIE et al. (1983a) with permission of the Scottish Medical Journal

In photographs of twins published by SIEMENS (1953) depigmentation and repigmentation occurred at similar sites over a period of 11 years suggesting that not only the anatomical pattern of vitiligo but also its sequence of development may be genetically determined. It should be noted that the similarity of patterns in monozygotic twins may be more apparent than real. There may be biased reporting in favour of concordance or the effect may be due to each pair sharing common melanocytotoxic environments. In view of the frequency of vitiligo it should be possible to clarify these important points by systematically comparing patterns in monozygotic and dizygotic twins. The occurrence of monozygotic twins discordant for vitiligo (as in the pair described by SCHACHTER (1947) in which one had vitiligo and thyrotoxicosis and the other was unaffected by either condition) furnishes information on the role of inheritance in the development of vitiligo but does not contribute evidence on the heritability of pattern.

In a study of 7 families with multiple cases of vitiligo and evidence of other forms of organ-specific autoimmunity (GOUDIE et al. 1983a), the first degree relatives had different patterns of depigmentation (Fig. 17) and the differences could not be explained on the basis of age or time-dependent progression or regression of the disease, or on external environmental factors. If, as seems likely from the reports on monozygotic twins mentioned above, vitiligo patterns are to some extent genetically determined, the positioning of lesions would thus appear to be multifactorial i.e. dependent on interactions between different polymorphic loci.

10.6 Vitiligo Simulating Internal Autoimmune Disease

GOUDIE et al. (1979) have noted that the skin patterns in vitiligo may mimic the anatomical distribution of the internal lesions of human autoimmune diseases, e.g. the front of neck and eyelids simulating the goitre and exophthalmos of thyrotoxicosis. Of 8 patients with this pattern, 2 actually suffered from thyrotoxicosis. The reciprocal pattern, subtotal vitiligo with residual pigmentation of the front of neck and eyelids, has also been described (MAGUIRE 1961).

Fig. 18 illustrates vitiligo localised mainly to the skin over the joints and simulating the distribution of rheumatoid arthritis in an 18 year old female. There are also symmetrical lesions over the posterior aspect of the shoulder joints, lateral apsects of hips and on the face. Thyroid autoantibody is present in her serum (indicative of subclinical focal autoimmune thyroiditis) but the girl is otherwise healthy. Interestingly, her father has rheumatoid arthritis and thyrotoxicosis raising the possibility that the daughter's vitiligo is superimposed on an anatomical pattern of joint disease inherited from her father.

10.7 Halo Naevi (KOPF et al. 1965)

In vitiligo simple pigmented naevi are frequently surrounded by depigmented macules up to several centimetres in diameter and may be the first manifestation

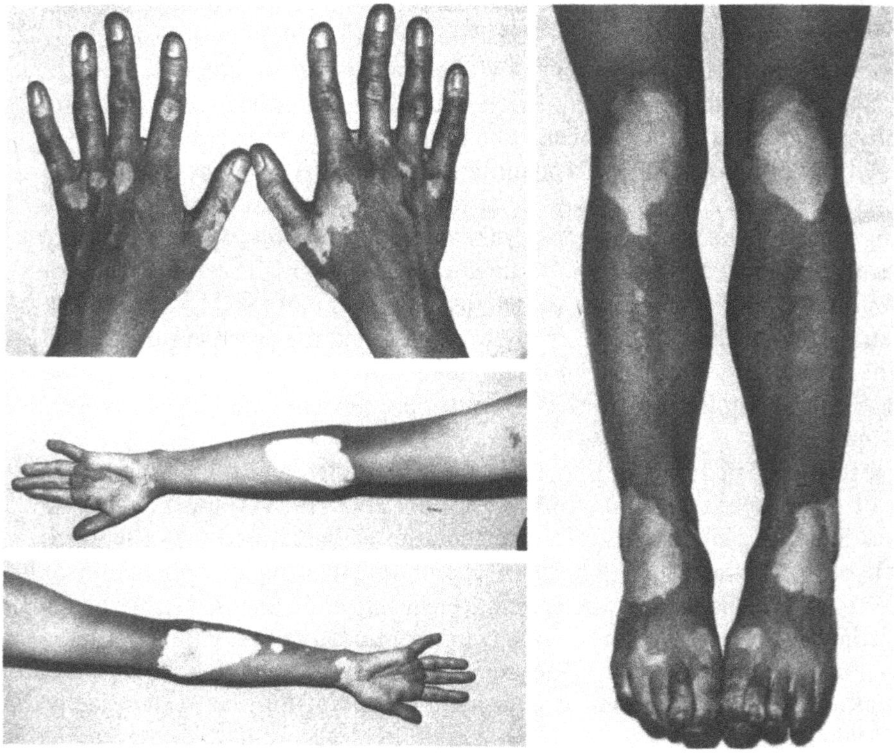

Fig. 18. Vitiligo pattern simulating joint disease in a girl whose father has rheumatoid arthritis and thyrotoxicosis

of the disease. In patients with multiple naevi some may have a halo while others are unaffected. Histologically, there is marked lymphoid infiltration of the central naevus but this may be absent in the surrounding melanocyte-deficient halo. Because of their importance in the initiation vitiliginous patches the structure and evolution of halo naevi deserve further detailed study. Halo naevi also develop in the absence of vitiligo and their association with melanocytic autoimmunity requires to be investigated.

10.8 Segmental Vitiligo

Approximately 1 in 20 cases of vitiligo has the segmental form of the disease (EL MOFTY and EL MOFTY 1980). It is unilateral with an anatomical distribution corresponding to all or part of one or more adjacent "dermatomes". As a rule it is not progressive, but occasionally it is followed by loss of pigment in other parts of the body, as in the twins shown in Fig. 14 (LUCHSINGER and HANHART 1949) who had lesions on the hands. The relationship between segmental vitiligo and antimelanocyte or other forms of organ-specific autoimmunity has yet to be investigated. It is generally assumed that the occurrence of lesions in a "dermatomal" distribution is determined by the local innervation of the skin (Scholtz and Williamson 1951) and there is an unconfirmed report of abnormal sympathetic function in the depigmented areas in segmental vitiligo (Koga 1977).

The segmental vitiligo in the monovular twins illustrated in Fig. 14 was accompanied by deafness and thus is probably due to a neural crest defect. It raises two points of great interest in relation to the genetics of pattern formation. (1) In each the same "dermatome" is involved – probably a unique illustration of programmed unilateral expression of a mutant germ line gene in one particular segment. (2) In keeping with the individual variation in all inherited abnormalities of pigmentation pattern already described the site of pigment loss in each twin is not the same within the affected segment.

Presumably a tendency to melanocyte loss inherited through the germ line is the cause of some other cases of segmental vitiligo. Yet others may be due to clones arising from somatic mutation (section 6) or acquired disease as in the case reported by Nellaus (1970) in which predominantly unilateral encephalitis was accompanied by vitiligo on the corresponding side of the head.

11. Conclusions

The patterned pigmentary disorders described above can be regarded as natural experiments involving variations on the theme of normal pattern formation.

The findings in human chimaerism resemble those in mouse chimaeras produced experimentally by fusion of early embryos. Cells of each genotype contribute to the pigment pattern on both sides of the body indicating considerable intermingling of cells during early development. Marked variation in pattern is seen in different individuals. Sometimes there are large blocks of dark and light pigmentation, sometimes fine stippling, depending on the cohesiveness of cells forming the basic banded pattern.

In 11 of 12 presumed skin pigment mosaics the abnormality is restricted to one side of the body (excluding minor encroachments on the midline). In this respect the mosaics are significantly different from chimaeras, perhaps because of the development of mosaicism comparatively late in embryogenesis. It is also possible that due to the wider genetic diversity of the component cells, the degree of mixing is greater in chimaeras and thus unrepresentative of what happens in normal development.

A remarkable harlequin pattern is described illustrating interchange of cells between corresponding positions on opposite sides of the midline early in development, with subsequent formation of a regular pattern by symmetrical clonal expansion and migration. It is unknown whether the harlequin pattern is merely a grotesque byproduct of normal melanocyte development or if it reflects the existence of a set of cells which contribute more fundamentally to the generally symmetrical pattern of most tissues of the body.

The inherited disorders of pigment pattern are genetically heterogeneous. From the pleiotropic effects of the various mutations it would appear that in piebaldism, Waardenburg's syndrome, the Ziprkowski syndrome, Woolf's syndrome and the monozygotic twins with segmental vitiligo described by LUCHSINGER and HANHART (1949), neural crest cells are the site of expression of the mutant genes. In each condition there is a characteristic pigmentation pattern though this varies in detail from case to case even in monozygotic twins. In addition, there is sometimes considerable pattern variation on the two sides of the body in individual cases and it would be interesting to know whether this is merely due to a peculiarity of abnormal melanocytes or if it is a property of mutations affecting pattern formation in other tissues.

Vitiligo is of particular interest in that it demonstrates an abnormal developmental process (patterned destruction of melanocytes) probably due to systemic immunity against the patient's own melanocytes, the local lesions being initiated in a variety of different circumstances including tissue injury, hamartomatous or neoplastic proliferation of melanocytes (halo naevi), or unknown intrinsic factors at least some of which are genetically determined.

References

Adamson D (1911) A case of unilateral pigmentary naevus. Br J Dermatol 23:77

Adamson ED, Gardner RL (1979) Control of early development. Br Med Bull 35:113–119

Addison T (1855) On the constitutional effects of the suprarenal capsule, Highly, London

Alberts B, Bray D, Lewis J, Raff M, Roberts K, Watson JD (1983) Molecular biology of the cell, Garland, New York and London

Bandler M (1960) Haemangiomatosis of the small intestine associated with mucocutaneous pigmentation. Gastroenterology 38:641–645

Bartholomew LG, Moore CE, Dahlin DC, Waugh JM (1962) Intestinal polyposis associated with mucocutaneous pigmentation. Surg Gynecol Obstet 115:1–11

Billingham RE (1948) Dendritic cells. J Anat 82:93–109

Birbeck MS, Breathnach AS, Everall JD (1961) An electron microscope study of basal melanocytes and high level clear cells (Langerhans' cells) in vitiligo. J Invest Dermatol 37:51–64

Blaschko A (1901) Die Nervenverteilung in der Haut in ihrer Bezeichnung zu den Erkrankungen der Haut. Beilage zu den Verhandlungen der Deutschen Dermatolischen Gesellschaft VII Congress, Breslau

Breathnach AS, Fitzpatrick TB, Wyllie LM-A (1965) Electron microscopy of melanocytes in human piebaldism. J Invest Dermatol 45:28–37

Brostoff J, Bor S, Feiwel M (1969) Autoantibodies in patients with vitiligo. Lancet 2:177–178

Capon D (1948) Case of unilateral lentigines with mental deficiency. Br J Dermatol 60:371–374

Chemke J, Rappaport S, Etrog R (1983) Aberrant melanoblast migration associated with trisomy 18 mosaicism. J Med Genet 20:135–137

Chevallier A, Kieny M, Mauger A (1977) Limb-somite relationships: origin of the limb musculature. J Embryol Exp Morphol 41:245–258

Comings DE, Odlands GF (1966) Partial albinism. JAMA 195:510–523

Corey MJ, Miller JR, MacLean JR, Chown B (1967) A case of XX/XY mosaicism. Am J Hum Genet 19:378–387

Crick FHC, Lawrence PA (1975) Compartments and polyclones in insect development: clones made in early development keep within certain fixed boundaries in the insect epithelium. Science 189:340–347

Cunliffe WJ, Hall R, Newall DJ, Stevenson CJ (1968) Vitiligo, thyroid disease and autoimmunity. Br J Dermatol 80:135–139

Davis BK, Verdol LD (1976) Expansion and contraction of hypomelanotic areas in human piebaldism. Hum Genet 34:163–170

Davis DG, Shaw MW (1964) An unusual human mosaic for skin pigmentation. New Engl J Med 270:1384–1388

Deol MS (1967) The neural crest and the acoustic ganglion. J Embryol Exp Morphol 17:533–541

Edelman GM (1983) Cell adhesion molecules. Science 219:450–457

El Mofty AM, El Mofty M (1980) Vitiligo, a symptom complex. Int J Dermatol 19:237–244

Findlay GH, Moores PP (1980) Pigment anomalies of the skin in the human chimaera: their relation to systematised naevi. Br J Dermatol 103:489–498

Fitzgerald PH, Donald RA, Kirk RL (1979) A true hermaphrodite dispermic chimaera with 46,XX and 46,XY karyotypes. Clin Genet 15:89–96

Fitzpatrick TB, Szabó G, Seiji M, Quevedo WC (1979) Biology of the melanin pigmentary system. In: Fitzpatrick TB, Eisen AZ, Wolff K, Freedberg IM, Austen KF (eds) Dermatology in general medicine, 2nd edn. McGraw-Hill, New York, p 131–163

Foley LM, Low NJ, Misheloff E, Tiwari JL (1983) Association of HLA – DR4 with vitiligo. J Am Acad Dermatol 8:39–40

Funderburk SJ, Crandall BF (1974) Dominant piebald trait in a retarded child with reciprocal translocation and small intercalary deletion. Ann J Hum Genet 26:715–722

Garrod AE (1909) Inborn errors of metabolism, Oxford University Press, London

Gorlin RJ, Anderson RC, Blaw M (1969) Am J Dis Child 117:652–662

Goudie BM, Wilkieson C, Goudie RB (1983a) A family study of vitiligo patterns. Scott Med J 28:338–342

Goudie BM, Wilkieson C, Goudie RB (1983b) Skin maps in vitiligo. Scott Med J 28:343–346

Goudie RB, Spence JC, Mackie R (1979) Vitiligo patterns simulating autoimmune and rheumatic diseases. Lancet 2:393–395

Goudie RB, Goudie DR, Dick HM, Ferguson Smith MA (1980) Unstable mutations in vitiligo, organ specific autoimmune diseases and multiple endocrine adenoma/peptic ulcer syndrome. Lancet 2:285–287

Goudie RB, Spence JC, Scothorne RJ (1980) Do vascular clones determine developmental patterns? Lancet 1:570–572

Grunnet I, Howitz J, Reymann F, Schwartz M (1970) Vitiligo and pernicious anaemia. Arch Dermatol 101:82–85

Hafez M, Sharaf L, Abd El - Nabi SM (1983) The genetics of vitiligo. Acta Derm Venereol (Stockh) 63:249–251

Hughes GS, Park HK, Jones BE (1983) Partial unilateral lentiginosis in a black patient with sickle cell anaemia. J Am Acad Dermatol 8:563–565

Jackson R (1976) The lines of Blaschko: a review and reconsideration. Br J Dermatol 95:349–360

Jacobson M (1978) Clonal origins of the central nervous system: towards a developmental neuroanatomy. Zoon 6:149–156

Jacobson M, Hirose G (1978) Origin of the retina from both sides of the embryonic brain: a contribution to the problem of crossing at the optic chiasma. Science 202:637–639

Jeghers H, McKusick VA, Katz KH (1949) Generalised intestinal polyposis and melanin spots of the oral mucosa, lips and digits. New Engl J Med 241:993–1005, 1031–1036

Katz SI, Tamaki K, Sachs DH (1979) Epidermal Langerhans cells are derived from cells originating in bone marrow. Nature 282:324–326

Kaufman MH, O'Shea KS (1978) Induction of monozygotic twinning in the mouse. Nature 276:707–708

Kimmig J, Janner M (1966) Colour atlas of dermatology. Saunders, Philadelphia, p 24

Koga M (1977) Vitiligo: a new classification and therapy. Br J Dermatol 97:255–261

Kopf AW, Morrill SD, Silverberg I (1965) Broad spectrum of leukoderma acquisitum centrifugum. Arch Dermatol 92:14–35

Lacassie Y, Thurmon TF, Tracy MC, Pelias MZ (1977) Piebald trait in a retarded child with interstitial deletion of chromosome 4. Am J Hum Genet 29:641–642

Leder P (1982) The genetics of antibody diversity. Sci Am 246: (No. 5) 72–83

LeDouarin N (1982) The neural crest, Cambridge University Press, Cambridge

Lerner AB (1959) Vitiligo. J Invest Dermatol 32:285–310

Lerner AB (1971) On the etiology of vitiligo and grey hair. JAMA 51:141–147

Luchsinger R, Hanhart E (1949) Über erhebliche Manifestationsschwankungen rezessiver Taubheit bei drei eineiigen Zwillingspaaren. Arch Vererbungsforsch Sozialanthropol Rassenhyg 24:417–436

Lyon MF (1961) Gene action in the X-chromosome of the mouse (Mus musculus L.). Nature 190:372–373

MacLeod JMH (1913) A case of pigmented naevi-like freckles. Br J Dermatol 25:191

Maguire A (1961) Acquired albinism with intraocular depigmentation. Proc R Soc Med 54:696–697

Mahakrishnan A, Srinivasan MS (1980) Piebaldness with Hirschprung's disease. Arch Dermatol 116:1102

McKelway JI (1904) Lentigo: unilateral distribution, report of a case. New York Med J 80:197–198

McKusick VA (1983) Mendelian Inheritance in Man, 6th edn. Johns Hopkins University Press, Baltimore, p 538–539

McLaren A (1976) Mammalian chimeras, Cambridge University Press, London

Meirowsky E (1942) Moles and malformations of the skin in their relationship to inheritance and phylogenesis (new and old investigations). Br J Dermatol 54:99–121, 129–153

Mintz B (1971) Clonal basis of mammalian differentiation. In: Davis DD, Balls M (eds) Control mechanisms of growth and differentiation XXV. Cambridge University Press, Cambridge, p 345–370

Mintz B, Sanyal S (1970) Clonal origin of the mouse visual retina mapped from genetically mosaic eyes. Genetics 64 (suppl): 43–44

Mohr J (1951) Vitiligo in a pair of monovular twins. Acta Genet Statist Med 2:252–255

Moores P (1973) Blood group and tissue mosaicism in a Natal Indian woman. Acta Haematol 50:299–304

Mosher DB, Fitzpatrick TB, Ortonne J-P (1979) Abnormalities of pigmentation. In: Fitzpatrick TB, Eisen AZ, Wolff K, Freedberg IM, Austen KF (eds) Dermatology in general medicine, 2nd edn. McGraw-Hill, New York, p 568–629

Muller SA and Winkelmann RK (1963) Alopecia areata: an evaluation of 736 patients. Acta Dermatol 88:290–297

Naughton GK, Eisinger M, Bystryn J-C (1983) Antibodies to normal human melanocytes in vitiligo. J Exp Med 158:246–251

Nellhaus G (1970) Acquired unilateral vitiligo and poliosis of the head and subacute encephalitis with partial recovery. Neurology (NY) 20:965–974

Norlund JJ, Lerner AB, Braverman IM, McGuire JS (1973) The multiple lentigines syndrome. Arch Dermatol 107:259–261

Norlund JJ, Lerner AB, Miller LH, Kennedy JA (1978) Proceedings of the First International Workshop on Vitiligo. J Invest Dermatol 7:165–166

Pearson K, Nettleship E, Usher CH (1911a) A monograph on albinism in man, Atlas part II. Dulau, London, Plate tau

Pearson K, Nettleship E, Usher CH (1911b) A monograph on albinism in man, Atlas part I. Dulau, London, Plate J

Peters RM, Markert CL (1979) Pigmentation pattern of a black – and – tan (a^t) black chimera. J Hered 70:65–67

Pickering JG (1973) Partial unilateral lentiginosis with associated developmental abnormalities. Guys Hospital Reports 122:361–370

Pinkus H (1959) Vitiligo – what is it? J Invest Dermatol 32:281–284

Polani PE, Moynahan EJ (1972) Progressive cardiomyopathic lentigines. Q J Med 41:205–225

Poole TW, Silvers WK (1976) The development of regional pigmentation patterns in black and tan (a^t) mice. J Exp Zool 197:115–120

Race RR, Sanger R (1975) Blood groups in man, 6th edn. Blackwell, Oxford

Rawles ME (1947) Origin of pigment cells from the neural crest in the mouse embryo. Physiol Zool 20:248–266

Rawles ME (1948) Origin of melanophores and their role in development of color patterns in vertebrates. Physiol Rev 28:383–408

Razin A, Riggs AD (1980) DNA methylation and gene function. Science 210:604–610

Sakurai T, Ochiai H, Takeuchi T (1975) Ultrastructural change of melanosomes associated with agouti pattern in mouse hair. Dev Biol 47:466–471

Sanderson KV (1960) Eruptive telangiectatic cellular naevi. Br J Dermatol 72:302–307

Sasaki M, Sonta S, Niikawa N, Hujita M (1972) A case of congenital asymmetry associated with trisomy 18 mosaicism. Jpn J Hum Genet 17:50–56

Schachter M (1947) Vitiligo généralisé chez un jumeau univitellin. Syndrome diencéphalo-pituitaire probable. Profil neuro-physiologique. Ann Paediatrie 169:337–344

Scholtz JR, Williamson C (1951) Vitiligo in (apparent) dermatomal distribution. Arch Dermatol 64:366–369

Scully RE (1970) Sex cord tumour with annular tubules – a distinctive ovarian tumour of the Peutz-Jeghers syndrome. Cancer 25:1107–1121

Searle AG (1968) Comparative genetics of coat colour in mammals, Logos, London

Searle AG (1978) Evidence for mutable genes concerning the origin of the germ line. In: Russell LB (ed) Genetic mosaics and chimeras in mammals. Plenum Press, New York, p 212

Selmanowitz VJ (1979) Pigmentary correction of albinism by autografts: II pathomechanism and pigment spread in piebaldism. Cutis 24:66–73

Shumate CA (1941) Pigmented unilateral naevus like lentigo. Arch Dermatol 43:410

Siemens HW (1953) Die Swillingspathologie der Vitiligo. Acta Genet Med Gemmellol (Roma) 2:118–125

Silvers WK (1979) The coat colors of mice, Springer, New York Heidelberg Berlin

Slack JMW (1983) From egg to embryo: determinative events in early development, Cambridge University Press, London

Snell RS (1967) Hormonal control of pigmentation in man and other mammals. In: Montagna W, Hu F (eds) Advances in biology of skin, vol 8. Pergamon, New York, p 447–466

Sundfor H (1939) A pedigree of skin spotting in man: 42 piebalds in a Norwegian family. J Hered 30:67–77

Sweet RD (1978) Vitiligo as a Köbner phenomenon. Br J Dermatol 99:223–224

Tarkowski AK (1961) Mouse chimeras developed from fused eggs. Nature 190:857–860

Telfer MA, Sugar M, Jaegar EA, Mulcahy J (1971) Dominant piebald trait (white forelock and leukoderma) with neurological impairment. Am J Hum Genet 23:383–389

Thiery J-P, Duband J-L, Rutishauser U, Edelman GM (1982) Cell adhesion molecules in early chicken embryogenesis. Proc Natl Acad Sci USA 79:6737–6741

Thomson GW, Diehl AK (1980) Partial unilateral lentiginosis. Arch Dermatol 116:356

Tippett P (1983) Blood group chimaeras, a review. Vox Sang 44:333–359

v. Mayenburg J, Vogt H-J, Ziegelmayer G (1976) Vitiligo bei einem eineiigen Zwillingspaar. Hautarzt 27:426–431

Vogel F, Dorn H (1964) Krankheiten der Haut – und ihrer Anhangsgebilde. In Becker PE (ed) Hum Genet. Thieme - Verlag, Stuttgart, p 414–416, 476–478

Weiss LW, Zelickson AS (1977) Giant melanosomes in multiple lentigines syndrome. Arch Dermatol 113:491–494

Weston JA (1982) Neural crest cell development. Prog Clin Biol Res 85:359–379

Whimster IW (1968) Morbid anatomy and the skin. Trans St John's Hospital Dermatol Soc 54:11–41

Whimster IW (1971) The group behaviour of pigment cells. Trans St John's Hospital Dermatol Soc 57:57–86

Whitten WK (1978) Combinational and computer analysis of random mosaics. In: Russell LB (ed) Genetic mosaics and chimaeras in mammals. Plenum Press, New York, p 449

Wolpert L (1978) Pattern formation in biological development. Sci Am 239: (No. 4) 124–137

Wolpert L (1981) Positional information, pattern formation, and morphogenesis. In: Connelly TG (ed) Morphogenesis and pattern formation, Raven Press, New York, p 5–20

Woolf CM, Dolowitz DA, Aldous HE (1965) Congenital deafness associated with piebaldness. Arch Otolaryngol 82:244–250

Zegarelli EV, Kutscher AH, Piro JD, Kupferberg N (1956) Oral melanin pigmentation in intestinal polyposis: histopathologic considerations. Am J Dig Dis 1:455–465

Zimmerman AA, Becker SW (1959) Melanoblasts and melanocytes in fetal negro skin. Illinois Monogr Med Sci 6:1–59

Ziprkowski L, Krakowski A, Adam A, Costeff H, Saae J (1962) Arch Dermatol 86:530–539

Zuelzer WW, Beattie KM, Reisman LE (1964) Generalised imbalanced mosaicism attributable to dispermy and probable fertilization of a polar body. Am J Hum Genet 16:38–51

Changes in Epidermal Cell Proliferation in Proliferative Skin Disease

N.A. WRIGHT

The epidermis is, of course, the largest expanse of squamous epithelium, and is often involved in disease states. There is now good evidence that changes in cell proliferation accompany several well-recognised skin diseases, and the term 'proliferative skin disease' is now well-ingrained in the dermatological literature; despite this, as yet the clinical impact of studies in epidermal cell proliferation has been muted, and this is probably related to the fact that, looked at critically, our knowledge of the kinetic organisation of the human epidermis, and of its changes in disease is, even at this stage of the game, rather poor, notwithstanding the clear-cut clinical fact that drugs which are effective in psoriasis uniformly depend on interference with cell proliferation; unlike cancer chemotherapy, which field is littered with premature attempts at kinetic optimisation of therapeutic schedules, with one notable exception (WEINSTEIN et al. 1971) there has been no real attempt to effect this in proliferative skin disease (WRIGHT and CAMPLEJOHN 1983).

Whatever the reason for this deficiency, and of course ethical constraints are high among these, we must side with GELFANT (1978b) to observe that the proliferative defect in psoriasis and similar diseases is an ideal situation where a concerted attack on the clinical aspects of cell proliferation could reap dividends.

The methods and concepts used in studying cell proliferation in human epidermis have recently been reviewed (see for example WRIGHT 1980a, b); I therefore intend, in this chapter, to attempt a distillation of current thought, and possible future directions, of the topic of proliferative skin disease.

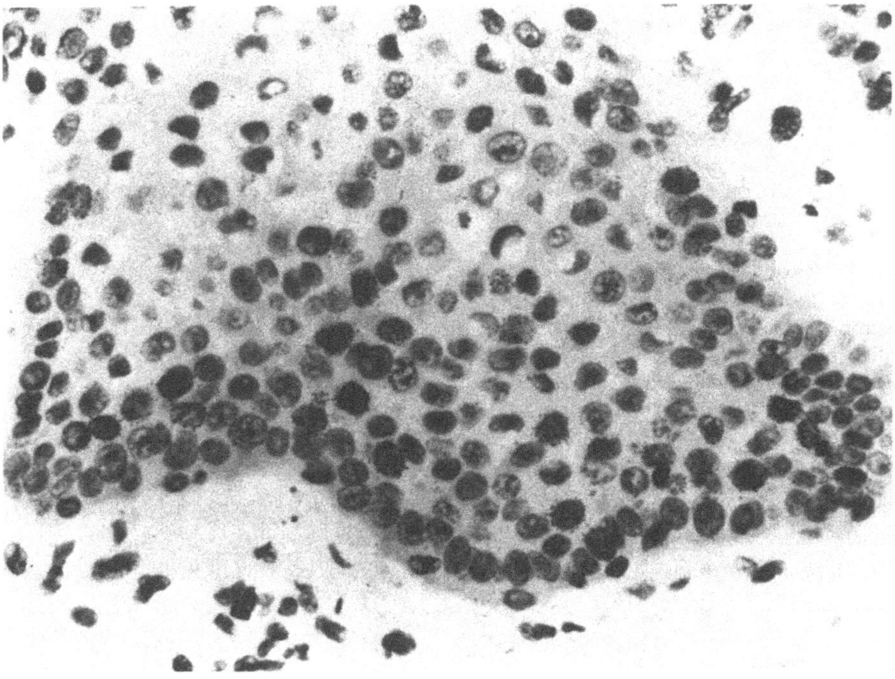

Fig. 1. The human epidermis in psoriasis; a rete peg from psoriatic epidermis which has been injected with ^{3}HTdR (10 μCi/site) and exposed for 28 days. Note the numerous labelled nuclei, many of which are in suprabasal cell positions, some 4 or 5 cell positions above the basal layer (× 600)

1. The Proliferative Defect in Psoriasis

Psoriasis is a skin condition which, in the U.K., effects some 2% of the population, and is as common as diabetes mellitus; it arises in various forms (ROOK et al. 1981), and despite recent advances in treatment, psoriasis remains a major dermatological problem.

There are now numerous *theories* concerning the aetiology and pathogenesis of psoriasis, both biochemical and immunological, largely outside the scope of this discussion, which tries to confine itself to observable phenomena (GUILDHOU et al. 1978). However, it is readily seen that the histological appearances in psoriasis are quite characteristic of a hyperplastic state (see Fig. 1), with elongation of the rete ridges, focal acanthosis and parakeratosis, in which nuclear remnants are found in the stratum corneum, due to incomplete differentiation (BERSAQUES 1966). There is also an increased number of cells per unit area, and an increase in the size of individual epidermal cells (GOODWIN et al. 1974). Our present interest arises in 1963 when Van Scott and Ekel observed a prominent increase in mitotic activity, which has frequently been confirmed.

1.1 Proliferative Indices in Psoriatic Epidermis

Two measurements which are useful in proliferative skin disease are the mitotic index (I_M), or the fraction of cells in mitosis, and the labelling index (I_S), the fraction of cells labelled in autoradiographs after local, intradermal injection of tritiated thymidine (^{3}HTdR); this shows the fraction of cells in DNA synthesis (the *S* phase); most workers are also agreed that there is an increase in the flash ^{3}HTdR labelling index in psoriatic epidermis, whether measured in biopsies taken after intradermal injection of ^{3}HTdR (DUFFILL et al. 1976; SHAHRAD and MARKS 1976), or by in vitro labelling (HELL and HODGSON 1966; PULLMAN et al. 1974), and also indicated by increased *S* phase fractions on integrating microdensitometry (GROVE et al. 1976) and flow cytometry (BAUER and DE GROOD 1975; BAUER et al. 1981), and by more simplistic methods such as scintillation counting (MARKS 1978); however, there is some dispute about the magnitude of this increase (GELFANT 1976 and see Table 1), and, in this respect, GELFANT (1976), who has exhaustively reviewed the reported proliferative index values in psoriasis, concludes that many labelling index values may be highly questionable. From Table 1 we can see that, while DUFFILL et al. (1976) and GOODWIN et al. (1973, 1974) have reported values of around 10 to 11% (compared with control values of about 3% in normal epidermis), results from Weinstein and his colleagues (WEINSTEIN and FROST 1968, 1969) indicate values in excess of 20%. The reason for this difference is interesting: WEINSTEIN and FROST (1968) considered that a correction factor should be employed to correct for the limited range of β-particles in tissue sections; most routine autoradiographers cut sections at what autoradiographers call 'infinite thickness', i.e. >2 μm, which means that they are thicker than the median range of the β-particles emanating from the ^{3}HTdR; consequently there may be some nuclei deep in the section, which are labelled, and although included in the interphase nuclear count, are not seen as labelled cells, since the β-particles do not reach the emulsion. SIMNETT (1968) has derived a correction factor of 1.4, based on considerations of β-particle track length and nuclear dimensions, by which the observed labelling index should be multiplied. Little work on the essentially practical need for this correction factor in epidermis has been done, but, from the few studies available, there is little evidence that section thickness has any influence on the magnitude of the labelling index; thus GELFANT (1962, 1976) compared the flash labelling index in human and mouse epidermis cut at a nominal thickness of 2 to 7 μm, and found no significant difference between them; this does not mean that the limited range of the β-particles has no influence on the accuracy of the estimate, but we are entitled to ask how large this source of error is likely to be, compared with other potential errors. Since WEINSTEIN and FROST (1968) used interphase nuclear counts which, in some instances, were as small as 850, the sampling error will also be considerable; moreover, it is interesting to note that, in numerous papers, WEINSTEIN is inconsistent in applying this correction factor (GELFANT 1976).

In addition to the questionable use of this correction factor, WEINSTEIN (1975) has accused other workers (namely GOODWIN et al. 1974) of including some 'non-germinative cells' in their interphase nuclear counts; in psoriasis the difficulty in recognising germinative cells is compounded by the multiple layers of proliferative cells (see Fig. 1), and by the fact that these cells are distributed unevenly, with many layers of proliferating cells in the rete pegs, but few above the papillae. Consequently we should not put too much weight

Table 1. Kinetic parameters in psoriatic epidermis

Growth fraction (%)	Duration of DNA synthesis (h)	Cell cycle time (h)	Turnover time (germinative cells) (h)	Flash labelling index (%)	Birth rate (cells/1000 cells/h)
100[a]	8.5	–	37.5	23	–
–	8.7–12.9	–	91	11	–
100[b]	7.7	56.5[c]	–	10	12.7[d]
	–	54.5[d]	–	–	–
In vitro					
–	–	50[e]	–	15[e]	–
–	14.4	–	114	13.6	–
74	6.5	53.2[c]	–	12	–
			–	13	–

[a] Psoriatic epidermis exposed to semicontinuous methotrexate for 36 h, then flashed with ^{3}HTdR; all germinative cells labelled

[b] Calculated from the ratio; experimental labelling index: theoretical labelling index

upon a single proliferative index; other workers have shown their faith in such single readings by using them to calculate the apparent cell cycle time or turnover time: the time taken to produce, by cell division, a number of cells equivalent to the total cellular content of the population – here the basal cell layer or germinative cell layer; in such calculations the vagaries of the labelling index estimation should be remembered, and measurements in which the definition of the population is less important (cf. the metaphase arrest method, see below) are perhaps to be preferred.

In vitro measurements also tend to give values of about 10 to 12% (see Table 1) for labelling indices carried out immediately after explanation, which of course is increased compared with normal values. However, Chopra and Flaxman (1974) report that I_S in outgrowths of normal and psoriatic epidermis do not differ a great deal. In the pustular variety of psoriasis, labelling indices are higher, up to 27% (Brassine and Conteaux-Dumont 1972), while very high indices are also seen in the outer root sheath of the hair follicle in psoriasis (Shahrad and Marks 1976). Having made these rather delicate points, it is perhaps discomforting to realise that, although some authors have suggested that psoriatic plaques are homogenous with respect to the spatial distribution of mitotic activity (Fry and McMinn 1970), there is substantial evidence that each psoriatic lesion is variable in its proliferative rate, both as a result of its being at different stages in its evolution and regression, and also because each psoriatic plaque has a definite kinetic architecture, with maximal proliferative indices seen at the periphery of the lesions, and lower values found towards the centre (Christophers and Braun-Falco 1970b; Soltani and Van Scott 1972; Van Scott 1972); therefore it is probably wise, when performing kinetic measurements, to biopsy similar areas in a plaque; our own practice is to use the peripheral portions exclusively (Duffill et al. 1976; Ralfs et al. 1981a).

However, this is not the overall situation; in developing psoriatic plaques,

Minimum transit time (viable cells) (days)	Transit time (S. corneum) (days)	Turnover time (viable cells) (hours)	Total turnover time (days)	Reference
2	–	–	–	WEINSTEIN and FROST (1968)
–	–	120	7	GOODWIN et al. (1974)
–	–	–	–	DUFFILL et al. (1976)
–	2.4	–	–	BAKER and KLIGMAN (1967)
–	–	–	–	BAUER and DE GROOD (1975)
–	–	–	–	PULLMAN et al. (1974)
–	–	–	–	CHOPRA and FLAXMAN (1974)
–	–	–	–	BRASSINE and CONTEAUX-DUMONT (1972)

[c] Derived from fraction of labelled mitoses data
[d] Derived from metaphase arrest experiments
[e] Derived from flow cytophotometry

at the stage of the early lesion, both epidermal thickness and I_S values are maximal at the centre of the lesion, and decrease towards the periphery (SOLTANI and VAN SCOTT 1972; CHRISTOPHERS, PARSEFALL and BRAUN-FALCO 1973); on the other hand, grain counts were reported as being lowest in the central area also, so that the significance of the regional variation in I_S is obscure; in general, cells with short S phase durations are said to have high grain counts, and vice versa (SHACKNEY 1975), and this may hint at an artefact effect associated with intradermal injection.

These results may indicate that the hyperplasia begins focally, and spreads centripetally, with the zone of most active proliferation maintained at the periphery, while central areas of the plaque, from a proliferative viewpoint at least, become less active.

Perhaps at this point, we should refer to a curious finding with respect to proliferative indices, which appears to apply only to human epidermis; in normal, non-lesional and lesional psoriatic epidermis there is a remarkable disparity between the number of labelled cells and of mitotic cells; in psoriasis the I_S:I_M ratio is 25:1, while in normal epidermis the ratio is as large as 400:1 (GOODWIN et al. 1973). This is not an isolated finding; CAMPLEJOHN et al. (1984), as a result of highly detailed studies on normal volunteers, found an I_S:I_M ratio of 105:1. If we were to try to explain this on the basis of differences in the length of the respective phases, this would indicate that the duration of DNA synthesis (t_S) was anything between 100 and 400 times the duration of mitosis (t_M) in normal epidermis and 25 times that in psoriasis. The available evidence (FISHER and WELLS 1968; FISHER 1968a, b; WEINSTEIN and FROST 1968; DUFFILL et al. 1976; GOODWIN and FRY 1977; RALFS et al. 1981a) indicates that, in normal epidermis, t_S is unlikely to exceed t_M by more than 12 to 16 times, in non-lesional epidermis by 11 to 12 times, and in psoriatic epidermis by 6 to 7 times. That this is not entirely a phase duration argument was

Table 2. Rates of entry into DNA synthesis and mitosis in psoriatic epidermis (After RALFS et al. 1981 a)

	Influx into S[a] (cells/1000 cells/h)	Influx into M[b] (cells/1000 cells/h)
(a) Studies on groups of patients	58 ± 11[c]	12.4 (17.8 / 7.1)[d,e]
(b) Studies on individual patients	47.5	7.7 (11.9 / 3.8)
	43.8	6.5 (10.7 / 2.5)
	40.3	9.1 (15.2 / 3.4)
	57.2	8.0 (12.4 / 4.3)

[a] From a double labelling method using two intradermal injections of ^{3}HTdR
[b] Using a metaphase arrest method with vincristine
[c] Mean ± SEM of 6 patients
[d] Group of 8 patients
[e] 95% confidence interval

further indicated, for lesional epidermis at least, by the results of RALFS et al. (1981 a), which are summarised in Table 2; they measured the rate of entry into DNA synthesis and mitosis, r_S and r_M, both in groups of different patients, and also in the same patient, by metaphase arrest and a double labelling technique with ^{3}HTdR, respectively. In each case, the flux into DNA synthesis was about 5 to 6 times the flux into mitosis (see Table 2). These observations are, of course, independent of phase duration considerations.

Now these data are hard to interpret: it could be that, in the double labelling experiment, the first injection of ^{3}HTdR is stimulating cells into the DNA synthesis phase, or depressing the mitotic index; however, the available evidence (GREULICH 1964; GIBBS and CASSERETT 1969; MØLLER et al. 1974) indicates that any action of ^{3}HTdR is much later (and about 4 h after injection) than the short period of the double labelling experiment. The difference is too large to be explained by differential fluxes into DNA synthesis and mitosis expected on the basis of the age distribution diagram, which in psoriasis, with a putative mean cell cycle time of 55 h, would only account for 1.4 times more cells entering DNA synthesis than mitosis if indeed the age distribution was exponential, as seems most likely (DUFFILL et al. 1977). Alternative explanations include: (*a*) a large flux to death between DNA synthesis and mitosis i.e. in G_2, for which there is, as yet, no morphological verification; however, we might note that CLAESSON and HARTMANN (1976) did find evidence of G_2 death in mouse small thymocytes; and (*b*) that cells are migrating during DNA synthesis and mitosis in both normal and psoriatic epidermis. Since most, if not all cells in suprabasal layers are diploid, this immediately means that such migrating cells must complete DNA synthesis and mitosis in the suprabasal layers. We will recall that, in normal human epidermis, labelled cells and mitoses are found above the basal layer, and it might be that these represent cells which have migrated in DNA synthesis and mitosis and are completing their cell cycle. However, this is unlikely to be the explanation in psoriatic epidermis, since suprabasal labelled cells and mitoses would automatically be regarded as germinative cells, and included in the labelling or mitotic count. We should also perhaps point out that the cause is unlikely to be a build up of cells in G_2 (GELFANT 1976), since this would have to be of such magnitude that (*a*) the system would run down, and (*b*) such cells would be present in increased numbers and would be detected by integrating (GROVE et al. 1976) or flow cytophotometry (BAUER et al. 1981).

On the other hand, making several assumptions, BAUER et al. (1981) concluded that their flow cytophotometric data did not support large labelling index: mitotic index ratios, and suggested that the increased numbers of labelled cells were most likely to be due to cells synthesising metabolic DNA. However, most labelled cells in human epidermis are heavily labelled, and moreover, do not need the prolonged exposure periods apparently necessary for the detection of metabolic DNA (APPLETON et al. 1969). The demonstration of different fluxes into DNA synthesis and mitosis (see Table 2) would also counter this argument.

We might conclude that this phenomenon, which only seems to be present in human epidermis, seems of singular importance, both operationally and theoretically, and certainly warrants more attention.

1.2 Turnover Times and Cell Cycle Times in Psoriasis

Naturally, the demonstration of increased proliferative activity is a long way from showing that psoriatic cells divide any faster than normal epidermal cells; nevertheless, several groups have calculated turnover times for psoriatic epidermis, using measurements of the duration of DNA synthesis, derived from the first peak of a composite fraction labelled mitosis curve (WRIGHT 1977) constructed from biopsies of several individuals, after intradermal injection of ^{3}HTdR (see Fig. 2), and flash ^{3}HTdR labelling indices, again the mean of several patients. These values have been euphemistically called 'cell cycle times', and have allowed WEINSTEIN and FROST (1968) and GOODWIN et al. 1974; GOODWIN and FRY 1977), with derived values of 37 and 91 h respectively, to compare these estimates with WEINSTEIN and FROST's (1969) value of 457 h for normal epidermis, and to propose a profound reduction in the cell cycle time in psoriatic epidermis.

But these values only reflect an increase in the cell production rate, and have little to do with cell cycle time (WRIGHT 1976, 1977, 1980a, b). There are, of course, three main reasons why this is so, which are perhaps worth examining; the presence of non-proliferating cells is, of course, most relevant for normal human epidermis, where present evidence indicates that the growth fraction may be as low as 20 to 30% (see Table 3), but we cannot even be certain of the situation in psoriatic epidermis. Here we might think that, because of the hyperproliferative state, all cells should be cycling. However, there have been only two experimental attempts to measure the growth fraction in psoriatic

Table 3. Population percentages of cells in various DNA classes and transformation to cell cycle phase durations in psoriatic and normal human epidermis (After GROVE 1979)

Reference	2C (%)	3C (%)	4C (%)	T_C[a] (h)	t_1[b] (h)	t_S[c] (h)	t_2[d] (h)
Involved Psoriatic epidermis							
GROVE et al. (1976)[e]	60	27	13	33	17	10	6
BAUER and DE GROOD (1975)[f]	58	39	12	35	17	12	6
BAUER and DE GROOD (1976)[f]	36	44	20	22	6	10	6
Normal and Uninvolved epidermis							
GROVE et al. (1976)[e]	90	8	2	270	233	29	8
BAUER and DE GROOD (1975)[f]	76	12	12	52	36	8	8
BAUER and DE GROOD (1976)[f]	82	10	8	76	58	10	8

[a] From $T_C = \dfrac{\ln 2\, T_C}{\ln(1+4C)}$

[b] From $t_1 = \dfrac{-T_C \cdot \ln\left(\dfrac{2C-2}{-2}\right)}{\ln 2}$

[c] From $t_S = \dfrac{T_C}{\ln 2} \cdot \ln \left[\dfrac{(3C/\ln 2\, t_2 + 1)}{e^{\,T_C}} \right]$

[d] From fraction labelled mitoses curves

[e] Flow cytophotometric measurements

[f] Microdensitometric measurements

epidermis in vivo: WEINSTEIN et al. (1971) reported that semi-continuous application of the cytotoxic drug methotrexate (which was held to arrest cells as the G_1/S boundary, or in S itself) for 36 h resulted in an almost complete labelling of the germinative cells by a short exposure to ^{3}HTdR at the end of the methotrexate treatment. It will be noted that the methotrexate was applied over the course of a putative cell cycle time, and this was interpreted as indicating that all cells in the 'germinative' compartment were proliferating. However, the cell injury and death produced by the methotrexate might be expected to bring into cycle any resting cells which were present, and which would then subsequently label. DUFFILL et al. (1976) used a different approach; they measured an experimental labelling index ($I_{S expt}$) of 10%, and calculated a theoretical labelling index $I_{S\ theor}$ (i.e. the labelling index expected if all cells were proliferating). This was also 10% and the equivalence of $I_{S\ theor.}$ and the $I_{S\ expt.}$ indicates that all cells in the 'germinative' compartment in psoriatic epidermis are proliferating. However, this does not help us in our comparisons of cell cycle times; even if the growth fraction *is* unity in psoriasis, we have no such yardstick to assess the growth fraction in normal epidermis, which, if small, could lead to a serious overestimate of the cell cycle time from stage-duration calculations.

The second potential error incurred from stage-duration calculations stems from the use of a single labelling index reading in the presence of duirnal synchrony; such variations do occur in normal human epidermis, but in psoriasis the evidence is conflicting; PULLMAN et al. (1974) showed periodic variations in the number of labelled cells in vitro, but without accompanying changes in the mitotic index (a most singular situation!), although circadian changes could not be confirmed by HELL and HODGSON (1966), also working with labelling indices in vitro, or by MILSTEIN and CORNELL (1973), who examined mitoses in psoriatic plaques in vivo.

The third problem in the choice of the age distribution, or distribution of cell ages in the germinative cell population (AHERNE et al. 1977); it has been shown that the correct form of the age distribution in tissues with multiple layers of proliferating cells is of *exponential type* (DUFFILL et al. 1977); consequently, to obtain a realistic value of the cell cycle time from a stage-duration calculation, an exponential age distribution should be used; even in psoriasis, this could decrease the estimate of GOODWIN et al. (1974) from 91 h to 62 h, but, in the case of the normal epidermis, a decrease from 457 to about 300 h would occur; a small growth fraction would bring this even closer to the quoted values for psoriatic epidermis.

There has been no little controversy about the difference between WEINSTEIN and FROST's 37 h and GOODWIN et al's 91 h (WEINSTEIN 1975; GOODWIN et al. 1975); we have seen that a basic difference between the methods lies in the use of the correction factor (see above) of 1.4 used by WEINSTEIN, which may be redundant. But of course, we should remember that the cell cycle time value has a distribution, and that the present values were obtained from a short-term experiment which was then extrapolated to the cell cycle time; therefore the confidence limits are likely to be wide (WRIGHT 1980b); we cannot therefore conclude that there is any basis for proposing a difference between these two sets of data (or indeed for proposing a difference between psoriasis and normal epidermis, for that matter).

Some idea of the variation in the cell cycle time in psoriatic epidermis can be adjudged from the work of DUFFILL et al. (1976); the cell cycle time was directly measured by applying the GILBERT (1972) computer program to an extended fraction labelled mitoses curve carried out on a single patient with psoriasis, over 45 h in vivo; ^{3}HTdR was injected intradermally into multiple sites in a stable psoriatic plaque (see Fig. 2C). The mean cell cycle time was 56.4 ± 2.9 (S.E.M.) hours, while the coefficient of variation was 75%, indicating considerable variation between individual cells, and highlighting the limited usefulness of a point estimate.

GROVE (1979) has reanalysed the three available FLM curves in psoriatic epidermis (i.e. those of WEINSTEIN and FROST 1968; GOODWIN et al. 1974; and DUFFILL et al. 1976) using the MENDELSOHN and TAKAHASHI (1971) computer method, and using an exponential age distribution to calculate the cell cycle time, realised values of 36.7, 64.0 and 61.0 h respectively. Noting that the curve of DUFFILL et al. (1976) was severely damped, Grove concluded that a reliable estimate of the total cell cycle duration could not be obtained; however, the format of the FLM curve depends so heavily on the variance of the cell cycle time; if the coefficient of variation of the cell cycle time is indeed 75%, this will not effect the accuracy of the estimate of the mean cell cycle time, only its precision; we would then disagree with Grove on this point.

By making assumptions about the duration of one phase, it is possible to perform a stage-duration type of calculation from cytophotometric data; assuming that all cells are proliferating, GROVE (1979) did this for his own data, and that of BAUER and DE GROOD (1975), using the duration of G_2 as the assumed variable, and the results are summarised in Table 3. The results for psoriasis would appear to indicate an underestimate compared with FLM stu-

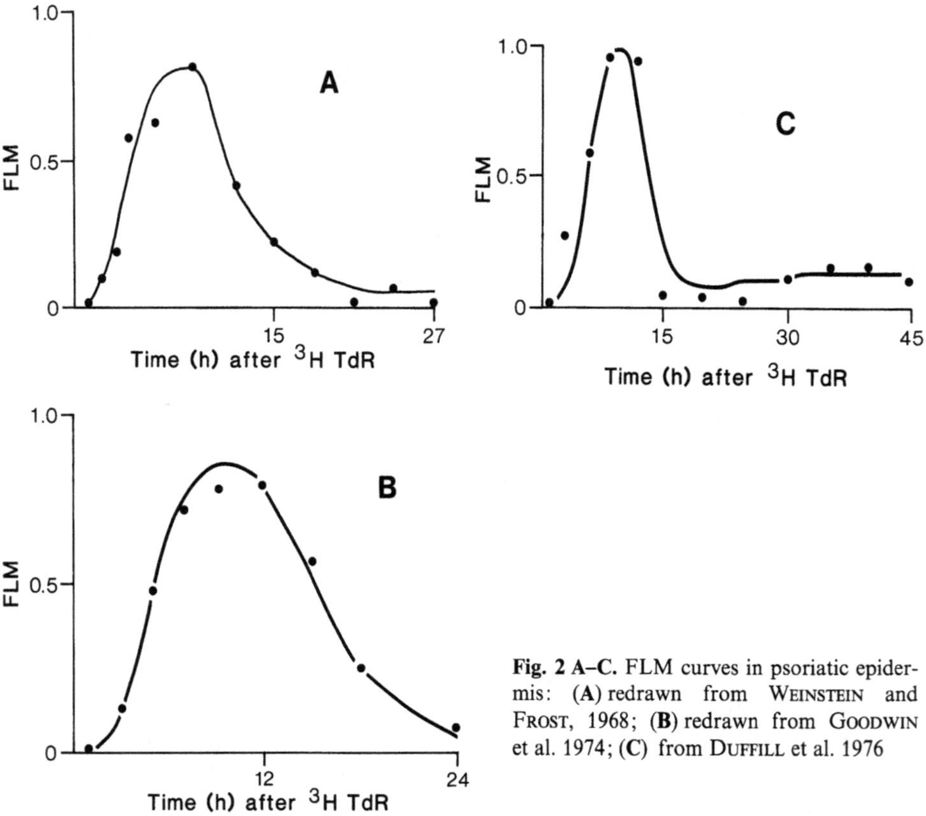

Fig. 2 A–C. FLM curves in psoriatic epidermis: (**A**) redrawn from WEINSTEIN and FROST, 1968; (**B**) redrawn from GOODWIN et al. 1974; (**C**) from DUFFILL et al. 1976

dies, but they do conform intrinsically in the same way. However, for normal or non-lesional epidermis, there is no good agreement. An important defect in this type of study is that no confidence interval is quotable for the cell cycle time, so that we cannot really comment on the reality of these changes.

BAUER et al. (1981) also made certain calculations of the cell cycle time from their flow data; unfortunately, in this, it was necessary to even make assumptions about the duration of DNA synthesis in order to calculate the total turnover time in the usual way; a value of 134 h was realised in psoriasis. To obtain the cell cycle time one must then assume equivalence between the proportion of cycling and differentiated cells to calculate, from this rather convoluted method, a value of 67 h for psoriatic epidermis, compared with a value of 131 h in normal epidermis.

As far as phase durations go, the duration of DNA synthesis, as determined from the fraction of labelled mitoses curves, appears to be shortened compared with normal epidermis (19 h, WEINSTEIN and FROST 1969), or non-lesional epidermis (11.4 h, GOODWIN and FRY 1977; see Table 1). However, Born (BORN and KALKOFF 1969; BORN 1977), on the basis of decreased mean interphase grain counts (obtained by flash labelling in vitro), maintains that the duration of DNA synthesis is lengthened in psoriasis; on the other hand, there is no *a priori* reason why the interphase grain count should be inversely correlated with the duration of the S phase; such a proposition assumes that ^{3}HTdR uptake is linearly related to time in the S phase, an assumption which is not born out by observation (WRIGHT and ALISON 1984). However, this concept of a shortened S phase is apparently confirmed by double labelling studies in vitro; PULLMAN (PULLMAN et al. 1974, 1977) not only confirmed the depressed grain count in psoriasis, but also claims that S phase durations as long as 19.9 ± 5.4 (S.E.M.) hours are seen in psoriasis, compared with control values of 7.2 ± 0.8 h in normal epidermis, and considers that this increase in the duration of DNA synthesis preceeds the hyperproliferation (STEIGLEDER and PULLMAN 1979). Moreover, BAUER et al. (1981) concluded that their flow cytometric data also supported this concept, although, since in this study no actual measurements of the duration of DNA synthesis were actually made, this conclusion is of course suspect. Even so, GALOSI et al. (1980) could not demonstrate any change in the duration of DNA synthesis as between the normal and lesional elbow epidermis. This disparity between double labelling and FLM methods warrants further investigation, particularly since the measurements of CHOPRA and FLAXMAN (1974), made using the fraction of labelled mitoses method in vitro, indicate a shortening of the duration of DNA synthesis from 11.5 h in controls to 6.5 h in psoriasis.

The mitotic duration is also subject to disparate reports; PULLMAN et al. (1974) reporting an increase from 1.2 to 1.3 h in controls to 3.5 h in psoriasis, while fraction labelled mitoses studies by WEINSTEIN and FROST (1968) indicate a shortened duration (1 and 0.76 h in normal and lesional epidermis respectively; the duration of G_2 appears to be considerably shortened, with estimates varying from 6 to 7 h to >14 h in normal epidermis, to around 4 h (WEINSTEIN and FROST 1968; DUFFILL et al. 1976) or 5 to 9 h (GOODWIN et al. 1974) in psoriasis, although it is interesting to note that GOODWIN and FRY (1977) reported values of about 14 h in non-lesional epidermis, indicating that this parameter only changes significantly in lesional psoriatic epidermis.

1.3 Metaphase Arrest Methods in Psoriasis

It is evident that the use of the stage-duration method in the study of psoriasis implies the usual limitations (WRIGHT 1976, 1977, 1980a, b), but such indirect methods can be shown to be consistent with the more cumbersome full fraction labelled mitoses method. DUFFILL et al. (1977) and RALFS et al. (1981a) have championed the use of the stathmokinetic method in psoriatic epidermis, and have shown that, with care, useful results can be obtained, but only in the more rapidly proliferating psoriatic state; injection of vincristine into multiple sites, followed by serial biopsy and enumeration of metaphases, gives the familiar metaphase arrest line, which can be carried out in both single patients (RALFS et al. 1981a) and in groups of patients (DUFFILL et al. 1976) (see Fig. 3); the method gives birth rate or cell production rate values of about 12.7 cells/1000 cells/hour, and, using the above calculated growth fraction of unity, an exponential age distribution, and also assuming asynchrony, we can calculate a cell cycle time of 54.5 h.

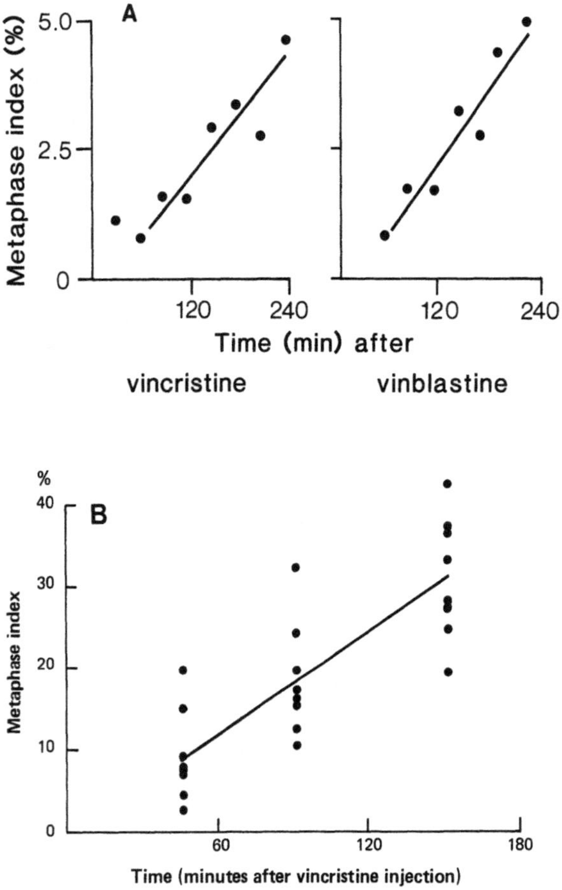

Fig. 3 A, B. Metaphase arrest lines in psoriatic epidermis (**A**) in individual patients and (**B**) in a group of 8 patients. In each case 1 μg was injected intradermally and the line is fitted assuming an exponential age distribution

There are four tenets which should be satisfied before these measurements are made: (*i*) the optimal dose of the stathmokinetic agent should be given; RALFS et al. carried out dose-response curves for both vincristine and vinblastine in psoriatic epidermis (Fig. 4), using the metaphase index at 2.5 h after intradermal injection as the end point. It is evident that a dose of 1 μg, given intradermally, represents the optimal dosage, although the format of the vincristine curve showed a sharp peak, which may indicate that metaphase degeneration is occurring before maximal metaphase indices are attained. However, this may be negated by the fact that the peak index with vincristine realised the same level as that attained by vinblastine; (*ii*) the avoidance of any delay before metaphase arrest is complete, and (*iii*), the demonstration of linearity of metaphase collection. Figure 5 shows that a latent period before complete metaphase arrest does exist in psoriatic epidermis, during which it would be incorrect to take cognisance of readings; moreover, both alkaloids appear to give linearity of metaphase collection over a 4 h period; finally, it is important to ensure that significant metaphase arrest should be avoided. The time of onset of metaphase degeneration was measured using the method described by RALFS et al.

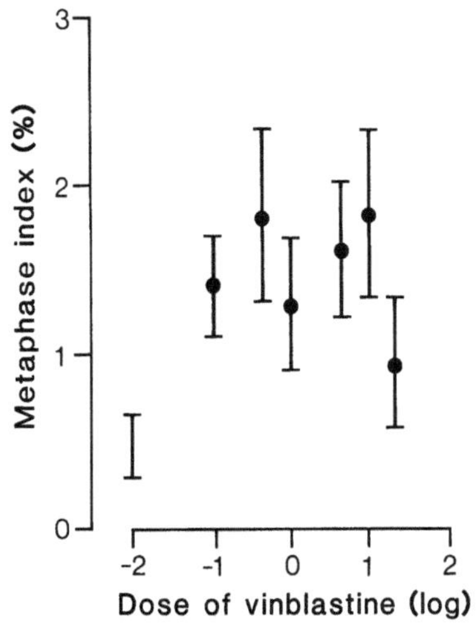

Fig. 4. A dose-response curve for vinblastine in psoriatic epidermis. Metaphase indices were measured at 2.5 h after injection

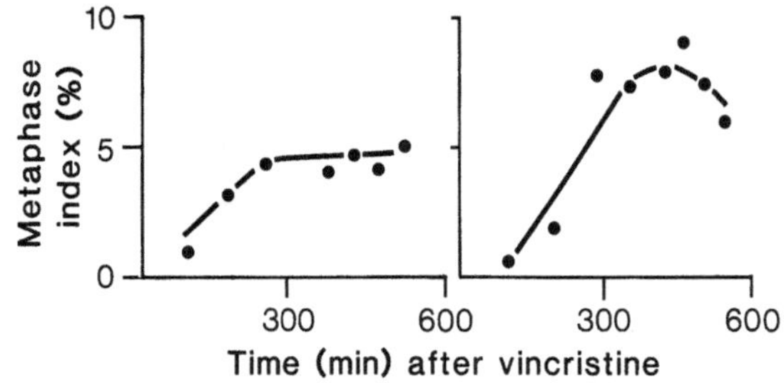

Fig. 5. Linearity studies with vincristine in psoriatic epidermis. The experimental conditions were as previously described

(1981 a) and Fig. 6 shows the results in two patients with psoriasis. The minimum lifetime of an arrested metaphase in psoriatic epidermis would appear to be about 4 h, and thus it would be unwise to continue these experiments beyond this point without compensating for the degeneration by using a correction factor, as suggested by Aherne and Camplejohn (1972). There is no doubt that Fisher (1968 b), Fisher and Wells (1968), Fisher and Maibach (1972) who used an arrest period of up to 12 h, incurred such errors in their experiments, which employed colcemid in cream form; Fisher reported a value for the birth rate in normal human epidermis of 0.027 cells/1000 cells/hour, using but a single reading at different times after application of colcemid cream; this value has been quoted many times now, but, if the criteria for metaphase degeneration described herein are also applicable to normal, human epidermis, then Fisher's value should be changed to 0.17 cells/1000 cells/hour, a considerable difference. However, in this context, we should note that Camplejohn et al. (1981) could not demonstrate any significant accumulation of arrested metaphases in normal human epidermis at up to 3 h after injection, even though metaphase arrest was complete, as judged by the absence of anaphase-telophase/

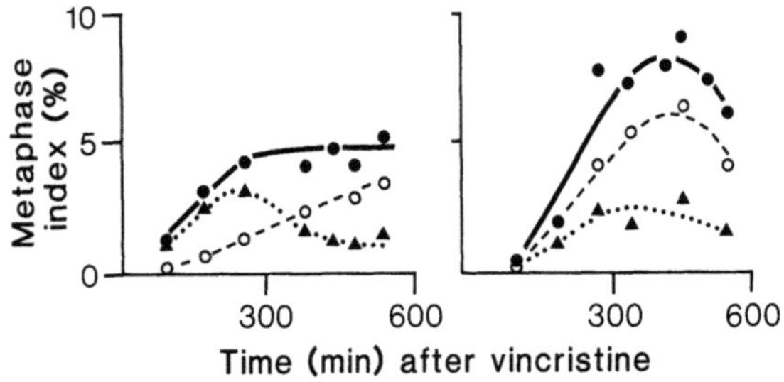

Fig. 6. The fate of arrested labelled and unlabelled metaphases in psoriatic epidermis. Vincristine (1 μg) and ^{3}HTdR (10 μCi) were injected intradermally at time 0. After 4 h, unlabelled metaphases, which represent cells originally in G_2 at the time of injection of vincristine and tritiated thymidine, begin to degenerate and disappear. This causes a plateau in the graph of total arrested mitoses, and would lead to considerable error if all the readings were included in an estimate of the birth rate or cell cycle time (●——● total mitoses; o---o labelled mitoses; ▲...▲ unlabelled mitoses)

pairs. It is interesting to note that, with the higher doses of vincristine, CAMPLEJOHN et al. saw a significant increase in the number of pyknotic cells, so it is possible that metaphase degeneration was occurring at an earlier time in normal epidermis. Of possibly greater import, however, is the possibility that the delay period before arrest is complete in normal epidermis is quite long, even as long as 2 h, which would explain the rise in metaphase index reported by FISHER (1968b), who used longer arrest periods, but not in the comparatively short arrest periods of 3 h used by CAMPLEJOHN et al. (1981). However, to extend the experimental period would be to invite errors due to metaphase degeneration.

It is thus evident that such indirect techniques can give results which compare with those given by an extended fraction labelled mitoses curve (see Fig. 2C), but only when the correct set of assumptions are used. With these assumptions, the 91 h of GOODWIN et al. (1974) becomes 65 h, while an independent measurement of 50 h comes from BAUER and DE GROOD (1975), using flow cytophotometry. We could also note that CHOPRA and FLAXMAN (1974) provided estimates of about 53 h, as measured from a fraction labelled mitoses curve for explants of psoriatic epidermis growing in vitro. However, the cell cycle time for normal epidermis, in the same conditions, was only 59 h; if these values also apply in vivo, then of course the proliferative defect cannot lie in the cell cycle time, but involves changes in the proliferating cell populations (see below).

Now all these estimates for the cell cycle time show a degree of consistency, but it should perhaps be emphasised that they should not be overinterpreted, regardless of the mean values, since there is a considerable spread of cell cycle times (WRIGHT 1977, 1980a, b). These comments apply equally well to the normal epidermis, and after critical analysis, we cannot be really sure that psoriatic epidermal cells are cycling any faster than normal epidermal cells. Stage-duration calculations based on duration of DNA synthesis and the labelling index values derived from in vitro studies (PULLMAN et al. 1974, 1977) indicate only a decrease from 280 to 114 h, and GELFANT (1976), from a review of the available published values, concluded that the difference in the cell cycle time was likely to be twofold, rather than twelvefold, as claimed by WEINSTEIN and FROST

(1968). We should, in all correctness, note that the 457 h 'cell cycle time' calculated by Weinstein from the duration of DNA synthesis value of 19 h, was actually the result of preliminary data, which has not been improved upon, or embellished; moreover, we must add the *caveat* that these are *turn-over times* rather than *cell cycle times*. Table 1 summarises these values and does indicate that they are mostly indirect calculations, with the inherent defects listed above. We would go further, and pronounce it premature to reach any conclusion at this time.

1.4 Proliferating Populations in Psoriatic Epidermis

If we can find no evidence for a decrease in cell cycle time, the other parameter which could account for the observed increase in proliferative indices is *the number of proliferating cells* (VAN SCOTT and FLAXMAN 1973); we do know that there is an absolute increase in proliferative cell number, with up to 3 layers of such cells in psoriatic epidermis (Fig. 1), but of course there is also room for a relative increase; if the growth fraction (i.e. the proportion of the epidermal cell population which is given over to cell proliferation – the fraction of proliferating cells) in normal epidermis is small, and of the order of 20 to 30% as indicated by the continuous labelling studies of GELFANT (1976), then a four or fivefold increase in the cell production rate would be possible merely by increasing the growth fraction to unity in the basal layer, even in the absence of any change in cell cycle time or three-dimensional expansion of the proliferative cell compartment. In this context, BORN and KALKOFF (1969), in probably the first such proposal, considered that the increased cell proliferation was due to a greater number of dividing cells per unit of skin surface; they also speculated that the cell cycle time was *increased* in duration in psoriasis. On the other hand, the only available measurements in vitro, made using the continuous labelling method, indicate little change in the growth fraction in psoriatic epidermis: CHOPRA and FLAXMAN (1974) report an increase from 66% in normal to 74% in psoriatic epidermis, while HARPER et al. (1978), also in vitro, reported no difference in the 'proliferative pool', as assessed by continuous labelling, between lesional and non-lesional epidermis; thus there is unlikely to be a difference in the growth fraction in the in vitro state, remembering the vagaries of the continuous labelling method (WRIGHT 1983), and the potential anomalies of the in vitro situation make definitive conclusions difficult.

In the light of these comments we should perhaps join GELFANT (1976, 1978b) in calling for more investigation of the mechanisms of cellular cycling and decycling in human epidermis. There is mounting evidence that the proliferative defect in psoriasis lies in changes in the absolute and relative numbers of proliferative cells, rather than in a reduction in the cell cycle time.

1.5 Turnover and Transit Times in Psoriasis

Whatever the mechanism of the elevated proliferative rate, the increased cell production rate ensures that the epidermal turnover time and the transit time, no matter for which population, are both decreased in psoriasis. We have seen that the turnover time of the germinative population is decreased, while GOODWIN et al. (1974) calculated a turnover time of 120 h for the viable cell population. Following the migration of ^{3}HTdR labelled cells, WEINSTEIN and FROST (1968) determined what was probably a *minimum* turnover time through the malpighian layer of about 2 days; with the transit time through the parakeratotic stratum corneum of 2 to 4 days (BAKER and KLIGMAN 1967), the total turnover time in psoriatic epidermis is of the order of 7 to 9 days. Many of these kinetic parameters are summarised in Table 1.

1.6 The Non-Lesional Epidermis in Psoriasis

There are various triggers which act to produce psoriatic lesions in the non-lesional epidermis of patients with psoriasis; for example, epidermal trauma will lead, after about 10 days, to the formation of a psoriatic lesion – the *Koebner phenomenon*. It is likely, therefore, that some defect exists even in non-lesional epidermis, and indeed HELL and HODGSON (1966), KAIDBY and KURBAN (1971), BRASSINE and CONTEAUX-DUMONT (1972) and GOODWIN et al. (1974) all reported increases in the labelling index in non-lesional epidermis compared with normal epidermis, while GROVE et al. (1976) have suggested that there is a slight increase in the microdensitometric DNA synthesis fraction in non-lesional epidermis; however, these changes could not be confirmed by WEINSTEIN and FROST (1968).

In this context, BRAUN-FALCO et al. (1971) and PULLMAN (1978) reported that tape stripping non-lesional epidermis gave rise to an elevated and prolonged regenerative response, indicating that the initial response to wounding in non-lesional epidermis is exaggerated, which of course may have some bearing on the nature of the Koebner phenomenon. This exaggerated proliferative response to wounding was confirmed by STEIGLEDER and PULLMAN (1979), who also showed that the response in non-lesional epidermis started earlier than in normal epidermis; this wounding response was apparently associated with a large increase in the duration of DNA synthesis as shown in a double labelling experiment. WILEY and WEINSTEIN (1979) reported that saline injection and tape stripping both induced a hyperproliferative response in non-lesional epidermis, and also that the β-blocker propanalol evoked excess cell proliferation in non-lesional epidermis. It is also possible to demonstrate a prominent proliferative response to stripping in non-lesional epidermis by measuring the rate of formation of corneocyte layers with dansyl chloride as a corneocyte marker (JOHANNESSON and HAMMER 1980). It is interesting to note that CHRISTOPHERS and BRAUN-FALCO (1970b) found that, after tape stripping, only the perilesional epidermis responded, and not the involved epidermis, perhaps indicating that maximal proliferative activity has been reached in the lesional epidermis; GROVE (1980) also reached this conclusion, having failed to elicit a proliferative response in lesional epidermis by injecting saline intradermally.

Perhaps the most detailed analysis of cell proliferation in non-lesional epidermis is due to GOODWIN and FRY (1977), who with considerable labour, constructed the first peak of a fraction of labelled mitoses curve; the duration of DNA synthesis was 11.4 h, and the labelling index was 4.9%, giving a turnover time of 230 h, which, however, is not a great deal different from many normal values (see Table 1), notwithstanding the general agreement that labelling indices are raised. If the increase in labelling index was due to an increase in the number of proliferative cells, as proposed by GOODWIN and FRY (1977), one might expect that the turnover time would also be decreased. The exact kinetic change in non-lesional epidermis must await the application of more powerful methods, but we might note that HARPER et al. (1978) could not detect any change in the kinetic behaviour of involved and non-involved psoriatic epidermis in vitro, while involved and non-involved epidermis growing in diffusion chambers in mice also show the same labelling indices (KARIENEMI 1974).

ROWE et al. (1978) compared a mitotic count (carried out per 20 cm of surface length) in non-lesional epidermis at 0900 h and 1500 h, and, observing an increase in the 1500 h biopsies, ascribed this change to the release of cells, blocked in the G_2 phase into mitosis; however, there was no direct measurement of the G_2 fraction (CLAUSEN et al. 1979) nor was there any attempt to relate this event to a previous wave of DNA synthetic activity; the duration of DNA synthesis was not measured, and interpretation of this study should perhaps be negated until further evidence is forthcoming.

2. Morphological and Kinetic Correlates in Proliferative Skin Disease

Generally speaking, the presence of parakeratosis is correlated with increased proliferative activity in skin disease, and is usually regarded as a result of incomplete differentiation, due to the decreased time available during transit. However, there is some debate on the exact relationship between parakeratosis and cell proliferation: although COX and WATSON (1971) obtained a good correlation between the degree of parakeratosis and mitotic counts, FRY and MCMINN (1968) reported that, with certain therapy, such as topical dithranol, the granular layer formed first (i.e. parakeratosis was lost) before the mitotic index fell, indicating a direct effect on the differentiation rate, rather than acting directly via mitosis. Moreover, CHRISTOPHERS and BRAUN-FALCO (1967) induced increased proliferative rate in guinea pig epidermis by both tape stripping and vitamin A treatment, but noting that neither was associated with parakeratosis, concluded that increased cell proliferation per se does not produce parakeratosis, but that there also has to be an associated defect in differentiation; this might indicate that, in psoriasis, there is an additional defect in differentiation, in addition to the proliferative lesion. However, we ought to note that JOHANNESSON and HAMMER (1980), studying lesional epidermis, have shown that the rate of formation of corneocyte layers, as measured with dansyl chloride, is highly correlated with the degree of parakeratosis; this would indicate a direct relationship between cell production rate and parakeratosis, although it does not, of course, exclude a role for a differentiation defect.

That this problem is not simple is indicated by the observation that during treatment of psoriatic epidermis with corticosteroids, the granular layer reforms at the same rate that the mitotic index falls, but still, one would expect that if increased mitotic activity was the root cause of parakeratosis, there should be a significant delay between the decrease in mitotic index and the emergence of a granular layer, and it would appear, on present evidence, that a defect in differentiation, rather than a simple relationship with enhanced cell proliferation, is the cause of parakeratosis in psoriasis.

There is evidence that increased epidermal thickness is associated with an elevated labelling index (CHRISTOPHERS 1972) in guinea pig tissues, and, expressing epidermal thickness as the ratio between the length of the basal lamina and the surface length in sections, MARKS and WELLS (1973) have found a linear relationship between this ratio and the flash labelling index in *lichen simplex*, indicating that a simple relationship exists in human epidermis.

It also seems as if the postulated relationship between proliferative rate and ordered structure may also hold in human epidermis; thus MENTON and EISEN (1971 b) reported good stacking in *ichthyosis vulgaris*, a condition associated with a low birth rate, but in conditions where the birth rate is increased, such as psoriasis and *lamellar ichthyosis*, there was much overlapping of surface corneocytes, with no stacking; it seems that elevated birth rates lead to loss of stacking in human epidermis.

3. The Action of Drugs in Psoriasis

Apparently, all agents which are of therapeutic value in psoriasis depend on the elevated proliferative rate for their beneficial effect in involved epidermis (FISHER and MAIBACH 1971; WEINSTEIN and MCCULLOUGH 1975); on the other hand, GELFANT (1976) has proposed that such drugs do not kill cells, but, by some direct or indirect action, cycling cells are removed into the non-cycling state, or into a G_1 and G_2 phase block. This is largely a theoretical argument at the moment, and is somewhat surprising in view of the same authors previous finding (SMITH and GELFANT 1974) that methotrexate and hydroxyurea, cytotoxic agents often used in antipsoriasis therapy, do cause the appearance of numerous damaged cells, as seen in sections; in the case of methotrexate, these appeared in relation to the dosage. Moreover, glucocorticoids, also widely used for treatment, act to inhibit the flow of cells from the G_1 phase into DNA synthesis in mouse epidermis (FRANKFURT 1968), and indeed steroids have also been shown to decrease the mitotic index in psoriatic and normal human epidermis (FRY and MCMINN 1968; BAXTER and STOUGHTON 1970; FISHER and MAIBACH 1971 a), while a screening test for potentially active steroids has been introduced which depends on the ability of the drug to inhibit the incorporation of ^{3}HTdR into DNA (DU VIVIER et al. 1976). However, such treatment of psoriatic epidermis is not accompanied by the appearance of histological evidence of damage and thus the steroid effect could be construed as a cytostatic rather than a cytotoxic effect.

Dithranol (anthralin) a coal tar product, decreased the labelling index in guinea pig epidermis at 12 h after application, and may act to inhibit DNA synthesis (SWANBECK and LIDEN 1966); anthralin certainly decreases the mitotic index in psoriatic epidermis (BAXTER and STOUGHTON 1970), and inhibits ^{3}HTdR incorporation in primary cultures of guinea pig epidermis, and also in the hyperproliferative epidermis of essential fatty acid deficient mice (WALTER et al. 1978). This action was interpreted as a primary block of cells in DNA synthesis (FISHER and MAIBACH 1975), while STEIGLEDER et al. (1973) found not only a decrease in labelling index after dithranol, but also a decrease in the duration of DNA synthesis, an action again construed as a primary effect inhibiting the passage of cells into DNA synthesis. In this context, it is interesting to note that anthralin decreases the elevated cyclic guanosine monophosphate (cGMP) content of psoriatic skin to normal levels after only five days of treatment, which, if elevated cGMP levels, or alternatively, altered cAMP (cyclic adenosine monophosphate): cGMP ratios are responsible for the hyperproliferative state, may be its mode of action (MARCELO and VORHEES 1980).

FISHER and MAIBACH (1975) carried out a detailed study of the effects of anthralin on cell proliferation in hairless mouse epidermis; topical pure anthralin, but not the dimer or the quinone, reduced mitotic activity, largely eliminating the circadian peak of the mitotic index; fraction labelled mitoses studies indicated a doubling of the duration of DNA synthesis and of G_2, and the action of anthralin was ascribed to the combination of a blocking effect and a prolongation of the DNA synhetic and G_2 phases.

The cytotoxic action of hydroxyurea, which inhibits the flow of cells into the DNA synthesis phase, and kills cells in DNA synthesis, is well known; WEINSTEIN (WEINSTEIN and FROST 1971; WEINSTEIN et al. 1971; WEINSTEIN and MCCULLOUGH 1975) considers that the action of methotrexate, which kills cells in the DNA synthesis phase, could be explained by a selective action on psoriatic epidermal cells, because of their increased proliferative rate; more cells are thus in DNA synthesis, and are present in the appropriate phase for methotrexate action. Certainly, giving methotrexate after prelabelling psoriatic epidermis leads to the presence of labelled, dying cells, which appear at 4 h, and peak at 8 to 10 h after treatment (WEINSTEIN and VELASCO 1972), and by timing the prelabelling procedure to obtain labelled cells mainly in G_1, G_2, and mitosis and DNA synthesis, WEINSTEIN and VELASCO reported that maximum killing of cells appeared to occur in the DNA synthesis phase. Additionally, psoriatic epidermal cells are held to have a greater individual susceptibility to methotrexate (WEINSTEIN and FROST 1971; WEINSTEIN and MCCULLOUGH 1975), since although methotrexate completely inhibited ^{3}HTdR labelling in psoriatic epidermis, this action was found to be only partial in normal epidermis. On the other hand, TAYLOR and HALPRIN (1977) found decreased uptake of methotrexate in psoriatic epidermis compared with normal epidermis, and it is probable that the higher DNA synthesis fraction in psoriasis can explain most, if not all, of the effects of methotrexate on lesional epidermis; the evidence that methotrexate has an additional selective action on psoriatic epidermal cells is, as yet, inconclusive.

Based on the putative cell cycle time of 37 h, WEINSTEIN (WEINSTEIN et al. 1971; WEINSTEIN and FROST 1971; WEINSTEIN and VELASCO 1972) designed a treatment schedule founded on three doses spread over the assumed cycle time (see also WEINSTEIN and MCCULLOUGH 1973; MCCULLOUGH and WEINSTEIN

(1979); however, if we take the 75% coefficient of variation of the cell cycle time of 56 h measured by DUFFILL et al. (1976) as indicative of the spread of cell cycle times, then as many as 62% of the germinative cells may not be meeting methotrexate during their DNA synthesis phase, using this schedule.

On the other hand, it should be noticed that FRY and MCMINN (1966) reported a decrease in mitotic index in psoriatic epidermis at 3 h after a systemic exposure to methotrexate; since the duration of G_2 is of the order of 4 to 5 h in psoriatic epidermis (DUFFILL et al. 1976), this might imply an additional action of methotrexate in G_2. The action of methotrexate is not simple: WEINSTEIN and VELASCO (1972) also reported a decrease in mitotic index at 2 h after methotrexate, and, despite its undoubted effect when given systemically, it appears to be ineffective when given topically, possibly due to poor penetration, although WEINSTEIN and MCCULLOUGH (1975) could find no effect on incubated epidermis; on the other hand, intradermal methotrexate does inhibit DNA synthesis.

Treatment with 8-methoxypsoralen and high intensity, long wave UV light (PUVA) is thought to specifically inhibit DNA synthesis in proliferating psoriatic cells, and lead to a clearing of psoriatic plaques (WALTER 1973). But HELL et al. (1979), who used only a single biopsy at 36 h after treatment to measure the effect, still felt able to conclude that no change in the labelling index occurred after PUVA therapy. Moreover, GOLDBERG et al. (1980) have claimed that there was no correlation between the pretreatment 'mitotic index' and the response to treatment, as assessed by the amount of irradiation given, or the number of treatments required to clear the lesions. However, there are a number of defects in this study; the mitotic index was the number of mitoses in some 12 mm length of epidermis; such a measurement has been heavily counselled against (WRIGHT 1977, 1983) and, particularly in psoriatic epidermis, where basement membrane length can be so variable, because of the variation in rete peg elongation, such a measurement is surely no basis for comparison. The subjective basis of clearing of lesions as an endpoint is one which needs a good deal more objective assessment. Consequently, the conclusions of GOLDBERG et al. (1980) are considered premature. In this context, BELL et al. (1983) have shown that PUVA treatment leads to a reduction in labelling and mitotic indices within 15 h; the pattern of response suggested an inhibitory action in the late DNA synthesis phase, and there was also demonstrable synchrony of cells in DNA synthesis some 24 h after exposure. PUVA would therefore appear to have considerable effects on cell proliferation. Moreover, HOFFMAN et al. (1980) have shown that there is a dose-related fall in the labelling index of psoriatic epidermis treated with PUVA, and the evidence from experimental animals indicates an action on DNA synthesising cells in both mouse (EPSTEIN and FUKUYAMA 1975) and guinea pig epidermis (PULLMAN et al. 1980). It is evident that a good deal more work is needed on this topic, both to establish the mode of action of PUVA on proliferating psoriatic cells, and to appreciate the post-treatment kinetics, with the possibility of optimally scheduling the treatment regime to catch the surviving cells in any phase which might be shown to be specifically sensitive to PUVA, such as the DNA synthesis phase (BELL et al. 1983).

We might conclude by proposing that the enhanced cell proliferation in psoriasis opens several avenues for therapeutic attack, and also offers a good opportunity for optimal scheduling: such optimisation can only be based on detailed kinetic studies.

4. Kinetic Parameters in Other Dermatoses

By and large the only measurements which have been made in most non-psoriatic dermatoses have been the labelling index and the minimum transit time. Thus in *lamellar ichthyosis* and *ichthyosiform erythroderma* the minimum transit time through the malpighian layer is decreased to about 4 days; the labelling index is also elevated in ichthyosiform erythroderma (FROST and VAN SCOTT 1966; FROST et al. 1966; FISHER and WELLS 1968; MARKS 1975), while the clinically milder forms of ichthyosis show no apparent abnormality. Virus and fungal infections of the skin also appear to increase proliferative rates in human epidermis (EPSTEIN et al. 1966; BERK et al. 1976), and despite the general impression that *lichen planus* is associated with a hypoproliferative state, MARKS et al. (1973) have reported increases in the labelling index in both lesional and perilesional epidermis in lichen planus; similar increases have been described in *lichen simplex* (MARKS and WELLS 1973), in *Dariers disease* (SATO et al. 1978), and large increases have been recorded in *discoid lupus erythematosus* (BRASSINE and PIERARD 1976); however, in the more common forms of dermatitis, BRUNNER (1976) could find little change in the labelling index in the epidermis of patients with *atopic* and *allergic dermatitis*.

There is also evidence that the epidermis in *pityriasis rubra pilaris* (PRP) is hyperproliferative; approximation of transit times using the labelled amino acid method gave results similar to those seen in psoriasis (PORTER and SHUSTER 1967), while measurements of the labelling index have indicated a considerable elevation (MARKS and GRIFFITHS 1973; NIEMI et al. 1976), which would also indicate a proliferative state comparable with psoriasis. This was confirmed by RALFS et al. (1981b), who reported an increase in the cell production rate, measured by the metaphase arrest method, similar to that seen in psoriatic epidermis. Interestingly enough, in this hyper-proliferative state the labelling index: mitotic index ratio was 14.5:1, which can most reasonably be explained by differences in the duration of mitosis and of DNA synthesis; measurements of the flux into DNA synthesis and mitosis showed approximately equal values, and the discrepancies so apparent in psoriasis were not evident. These diseases, although sharing a hyperproliferative state, do appear to differ in this respect.

5. The Mechanism of Increased Cell Proliferation in Psoriasis

There is considerable evidence that a defect in cyclic nucleotide metabolism exists in psoriatic epidermis, and, since changes in cyclic nucleotide levels are associated with variations in proliferative rate, there is often assumed to be a causal relationship between the two. This rather complex topic is outwith the scope of this chapter, and is discussed elsewhere (WRIGHT and ALISON 1984).

There is, however, some indication that extracts of psoriatic epidermis stimulate cell proliferation in organ cultured human epidermis (HELL and HODGSON 1978), although we should note that, since for some reason a 4 h continuous labelling period was used, because of the possible interference by labelled cells dividing in the labelling period, we cannot say anything about mechanisms (WRIGHT and SALTER 1979). Moreover, STANKLER (1969) has claimed that a factor present in the dermis of active psoriatic lesions was capable of stimulating the development of psoriatic lesions in uninvolved epidermis, while serum from patients at the stage of recovery from active psoriasis can apparently inhibit the development of the Koebner phenomenon, and has a healing effect on an active lesion. These studies are not, as yet, kinetically based, and we have no inkling of the nature of the substances involved; more work is evidently needed.

6. Conclusions

So how can we conclude? We are faced with a known increase in proliferative rate, but without an agreed kinetic mechanism. Weinstein would have us believe that a decrease in the cell cycle time would explain the data, but, as we have seen, we are uncertain enough about the cell cycle time in normal epidermis as to be unsure if indeed such differences are indicated by the measurements. GELFANT (1976, 1978b) would advocate instead a change induced wholly by the growth fraction, possibly by release of cells blocked in G_1 or G_2 phases, or in a putative resting G_0 compartment, although the small number of G_2 cells in normal human epidermis would appear to negate the role of that phase, at least, as an important population (GROVE 1979). We can, however, conclude reasonably safely, that (*a*) the *relative* growth fraction is raised in the basal layer, and (*b*) that there is an *absolute* increase in the number of proliferating cells. Can such changes be responsible for the increase in the cell production rate? The answer is probably, yes. It would appear as if changes in the fraction of cells in the epidermis which are committed to proliferation is likely to be the causative parameter, in which case there maybe no need to propose cell cycle time changes. We are forced to the conclusion that, this far, the data are not good enough for a reasonable decision, either way.

References

Aherne WA, Camplejohn RS, Wright NA (1977a) An introduction to cell population kinetics. Edward Arnold, London

Aherne WA, Al-Wiswazy M, Ford D, Keller AM (1977b) Assessment of inherent fluctuations of mitotic and labelling indices of human tumours. Br J Cancer, 36:577–591

Aherne WA, Camplejohn RS (1972) On correcting the error due to metaphase degeneration in stathmokinetic studies. Exptl Cell Res 74:496–502

Appleton TC, Pelc SR, Tarbit MH (1969) Formation and loss of DNA in intestinal epithelium. J Cell Sci 5:45–53

Baker H, Kligman A (1967) Techniques for estimating turnover time of human stratum corneum. Arch Derm 95:405–411

Bauer FW, Grood RM de (1975) Impulse cytophotometry in psoriasis. Br J Derm 93:225–228

Bauer FW, Crombag NHCMN, Boezemann JBM, Grood RM de (1981) Flow cytometry as a tool for the study of cell kinetics in skin. 2. Cell kinetic data for psoriasis. Br J Derm 104:271–276

Bauer FW, Grood RM de (1975) Impulse cytophotometry in psoriasis. Br J Dermatol 93:225–228

Baxter DL, Stoughton RB (1970) Mitotic index of psoriatic lesions treated with anthralin, glucocorticoid and occlusion only. J Invest Dermatol 54:410–412

Bell C, Ralfs I, Wright A (1983) The effect of PUVA on cell proliferation in psoriatic plaques; an approach to synchronisation therapy in human epidermis. In: Wright NA, Camplejohn RS (eds) 'Psoriasis: Cell Proliferation'. Churchill Livingstone, pp 355–359

Berk HS, Penneys NS, Weinstein GD (1976) Epidermal activity in annular dermatophytoses. Arch Dermatol 112:485–488

Bersaques J de (1966) Deoxyribonucleic acid in epidermis. J Invest Dermatol 46:40–41

Born W, Kalkoff KW (1969) Zur DNS syntheses der psoriatischen Epidermiszelle. Arch Klin exp Derm 236:43–52

Born W (1977) Proliferation kinetic model for the understanding of the epidermal cell cycle in psoriasis. Fortschr Med 95:1395–1402

Brassine MF, Conteaux Dumont CM (1972) Tritiated thymidine labelling of epidermis in pustular psoriasis. Arch Derm 106:768–769

Brassine MF, Pierard P (1976) Cell renewal in discoid lupus erythematosus. J Cutan Pathol 3:175–179

Braun-Falco O, Burg G, Schoefinius HA (1971) Über die Wirkung von Dithranol (Cignolin) bei Psoriasis vulgaris. Cyto- und Untersuchungen. Arch Dermatol Forsch 741:217–237

Brunner R (1976) Cytokinetics of dermal and epidermal cells in allergic contact dermatitis and atopic dermatitis. Arch Derm Res 255:297–304

Burholt DR, Schultze B, Maurer W (1976) Mode of growth of the jejunal crypt cells of the rat; an autoradiographic study using double labelling with 3H- and 14C-thymidine in lower and upper parts of the crypt. Cell Tissue Kinet 9:107–117

Burns FJ, Tannock IF (1970) On the existence of a G_0 phase in the cell cycle. Cell Tissue Kinet 3:321–334

Camplejohn RS, Gelfant S, Chalker D (1981) An attempt to use vincristine and colcemid to measure proliferative rates in normal human epidermis in vivo. Brit J Dermatol 104:243–247

Camplejohn RS, Gelfant S, Chalker D (1984) Circadian and seasonal variation in labelling and mitotic indices in human epidermis. Cell & Tissue Kinetics (in press)

Chopra DP, Flaxman R (1974) Comparative proliferation kinetics of cells from normal human epidermis and benign epidermal hyperplasia (psoriasis) in vitro. Cell Tissue Kinet 7:69–76

Christophers E (1972) Correlation between column formation, tissue size and new cell production in guinea pig epidermis. Virchows Arch Path 10:286–292

Christophers E, Braun Falco O (1967) Mechanisms of parakeratosis. Brit J Dermatol 82:268–276

Christophers E, Braun-Falco O (1970a) The architecture of the stratum corneum after wounding. J Invest Dermatol 54:437–440

Christophers E, Braun-Falco O (1970b) Psoriatic hyperplasia – some measurements. Brit J Dermatol 83:63–68

Christophers E, Laurence EB (1973) Regional variations in mouse skin; quantitation of epidermal components in two different body sites. Virchows Arch Cell Path 12:212–223

Christophers E, Parsefall E, Braun-Falco O (1973) Initial events in psoriasis: quantitative assessment. Brit J Dermatol 89:327–334

Claesson MH, Hartmann NR (1976) Cytodynamics in the thymus of young mice: a quantitative study on the loss of thymic blast cells and nonproliferating small thymocytes. Cell Tissue Kinet 9:273–291

Clausen OPF, Thorud E, Bjerknes R, Elgjo K (1979) Circadian rhythms in mouse epidermal cell proliferation. Variations in compartment size, flux and phase duration. Cell Tissue Kinet 12:314–337

Cox AJ, Watson IV (1971) Histological evidence on the nature of psoriasis. In 'Psoriasis' Ed. Farber EM and Cox AJ. Stanford University Press, pp 151–159

Duffill M, Wright NA, Shuster S (1976) The cell proliferation kinetics of psoriasis examined by three different in vivo techniques. Brit J Derm 94:366–363

Duffill M, Appleton DR, Shuster S, Dyson P, Wright NA (1977) The measurement of the cell cycle time in squamous epithelium using the metaphase arrest method with vincristine. Brit J Dermatol 96:493–502

Du Vivier A, Bible R, Mikiuriyn RK, Stoughton R (1976) An animal model for screening drugs for anti-psoriatic properties using hydroxyapatite to isolate DNA rapidly from the epidermis. Brit J Dermatol 94:1–6

Epstein JH, Conant MA, Krasnobrod H (1966) Molluscum contagiosum; normal and virus infected epidermal cell kinetics. J Invest Dermatol 46:91–103

Epstein JH, Fukuyama K (1975) Effects of 8-methoxypsoralen-induced phototoxic effects of mammalian epidermal macromolecular synthesis in mice. Photochem Photobiol 21:325–330

Fisher LB (1968a) Determination of the normal rate and duration of mitosis in human epidermis. Br J Derm 80:24–33
Fisher LB (1968b) The diurnal mitotic rhythm in the human epidermis. Brit J Derm 80:75–80
Fisher LB, Maibach AI (1971) The effect of corticosteroids on human epidermal mitotic activity. Arch Derm 103:39–44
Fisher LB, Maibach AI (1972) The effect of occlusive and semipermeable dressings on the cell kinetics of normal and wounded epidermis. In: Maibach HI, Rovel D (eds) 'Epidermal Wound to Healing'. Year Book Publishers, pp 113–131
Fisher LB, Maibach HI (1975) The effect of anthralin and its derivates on epidermal cell kinetics. J Invest Dermatol 64:338–341
Fisher LB, Wells GC (1968) The mitotic rate and duration in lesions of psoriasis and ichthyosis. Brit J Dermatol 80:235–240
Frankfurt OS (1968) Effect of hydrocortisone, adrenalin and actinomycin D on transition of cells to the DNA synthesis phase. Exp Cell Res 52:222–232
Frost P, Weinstein GD, Van Scott FJ (1966) The ichthyosiform dermatoses II. Autoradiographic studies of epidermal cell proliferation. J Invest Dermatol 47:561–565
Frost P, Van Scott E (1966) Ichthyosiform dermatoses. Arch Derm 94:113–126
Fry L, McMinn RMH (1968) The action of chemotherapeutic agents on psoriatic epidermis. Brit J Dermatol 82:19–22
Fry L, McMinn RMH (1970) Observations on mitosis in psoriatic epidermis. Brit J Dermatol 82:19–22
Galosi H (1980) Abnormal cell proliferation on the elbow in psoriatic and normal skin. Arch Dermatol Res 267:105–107
Gelfant S (1962) Initiation of mitosis in relation to the cell division cycle. Exp Cell Res 26:395–403
Gelfant S (1976) The cell cycle in psoriasis: a reappraisal. Brit J Dermatol 95:577–590
Gelfant S (1978a) Tissue and Tumour Cell Proliferation. In: Dirksen ER, Prestcott D, Fox M (eds) 'Cell Reproduction'. Academic Press, pp 689–699
Gelfant S (1978b) Understanding chemotherapy of psoriasis in terms of epidermal cell proliferation. Cell Tissue Kinet 11:577–578
Gibbs S, Casserett G (1969) Influences of a circadian rhythm and mitotic delay from tritiated thymidine on cytokinetic studies in hamster cheek pouch epithelium. Radiation Res 40:588–600
Gilbert CW (1972) The labelled mitoses curve and the estimation of the parameters of the cell cycle. Cell Tissue Kinet 5:53–63
Goldberg H, Cox AJ, Abel EA (1980) The mitotic index in psoriatic plaques and their response to PUVA therapy. Brit J Dermatol 10:401–405
Goodwin PG, Hamilton S, Fry L (1973) Comparison between DNA synthesis and mitosis in uninvolved and involved psoriatic epidermis and normal epidermis. Brit J Dermatol 89:619–628
Goodwin PG, Fry L (1974) Turnover times in psoriasis. Proc R Soc Med 67:598–600
Goodwin PG, Hamilton S, Fry L (1974) The cell cycle time in psoriasis. Brit J Dermatol 90:517–525
Goodwin PG, Hamilton S, Fry L (1975) On the cell cycle time in psoriasis. Brit J Dermatol 92:231–232
Goodwin PG, Fry L (1977) The cell cycle time in psoriasis. The uninvolved epidermis. Clin Exp Dermatol 2:259–264
Greulich RC (1964) Aspects of cell individuality in the renewal of stratified squamous epithelium. In: Montagna W, Lobitz WC (eds) 'The Epidermis'. Academic Press, New York, pp 117–133
Grove GL, Anderton RL, Graham Smith J (1976) Cytophometric studies of epidermal proliferation in psoriatic and normal skin. J Invest Dermatol 66:236–239
Grove GL (1979) Epidermal cell kinetics in psoriasis. Int J Dermatol 18:111–122
Grove GL (1980) Proliferative response to fluid injection in psoriatic and normal epidermis. Brit J Dermatol 102:281–283
Guildhou JJ, Meynadier J, Clot J (1978) New concepts in the pathogenesis of psoriasis. Brit J Dermatol 98:585–592
Harper RA, Flaxman BA (1974) Mitotic index of normal and psoriatic keratinocytes in vitro to compounds known to affect intracellular cAMP. J Invest Dermatol 62:384–387
Harper RA, Rispler J, Urbaulk WR (1978) DNA synthesis among involved and uninvolved epidermal cells in vitro. I Invest Dermatol 70:254–256
Hell E, Hodgson C (1966) The uptake of 3H-thymidine by epidermal cells in normal and psoriatic subjects. Brit J Dermatol 78:262–268

Hell E, Hodgson C (1978) Human epidermal stimulants, normal and psoriatic. Clin Exp Dermatol 3:269–278

Hell E, Hodgson C, Manna V (1979) Psoralen photochemotherapy of psoriasis. Brit J Dermatol 101:293–298

Hoffman C, Landthaler M, Plewig G, Braun-Falco O (1980) In vivo autoradiography and planimetry of epidermis in psoriatics under PUVA therapy. Arch Dematol Res 267:61–70

Johannesen A, Hammar H (1980) The rate of formation of corneocyte layers after stripping the non-involved psoriatic skin and its relation to parakeratosis and epidermal enzyme levels. J Invest Dermatol 74:226–229

Kaidbey KH, Kurban R (1971) Mitotic behaviour of the buccal mucosal epithelium in psoriasis. Brit J Dermatol 85:162–166

Karienemi AL (1974) Culture of psoriatic and uninvolved human skin in diffusion chambers in mice. J Invest Dermatol 63:388–391

Marcelo CL, Vorhees JJ (1980) Cyclic nucleotide control of psoriatic cell function. Adv Cyclic Nucleotide. Res 12:129–137

Marks F (1975) Isolation of an endogenous inhibitor of DNA synthesis (G_1 chalone) from pig skin. Hoppe Seylers Z Physiol Chem 356:1989–1992

Marks F (1978) Homeostatic regulators of epidermal cell proliferation. Bull Cancer (Paris), 65:207–222

Marks R (1975) Is there a relationship between clinical morphology and epidermal cell kinetics? Proc Roy Soc Med 68:161–167

Marks R, Boghel B (1973) Scanning electron microscopy of the normal epidermis in vitro. Brit J Dermatol 90:387–396

Marks R, Griffiths A (1973) The epidermis in pityriaris rubra pilaris: a comparison with psoriasis. Brit J Dermatol 89:Suppl 9, 19–24

Marks R, Wells GC (1973) Lichen Simplex: morphodynamic correlates. Br J Dermatol 88:249–256

Marks R, Black M, Wilson Jones E (1973) Epidermal cell kinetics in lichem planus. Brit J Dermatol 88:37–45

McCullough JL, Weinstein GD (1979) The role of cell kinetics in the chemtherapy of hyperproliferative skin disease. Pharmacol Ther 4:601–615

Mendelsohn ML, Takahashi M (1969) A critical evaluation of the labelled mitoses method as applied to the analysis of tumours and other cycles. In: Baserga R (ed) 'The Cell Cycle and Cancer'. Marcel Dekker, New York, pp 73–91

Menton DN, Eisen AZ (1971a) Structure and organisation of mammalian stratum corneum. Ultrastruct Res 35:247–264

Menton DN, Eisen AZ (1971b) Structural organisation of the human corneum in certain scaling disorders. J Invest Dermatol 51:296–307

Milstein H, Cornell R (1977) Diurnal mitotic studies of psoriatic epidermis. J Invest Dermatol 61:180–183

Møller U, Larsen JK, Faber M (1974) The influence of injected tritiated thymidine on the mitotic circadian rhythm in the epithelium of the hamster cheek pouch. Cell Tissue Kinet 7:231–239

Niemi KM, Konsa M, Storgards K (1976) Pityriasis rubra pilaris: a clinicopathological study with special reference to autoradiography and histocompatibility antigens. Dermatologica 152:169–182

Porter D, Shuster S (1967) A new method for measuring replacement of epidermis and s corneum in human skin. J Invest Derm 49:251–256

Pullman H (1978) Pathogenesis of psoriasis. Fortschr Med 96:1335–1338

Pullman H, Lennartz KJ, Steigleder GK (1974) In vitro examination of cell proliferation in normal and psoriatic epidermis with special regard to diurnal variations. Arch Derm Forsch 250:177–184

Pullman H, Lennartz KJ, Steigleder GK (1977) Disturbance of DNA synthesis in early psoriasis. Arch Derm Res 258:211–218

Pullman H, Steigleder GK, Lennartz KJ (1980) Effects of selective UV phototherapy (SUP) and local PUVA treatment on DNA synthesis in guinea pig skin. Arch Derm Res 267:37–45

Ralfs I, Dawber R, Ryan T, Duffill M, Wright NA (1981) The kinetics of metaphase arrest in human psoriatic epidermis; an examination of optimal experimental conditions for determining the birth rate. Brit J Dermatol 104:231–242

Ralfs I, Dawmer R, Ryan T, Wright NA (1981b) Pityriasis rubra pilaris: epidermal cell kinetics. Brit J Dermatol 104:249–253

Rook A, Wilkinson DS, Ebling FJG (eds) (1981) Textbook of Dermatology

Rowe L, Dixon WJ, Forsythe A (1978) Mitoses in normal and psoriatic epidermis. Brit J Dermatol 98:293–299
Sato A, Anton-Lamprecht I, Schuyder UW (1978) 3H thymidine labelling of epidermis in morbus Darier. J Cutan Path 5:142–144
Shackney SE (1975) The radioautographic transfer function and its implications for radioautographic methodology. J Natl Cancer Inst 55:811–820
Shahrad P, Marks R (1976) Hair follicle kinetics in psoriasis. Brit J Dermatol 94:7–12
Simnett JD (1968) The measurement of mitotic incidence and radioautographic labelling index from tissue sections: some mathematical considerations. J Roy Microscop Soc 88:371–382
Smith C, Gelfant S (1974) Effects of methotrexate and hydroxyurea on psoriatic epidermis. Preferential cytotoxic effects on psoriatic epidermis. Arch Derm 110:70–72
Soltani K, Van Scott EJ (1972) Pattens and sequence of tissue changes in incipient and evolving lesions of psoriasis. Arch Dermatol 166:484–490
Stankler L (1969) Blood tissue factors influencing Koebner reaction in psoriasis. Br J Derm 81:207–212
Steigleder GK, Pullman H (1979) Cell proliferation in psoriasis. Acta Derm Vener Suppl 87:64–66
Steigleder GK, Schumann H, Lennartz KJ (1973) Autoradiographic in vitro examination of psoriatic skin before, during and after dithranol treatment. Arch Derm Forsch 246:231–235
Swanbeck C, Liden S (1966) The inhibitory effect of dithranol on DNA synthesis. Acta Derm Vener, Stockholm 46:228–230
Taylor JR, Halprin KM (1977) Metrotrexate uptake by psoriatic epidermis. Brit J Dermatol 96:167–170
Van Scott EJ (1972) Tissue compartments of the skin lesion of psoriasis. J Invest Dermatol 59:4–6
Van Scott EJ, Flaxman BA (1973) Lesion kinetics in psoriasis. Acta Derm Vener Suppl 73:75–82
Walter JF (1973) Psoralen plus black light inhibits epidermal DNA synthesis. Arch Dermatol 107:861–865
Walter JF, Stoughton RB, De Quoy P (1978) Supression of epidermal proliferation by ultraviolet light, coal tar and anthralin. Brit J Dermatol 99:89–96
Weinstein GD (1975) On the cell cycle of psoriasis. Brit J Derm 92:229
Weinstein GD, Frost P (1968) Abnormal cell proliferation in psoriasis. J Invest Dermatol 50:254–259
Weinstein GD, Frost P (1969) Cell proliferation kinetics in benign and malignant skin disease in humans. Nat Cancer Inst Monogr 30:225–246
Weinstein G, Frost P (1971) Methotrexate for psoriasis. Arch Dermatol 103:33–41
Weinstein G, Goldfaben G, Frost P (1971) The effect of methotrexate on DNA synthesis in psoriasis. Arch Dermatol 164:236–248
Weinstein GD, Velasco J (1972) Selective action of methotrexate on psoriatic epidermal cells. J Invest Dermatol 59:122–128
Weinstein GD, McCullough JL (1973) Cytokinetics in diseases of epidermal hyperplasia. Ann Rec Med 24:345–352
Weinstein G, McCullough JL (1975) Effects of methotrexate esters on normal and psoriatic skin. Arch Dermatol 111:471–475
Wiley HE, Weinstein GD (1979) Abnormal proliferation of uninvolved psoriatic epidermis. Differential induction by saline, propanolol and tape stripping in vivo. J Invest Dermatol 73:545–547
Wright NA (1976) A new look at epidermal cell kinetics in psoriasis and other dermatoses. Clin Exp Dermatol 1:275–278
Wright NA (1977) Cell population kinetics in human epidermis. Int J Dermatol 16:449–463
Wright NA (1980a) The kinetics of human epidermal cell populations in health and disease. In: Rook A, Hunter J (eds) 'Recent Advances in Dermatology' Churchill Livingstone, pp 317–343
Wright NA (1980b) A methodological approach to epidermopoiesis. In: Markes R, Christophers E (eds) 'Epidermis in Disease'. MTP Press, pp 139–153
Wright NA (1983) Discussion: Statistical and operational problems in cell kinetic methodology in human epidermis. In: Wright NA, Camplejohn RS (eds) 'Psoriasis: Cell Proliferation'. Churchill Livingstone, Edinburgh, Oxford, pp 117–123
Wright NA, Camplejohn RS (1983) Psoriasis: cell proliferation. Churchill Livingstone Edinburgh
Wright NA, Salter D (1979) Human epidermal stimulants, normal and psoriatic. Clin Exp Derm 4:545–547
Wright NA, Alison M (1984) Biology of Epithelial Cell Populations. University Press, Oxford vol I, p 468

Mycosis fungoides *

W. Sterry

1. Definition

Mycosis fungoides is a T-cell lymphoma of low grade malignancy that most probably originates in the skin; it was described in France by Alibert as early as 1806. The skin changes are characterized by a sequence beginning with eczematous patches that develop into infiltrated plaques and terminate in ulcerating tumours; its natural course ranges from 10 to 15 years. Mycosis fungoides affects predominantly elderly people with a slight male preponderance. Although

* Dedicated to Prof. Dr. med. G.K. Steigleder for his 60th anniversary.

the term chosen by ALIBERT clearly is ethymologically and aetiologically a misnomer, it was rapidly accepted and is still used today.

Sézary syndrome is a T-cell lymphoma of intermediate grade malignancy. The natural course is approximately between one and three years. Clinical findings include initial erythroderma, lymphadenopathy and a leukaemic blood picture. The Sézary syndrome is related to mycosis fungoides because of similar skin histology, ultrastructure and immunological characteristics of the malignant lymphocytes. It differs from mycosis fungoides by the more aggressive clinical course, initial leukaemia and initial erythroderma (KERL 1981).

Mycosis fungoides and Sézary syndrome have been described in central Europe, where they are still observed in their typical expression, whereas atypical presentations are rare. In the United States, there are many patients with intermediate clinical pictures, so that SCHEIN, MACDONALD and EDELSON (1976) proposed that they should discard this "archaic" nomenclature and regard these disorders as variations of "cutaneous T cell lymphoma" (CTCL). They stated that "both disorders result from the proliferation of malignant thymus-derived lymphocytes with progressive involvement of skin, lymph nodes, and visceral organs" and included mycosis fungoides, Sézary syndrome, lymphomatoid papulosis and pagetoid reticulosis (see PATTERSON and EDELSON 1983).

It is increasingly evident that in different parts of the world distinct lymphomas exist that are specific for the respective area, for example Japanese adult T-cell leukaemia. Although these disorders have well defined characteristics, they would also fit into the definition of "cutaneous T-cell lymphoma". We feel therefore that instead of clarifying the situation by introducing the term CTCL, it was a step backwards. It forces probably different lymphoma entities into a single disease spectrum and thus inhibits attempts to separate further distinct lymphomas with perhaps differing aetiology, pathogenesis or therapeutic response. The same opinion was recently expressed by KERL et al. (1984).

The fact that investigators from the United States and from Europe have differing views on cutaneous lymphomas is not new, since Symmers in New York (1932) described mycosis fungoides as "clinical and pathologic nonexistant"; the european point of view was formulated by ROBB-SMITH (1942), who writes that "through all the varying accounts one gains the impression there is a distinct clinical entity with a characteristic histology, and that if really critical observation and histology were applied to these disorders (reticuloses), mycosis fungoides would stand out even more certainly as a disease with a characteristic natural history and pathology."

In this review, only the classical disease entity of mycosis fungoides will be described.

2. Epidemiology

Mycosis fungoides is a rare disease. Retrospective studies from cancer registries suggest an annual incidence of less than five per million inhabitants (United States Bureau of the Census, 1960). These figures correspond well to the personal experience of the author for Western Germany. Other types of malignant T-cell lymphomas originating or predominantly presenting within the skin seem to be twice as common in the United States (EDELSON 1979).

Analyzing data that had been collected by the Mycosis Fungoides Cooperative Study Group (1975) and by the county-by-county survey of cancer mortality conducted by the National Cancer Institute (1973), GREENE et al. (1979) published a large, epidemiological study on mycosis fungoides, including 429 patients. 64% of those affected were males, with manifestation of the disease between 45 and 69 years of age in the majority of the patients; the average age at diagnosis was 52 years. The incidence is similar in blacks and whites (BRODER and BUNN 1980).

Allergic skin diseases were found in the histories of 56% of these patients; susceptibility to fungal or viral infections of the skin were observed in 64% in this series. Only 16% of patients with proven mycosis fungoides had dermatoses that are thought to be possible precursors of mycosis fungoides like parapsoriasis, poikiloderma or alopecia mucinosa (GREENE et al. 1979). 10 patients had suffered from another malignancy before the development of mycosis fungoides; two patients had cancers following the diagnosis of mycosis fungoides (see chapter 3.2.5.).

3. Clinical Features

3.1 Cutaneous Findings

Skin changes caused by mycosis fungoides were described as early as 1806 by ALIBERT. Three types of skin lesions occur sequentially: eczematoid patches, infiltrated plaques and tumours. This sequence of lesions is called "classical mycosis fungoides" and BAZIN (1870) was the first to recognize this course. So-called "atypical" cases, for example initial development of tumours (d'emblée-type of VIDAL and BROCQ 1885), or presentation with initial erythroderma (BESNIER and HALLOPEAU 1892) most probably represent other disease entities that need further careful immunological work-up (see chapter 1) (see also BLUEFARB 1954).

3.1.1 Macroscopic and Microscopic Skin Changes

The first visible skin lesions are either flat, light red, slightly scaling patches of several centimeters in diameter (Fig. 1) or large atrophic lesions with teleangiectasies and hypo- and hyperpigmentation. The first type of lesions is often elongated and arranged along the skin extension lines and thus acquires a digitate appearance. Pruritus may be pronounced. The second corresponds to the large variant of parapsoriasis en plaques, which frequently evolves into mycosis fungoides (SAMMAN 1972; HEID et al. 1976). Pruritus is nearly always present.

The histology of the nonatrophic patches shows a nearly normal epidermis with slight hyperkeratosis and a mild to moderate infiltrate of lymphocytes

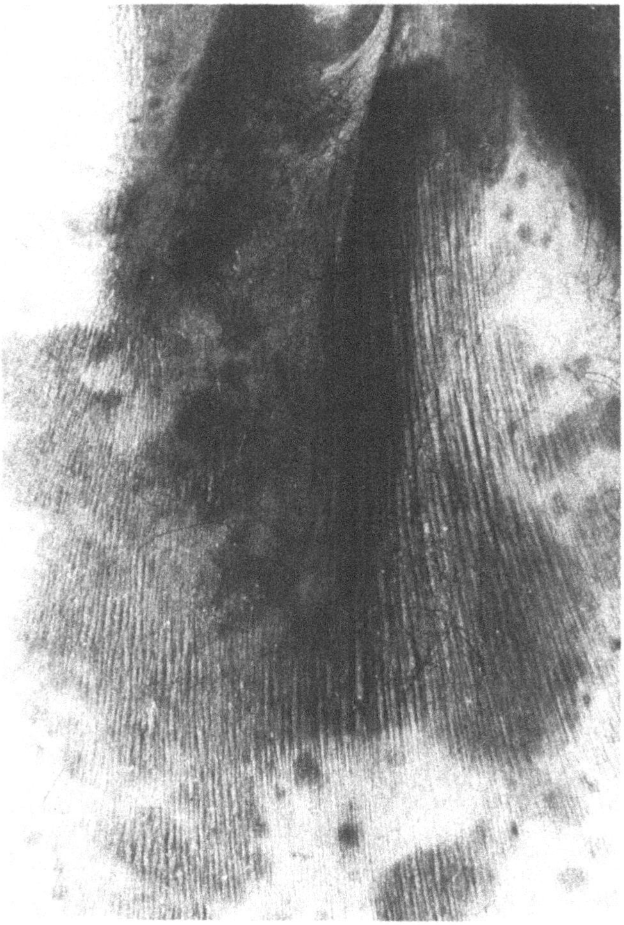

Fig. 1. Eczematous lesions with slight scaling and variable, minimal infiltration

and histiocytes around the vessels of the upper dermal plexus. Some of the lymphocytes enter the epidermis without signs of spongiosis (ACKERMAN et al. 1974; SANCHEZ and ACKERMAN 1979; LEVER and SCHAUMBURG-LEVER 1983); this phenomenon is called epidermotropism (Fig. 2). Atrophic plaques show epidermal atrophy, dilatation of capillaries in the upper dermis, extravasation of erythrocytes, and melanophages in the papillary dermis. In routine histology, the diagnosis often cannot be firmly established but can only be suscepted, even if strict criteria are used (CIVATTE and KAPETIS 1977; LEFEBER et al. 1982).

Palpable and visible infiltration gives rise to plaques with more or less pronounced scaling (Fig. 3). Pigmentation may be present, but more often plaques are reddish. Scratching leads to irritation of the plaques.

Histologically, plaques exhibit the most characteristic findings of mycosis fungoides:

- within the epidermis, numerous small lymphocytes with convoluted nuclei (Lutzner-cells; Sézary-cells) are scattered; aggregates of several of these lym-

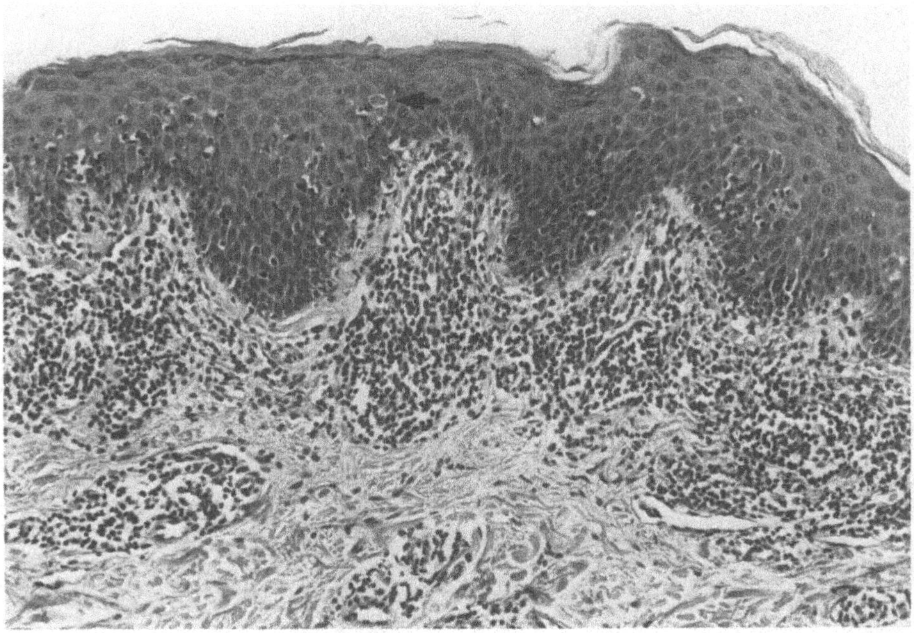

Fig. 2. Single cell epidermotropism with numerous lymphocytes invading the epidermis; note the absence of spongiosis. Single necrotic keratinocytes (*arrow*). Dense infiltrate in the papillary body with confluence to a bandlike appearance. Dilated capillaries

phocytes within the epidermis are highly characteristic forming Pautrier's microabscesses. Due to more pronounced shrinkage of the lymphocytes when compared with the keratinocytes the cells within the Pautrier's microabscesses are surrounded by a clear halo (Fig. 4). The papillary body and the upper dermis are occupied by a bandlike infiltrate, consisting of the same cerebriform lymphocytes found within the epidermis, sometimes large lymphocytes with dark irregular nuclei (socalled mycosis cells), and histiocytes.

- in longstanding plaques the epidermis shows psoriasiform acanthosis with parakeratosis and elongation of the rete ridges.
- two types of cells are present in varying amounts from patient to patient and give the impression of an inflammatory infiltrate: eosinophils and plasma cells. Plasma cells are often found in nests at the lower edge of the infiltrate.

The development of tumours is seen in more advanced disease after long duration: usually, the tumours vary from two to five centimeters in diameter with skin coloured or red surfaces (Figs. 5, 6). Central ulceration occurs frequently.

The histological picture is characterized by large infiltrated dermal areas which may extend into the subcutaneous tissue (Fig. 7); due to previous therapy or to the natural course, epidermotropism may be absent (Fig. 7). The cytological features are extremely variable; in most instances, the cells will exhibit signs of atypia including atypical mitoses and nuclear and cellular polymorphism. Cytology at high power magnification frequently shows immunoblasts, i.e. large

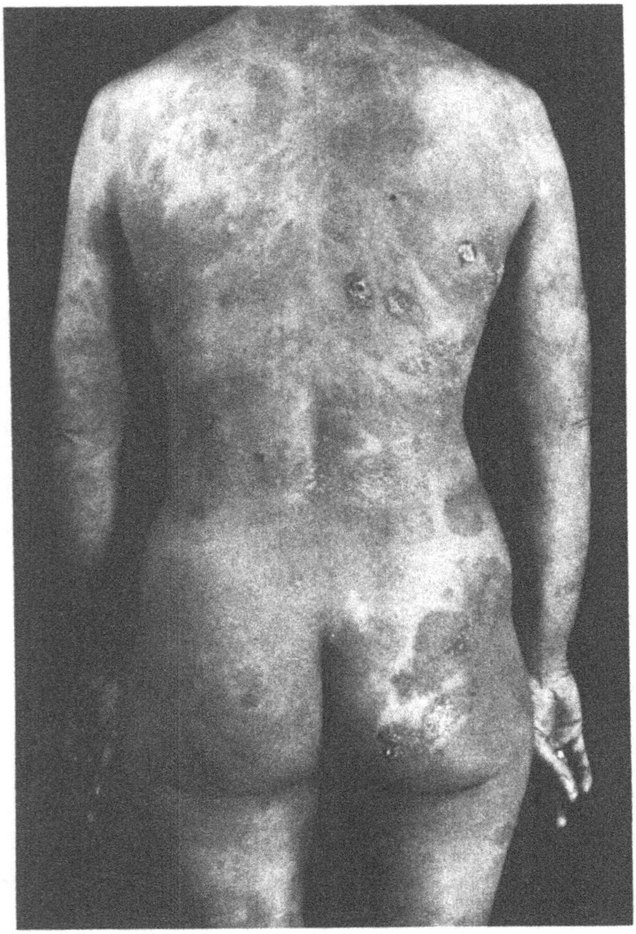

Fig. 3. Generalized eczematous lesions and plaques (T2). The plaques are covered by scales and crusts, partually due to irritation by scratching

lymphocytes with a prominent central nucleus and broad basophil cytoplasm best seen in Giemsa staining (Fig. 8).

In tumours, epidermotropism may be lost (Fig. 7). The loss of epidermotropism also was observed in a follow up study by EDELSON (1980). This phenomenon must, however, be strictly separated from the absence of epidermotropisms at initial presentation, because these patients clearly show a different age distribution and a poor prognosis (YAMAMURA et al. 1984).

Recently, a histopathological classification has been proposed by KERL et al. (1984). This classification divides the disease into four subtypes:

- lymphocytic type
- mixed cell type
- atrophic sclerosing type (medium sized)
- immunoblastic type

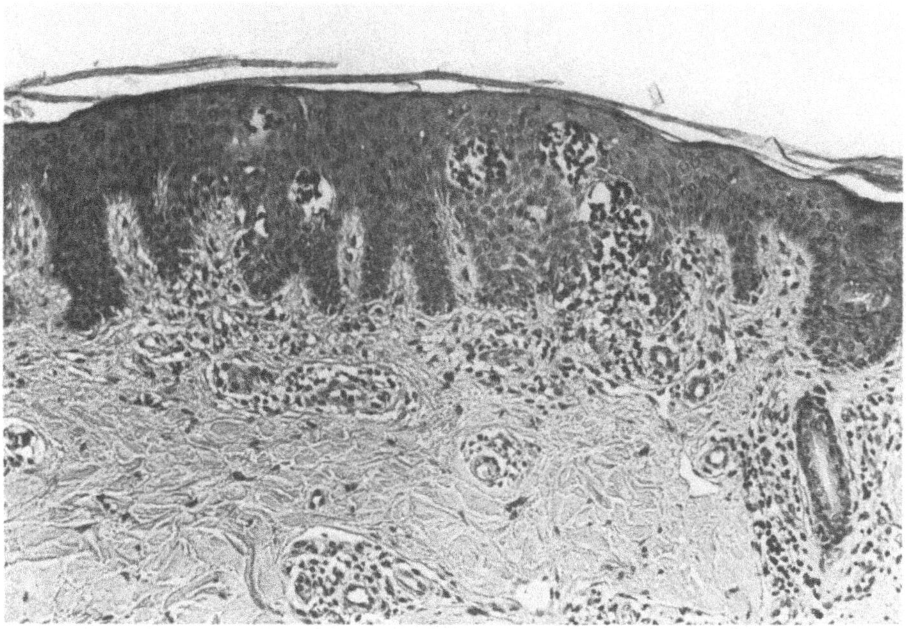

Fig. 4. Several aggregates of small hyperchromatic lymphocytes in close adjunction to single keratinocytes and Langerhans cells within the epidermis are surrounded by a clear halo: Pautrier's microabscesses. Sparse perivascular lymphocytic infiltrate in the upper dermis. This histological picture with lack of spongiosis is diagnostic of mycosis fungoides

The first two types are characterized by a chronic course, whereas the last two correspond to an aggressive clinical behaviour. The value of such a classification will have to be confirmed.

Scanning electron microscopy of isolated lymphocytes from dermal infiltrates in mycosis fungoides showed several signs of atypia that are not found in benign lymphocytic infiltrates; among these are loss of the round cell shape, irregular distribution of microvilli and variations in the thickness of microvilli (Fig. 9) (STERRY et al. 1981 b; STERRY et al. 1981 c).

The microtubular system of the dermal lymphocytes in mycosis fungoides seems to be altered, as indicated by an elevated colchicine sensitivity (STERRY et al. 1980 b).

On occasion, mycosis fungoides may present with morphological variants, which may cause difficulties in differential diagnosis and should therefore be mentioned. Pustulation within mycosis fungoides plaques, which may be regarded as macroscopically visible Pautrier's microabscesses (ACKERMAN et al. 1966), bullae formation within plaques (Fig. 10) (ROENIGK and CASTROVINCI 1971) and hyperkeratotic and verrucous epidermal hyperplasia (PRICE et al. 1977) are such rare clinical findings. Bulla formation seems to be mediated by eosinophils. Hypopigmented patches in mycosis fungoides have been repeatedly observed in patients with coloured skin (BREATHNACH et al. 1982).

Further information about the morphology of the infiltrating lymphocytes and their significance was obtained using semithin and ultrathin sections. Semi-

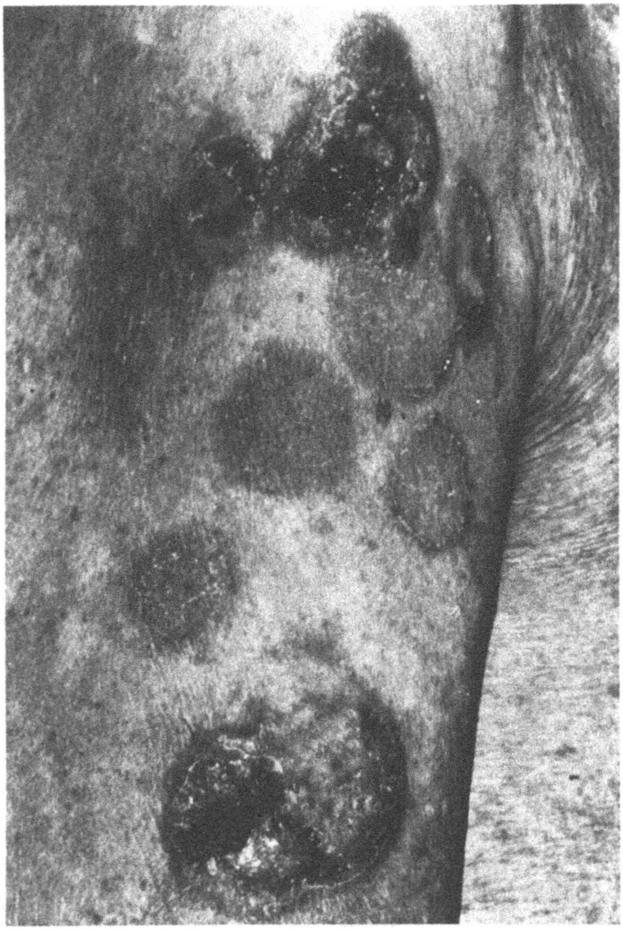

Fig. 5. Several plaques with minimal scaling and raised borders; in some of the plaques transition to tumours with central ulceration can be seen

thin sections permit better identification of the nuclear details of the infiltrating cells, particularly of lymphocytes with convoluted nuclei and of immunoblasts (SCHMOECKEL et al. 1979; VAN DER PUTTE and VAN DER MEER 1981).

Numerous electron microscopic studies of skin infiltrates consistently reveal the presence of lymphocytes with highly convoluted nuclei (Fig. 11 and 12) (BONNEAU and COSARINI 1967; BROWNLEE and MURAD 1970; FISHER et al. 1972; LUTZNER et al. 1971; for review see PAYNE et al. 1984). Interactions between convoluted lymphocytes, Langerhans cells and keratinocytes have been observed at the ultrastructural level; keratinocytes degenerate within the Pautrier's microabscesses (SCHMITT and THIVOLET 1980).

The nonspecificity of lymphocytes with convoluted nuclei for mycosis fungoides soon became evident, because similar cells were described in several benign dermatoses (FLAXMAN et al. 1971; for review see PAYNE et al. 1984), after in vitro stimulation with PHA (YECKLEY et al. 1975) and in normal spleens and reactive lymph nodes (ROSAS-URIBE et al. 1974). ROSAS-URIBE et al. (1974)

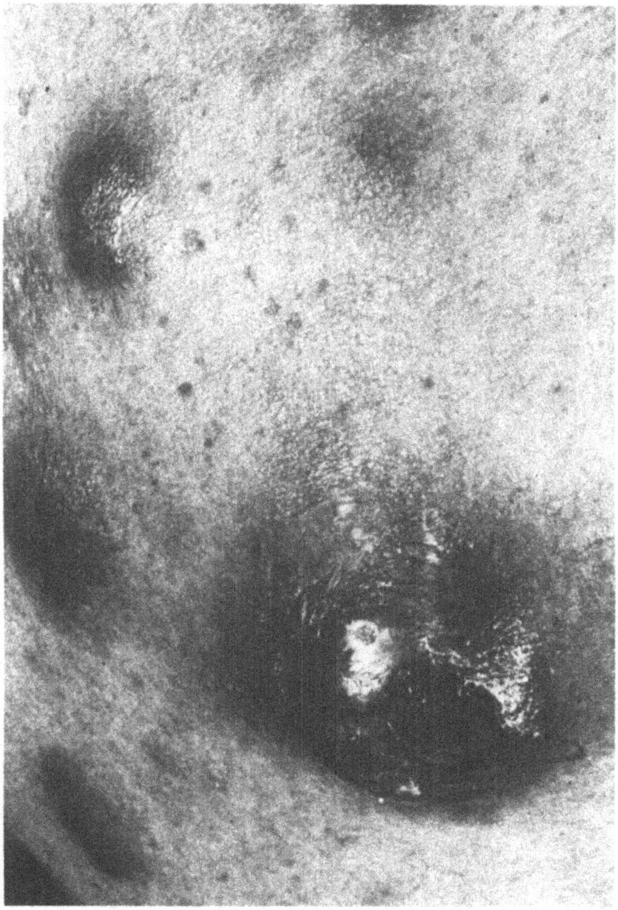

Fig. 6. Tumours of varying size in mycosis fungoides; some show central ulceration

pointed out, however, that the appearance of clusters of lymphocytes with convoluted nuclei could be regarded as specific for mycosis fungoides. This view cannot be accepted today, especially after the study of PAYNE et al. (1984) who found such clusters in various benign skin disorders. Moreover, CHU et al. (1983b) demonstrated that cerebriform lymphocytes are not specific for a single disease or a particular T-cell-population, as these cells can be found in actinic reticuloid and there show OKT 8 phenotype.

Quantitative ultrastructural techniques for assessment of the degree of nuclear convolution were introduced as a diagnostic tool by MEIJER et al. (1978). They showed that the frequency distribution of a nuclear shape parameter (nuclear contour index: NCI) permitted correct classification into malignant or benign disorders (MEIJER et al. 1980; VAN DER LOO et al. 1981); the finding was confirmed by others (MCNUTT and CRAIN 1981). NCI provides far better information about prognosis than DNA-cytophotometry. The disadvantage of this technique is the time it takes and the technical difficulties. PAYNE et al. (1984) presented a more exact and much easier technique for assessing the

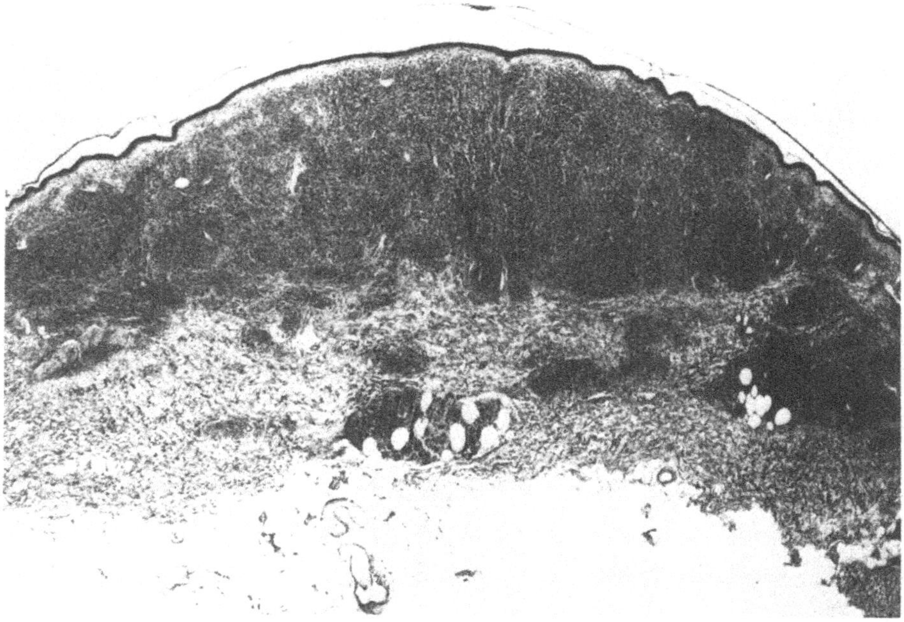

Fig. 7. Tumour in mycosis fungoides. Large areas of the papillary and reticular dermis are occupied by a dense infiltrate; sometimes the infiltrate penetrates into the subcutaneous fat. Epidermotropism is absent

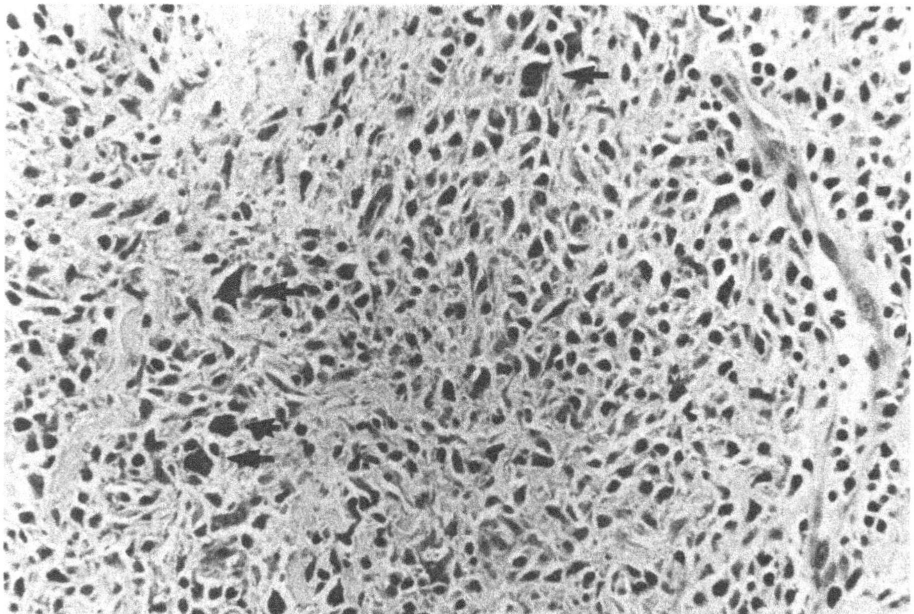

Fig. 8. High power magnification of figure 7. Note several immunoblasts (*arrows*) that are intermingled between the small and medium sized, pleomorphic lymphocytes and numerous histiocytes

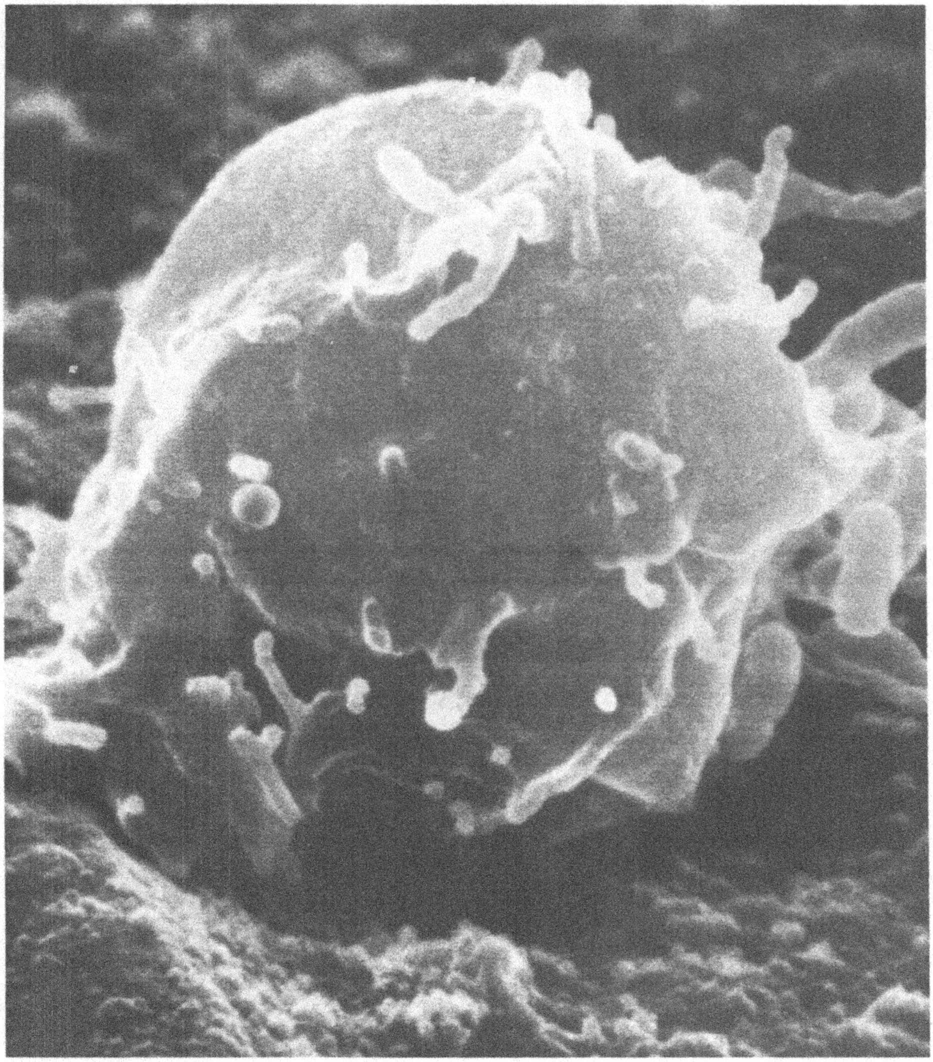

Fig. 9. Scanning-electron micrograph from an isolated lymphocyte of the dermal infiltrate in mycosis fungoides. Note the loss of the round cell shape as well as the irregular distribution and thickness of the microvilli. (From STERRY et al. 1981 b)

degree of nuclear convolution: the enumeration of sharply angled nuclear invaginations per lymphocyte at electron microscopic examination. This technique may be very useful in patients with early mycosis fungoides and equivocal histological and immunological findings.

3.1.2 Immunological Characterization of the Cutaneous Infiltrate

The development of our understanding of the immunological nature of the infiltrating cells in mycosis fungoides can be divided into three steps:

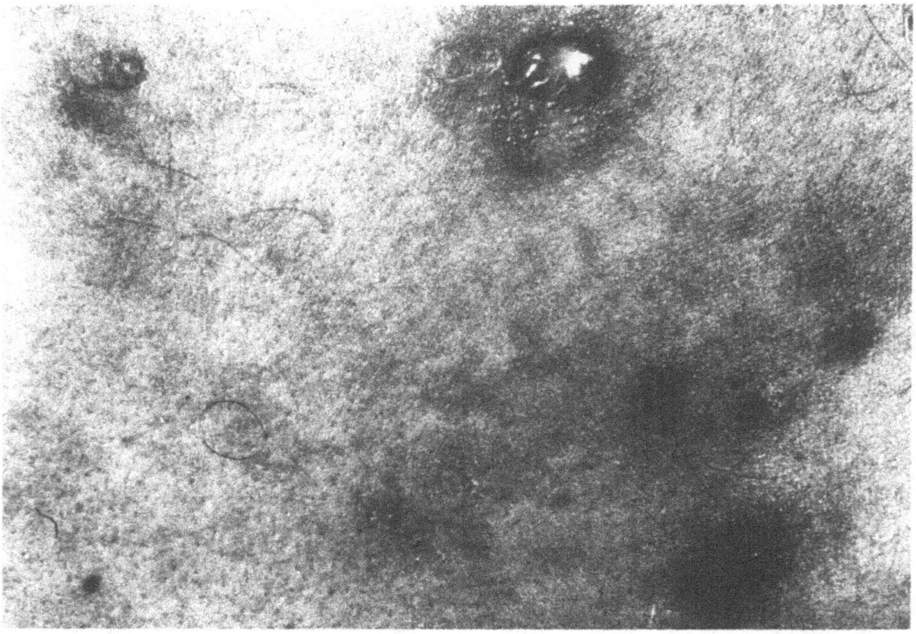

Fig. 10. Bulla formation within a plaque of mycosis fungoides; 45 year old male caucasian patient. Histologically, numerous eosinophils are present at the dermoepidermal junction

1. identification of the majority of the infiltrating cells as T-lymphocytes by E-rosetting
2. confirmation of these findings by demonstration of *h*uman-*T*-*l*ymphocyte-*a*ntigen (HTLA)
3. application of broad series of monoclonal antibodies directed against various antigens present on human lymphocytes.

Summarizing the results obtained with these three principal techniques, it has been demonstrated that in plaques of mycosis fungoides most of the infiltrating cells are T-lymphocytes with membrane properties corresponding to normal peripheral T-lymphocytes. During progression of the disease, the infiltrating lymphocytes show a loss of such typical markers together with the appearance of immature phenotypes. Additionally, the functional capacity of lymphocytes isolated from tumours is increasingly impaired.

EDELSON et al. were the first to show that the majority of the infiltrating cells of the mycosis fungoides are T-lymphocytes by E-rosette studies (EDELSON et al. 1974); an example of an isolated dermal lymphocyte from mycosis with an E-rosette is given in Fig. 13. In the same study the authors provided evidence that malignant T-lymphocytes exhibit a pronounced affinity for the skin; they found that patients, in whom initially chronic lymphatic leukaemia had been diagnosed and which presented with erythroderma, suffered from a T-lymphocyte neoplasm. In contrast, patients with B-chronic lymphatic leukaemia had no skin involvement. These observations were the starting point of the unifying concept of cutaneous T-cell lymphomas (LUTZNER et al. 1975; SCHEIN et al. 1976). It has already been stressed that although such a concept has certain

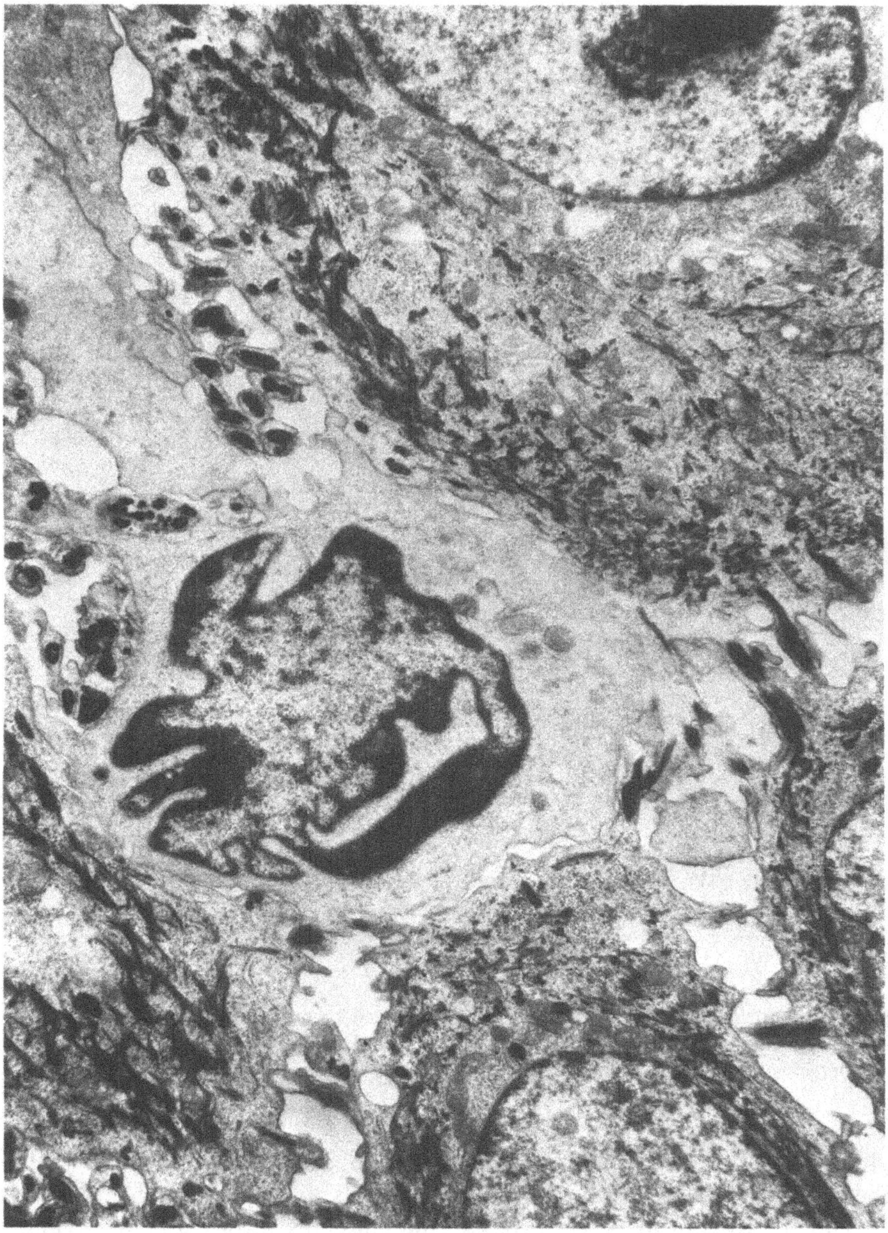

Fig. 11. Lymphocyte with a highly convoluted nucleus between several keratinocytes within the epidermis. Numerous cellular contacts between the lymphocyte and the keratinocytes can be seen. ×17000

advantages, it partially inhibits the recognition of lymphoma entities with distinct prognostic characteristics and therapeutic requirements because of their inclusion into a single disorder.

E-rosetting was later performed by VAN LEEUWEN et al. (1975) and BURG and BRAUN-FALCO (1975); both found that in plaques about 50% of the isolated

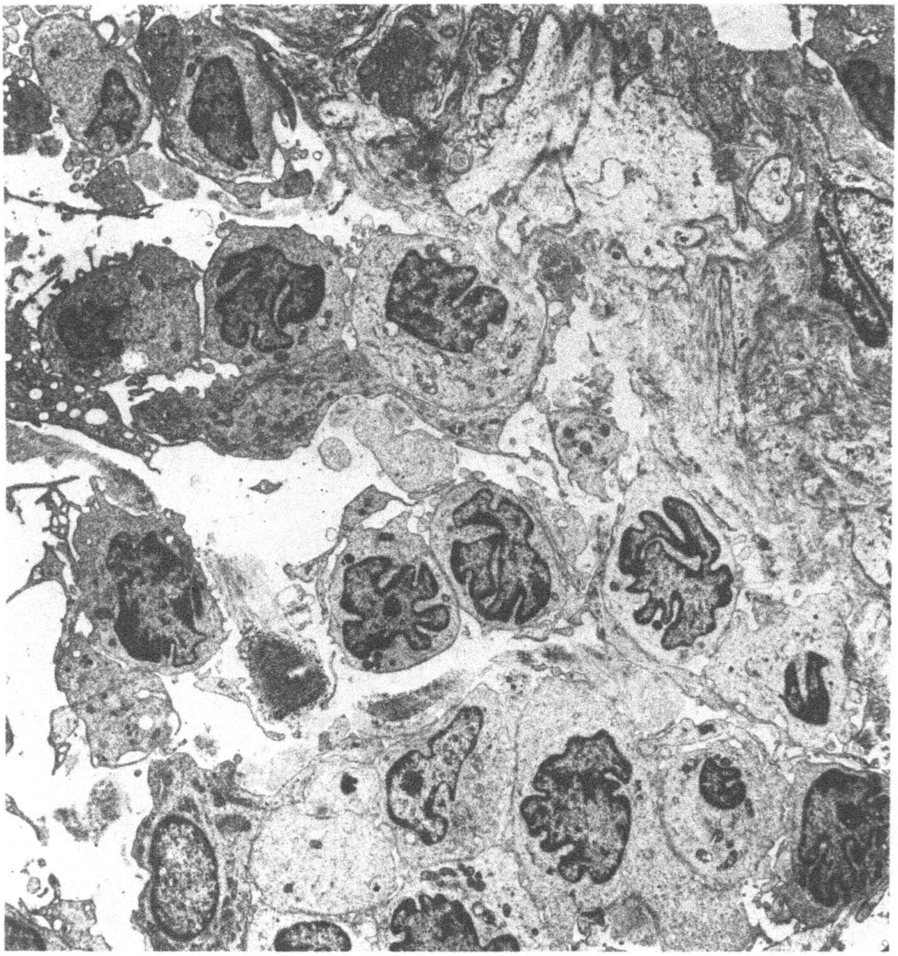

Fig. 12. Dermal infiltrate in mycosis fungoides. Numerous small lymphocytes with highly convoluted nuclei are seen intermingled between the collagen bundles. Additionally, histiocytes can be seen in close contact with the lymphocytes. × 7,000

lymphocytes express E-receptors, whereas in cells isolated from tumours this number decreases below 5%. An increase of cells exhibiting an Fc-receptor for IgG in the tumour stage of mycosis fungoides was shown by STINGL and KNAPP (1977), probably indicating an increased stimulation of these lymphocytes.

The second step in the investigation of the immunology of the cutaneous infiltrate in mycosis fungoides came with the development of heterologeous antiserum against a specific T-lymphocyte antigen (ALBIN and MORRIS 1973; SMITH et al. 1973). Subsequently, this surface antigen was named human-T-lymphocyte-antigen (HTLA) by TOURAINE et al. (1974). Using anti-HTLA-serum, the T-cell nature of the epidermal and dermal infiltrate in mycosis fungoides was further established using isolated cells (SCHMITT et al. 1977; CLAUDY

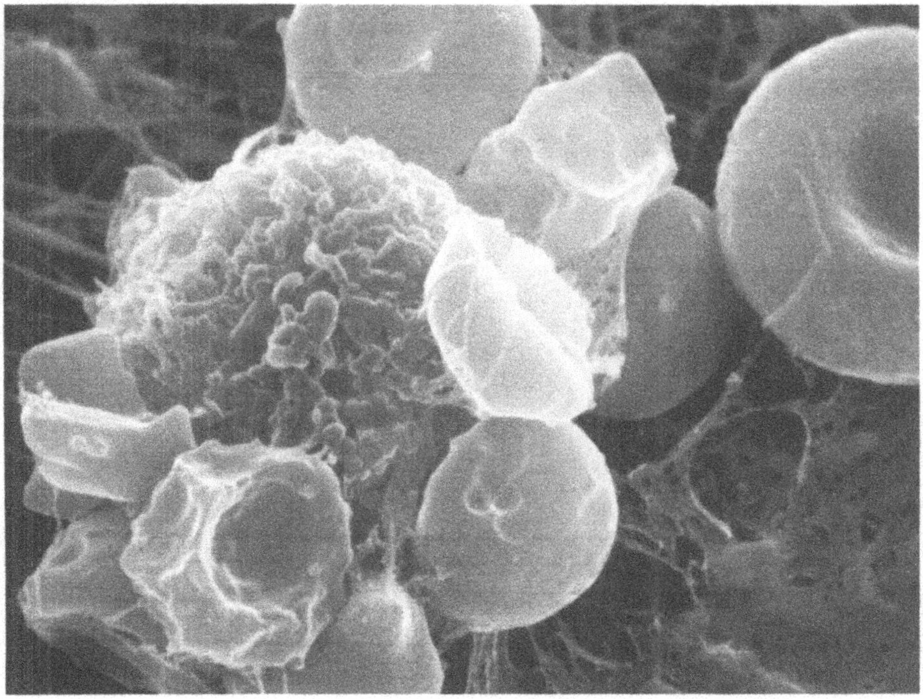

Fig. 13. Isolated lymphocyte from the dermal infiltrated of mycosis fungoides. Demonstration of sheep erythrocyte receptors; these have formed an E-rosette around the lymphocyte, thus demonstrating its T cell nature. Note the larger human erythrocyte on the right edge of the picture. (From STERRY et al. 1981 b)

et al. 1977; BURG et al. 1978), tissue sections with immunoperoxidase (CLAUDY et al. 1977; CHU and MACDONALD 1979) and immunofluorescence (BRAATHEN et al. 1979; DAVID et al. 1980) as well as by applying immunoelectron microscopy techniques (SCHMITT et al. 1977; CHU et al. 1980). Moreover, it was established that in mycosis fungoides T-cells show cerebriform nuclei both in the epidermis and in the dermis (CHU et al. 1980).

The development of monoclonal antibodies against various subtypes of lymphocytes gave further insight into the pathology of mycosis fungoides. Along with the increasing understanding of normal lymphocyte maturation and function (for review see SCHLOSSMAN and REINHERZ 1984), it was possible to define distinct steps in the intra- and extrathymic life of lymphocytes that are defined by combinations of cell surface antigens; such a maturation sequence has been proposed by REINHERZ et al. (1980). Our group currently divides five types of T-lymphocyte surface antigens: 1. maturation antigens, which are expressed during distinct stages of intra- and extrathymic maturation;
2. differentiation antigens, which are associated with functional differentiation;
3. activation antigens, which are expressed during activation of T-lymphocytes;
4. proliferation antigens, which are present when cells are not in G_0 of the cells cycle (GERDES et al. 1983; GERDES et al. in press a and b) and
5. tumour-associated antigens which are expressed on lymphocytes in mycosis

Table 1. List of monoclonal antibodies currently used in the analysis of the infiltrating lymphocytes in mycosis fungoides

Maturation
Antigens expressed during distinct stages of intra- or extrathymic maturation
OKT 10 T 6 (Leu 6, OKT 6) 3A1 / Tü 14 Leu 8
Differentiation
Antigens associated with functional differentiation
Pan T OKT 1 / Leu 1 OKT 3 / Leu 4 / T 28
helper T OKT 4 / Leu 3a
suppressor T OKT 8 / Leu 2a
natural killer cells Leu 7
Activation
Antigens expressed during activation of T-lymphocytes (and other cells)
Transferrin receptor (OKT 9/5 E 9); HLA-DR (OK Ia1, Leu anti HLA-DR); HLA-DS (Leu 10)
Proliferation
Nuclear antigens expressed during cell proliferation
Ki 67
Tumor-associated antigens
Antigens only expressed on lymphocytes in mycosis fungoides and Sézary-syndrome but not normal T-lymphocytes
BE 1 / BE 2

fungoides and Sézary's syndrome (Berger et al. 1982). The antibodies most commonly used are summarized in Table 1.

Several groups, including our own, have applied a panel of these antibodies to characterize the phenotype of the lymphocytes of the dermal and epidermal infiltrate in mycosis fungoides. Recently, Chu (1983) has reviewed these studies excellently; Tables 2 and 3 give an overview of the studies published up to the time of writing (June 1984) and have been modified after the review of Chu.

Lymphocytes infiltrating the epidermis show pan-T-antigens (Fig. 14) and are predominantly helper T-lymphocytes (Table 2). Suppressor-T-cells are rarely present within the epidermis; in our studies the helper/suppressor- ratio in the epidermis was higher than 10:1 in all cases.

Monoclonal antibody OKT6 reacts with the cortical thymocyte antigen

Table 2. Lymphocyte phenotype in the epidermal infiltrate. (Modified after CHU 1983, with kind permission of the author)

	No. of patients	Pan T-cell	Leu 3a/ OKT 4	Lue 2a/ OKT 8	OKT 6	OKT 10	OKT 9	3A1/ Tü14	Leu 8
MCMILLAN et al. 1982a	5	most	many	∅ in 4/5	in-creased	n.d.	n.d.	n.d.	n.d.
THOMAS et al. 1982	7	n.d.	4/7 75% 3/7 few or absent	25% 3/7 most	present	n.d.	n.d.	n.d.	n.d.
MACKIE and TURBITT 1982	17	most	n.d.	n.d.	n.d.	n.d.	n.d.	n.d.	n.d.
HAYNES et al. 1982a	11	80%	80% 7/11 20% 4/11	20% 10/11 80% 1/11	20%	n.d.	n.d.	80% 7/11 10% 3/11	n.d.
HOLDEN et al. 1982a	5	most	all	∅	in-creased	n.d.	n.d.	n.d.	n.d.
MCMILLAN et al. 1982c	4	n.d.	n.d.	n.d.	n.d.	n.d.	"posi-tive"	n.d.	n.d.
SCHMITT et al. 1982	10	most	most	∅	present	n.d.	n.d.	n.d.	n.d.
HAYNES et al. 1982b	4	n.d.	n.d.	n.d.	n.d.	n.d.	positive in 2/4	n.d.	n.d.
CHU et al. 1982d	91	many	many	some in 24/91	present	∅	n.d.	n.d.	n.d.
FELLER and STERRY (submitted)	25	many	many	few to ∅	in-creased	n.d.	n.d.	present if there are many in the dermal infiltrate	

HTA-1 (REINHERZ et al. 1980); HTA-1 is acquired by the cortical thymocyte stage II and expressed until early stage III. There is a short phase of intrathymic differentiation in which OKT6 and OKT3 are expressed simultaneously. OKT6 positive cells are not present in normal peripheral blood. It must be mentioned that OKT6 does not react exclusively with thymocytes, as the same antigen has also been found on human Langerhans cells and is today frequently used for their identification. OKT6 positive dendritic epidermal cells have been found in increased numbers in nearly all studies; MCMILLAN et al. (1982b), HAYNES et al. (1982a) and CHU et al. (1982c) demonstrated OKT6 positive cells within Pautrier microabscesses in contact with lymphoid cells (see Fig. 15).

The dermal infiltrate in mycosis fungoides is composed of T-lymphocytes with a predominantly helper-phenotype (see Table 3); however, suppressor T-lymphocytes may make up a considerable proportion in our cases. OKT6 positive dendritic cells are surprisingly frequent and make up about 10% of all infiltrating cells. Some of the OKT6 positive cells in the dermal infiltrate are rather rounded than dendritic and thus appear to be lymphoid; double labelling studies (CHU et al. 1982c; MACKIE and TURBITT 1982; THOMAS et al. 1982) have shown so far however that dermal OKT 6-positive cells are negative for

Table 3. Lymphocyte phenotype in the dermal infiltrate (modified after CHU 1983, with kind permission of the author)

	No. of patients	Pan T-cell	Leu 3a/ OKT 4	Leu 2a/ OKT 8	OKT 6	OKT 10	OKT 9	3A1/ Tü14	Leu 8
CHU et al. 1982c	23	n.d.	n.d.	n.d.	1–5%	n.d.	n.d.	n.d.	n.d.
MCMILLAN et al. 1982b	5	n.d.	n.d.	n.d.	5–10%	n.d.	n.d.	n.d.	n.d.
MCMILLAN et al. 1982a	5	50%	most	∅ in 2/5 few in 3/5	present	n.d.	n.d.	n.d.	n.d.
THOMAS et al. 1982	7	many	80–90%	10–20%	few	n.d.	n.d.	n.d.	n.d.
MCKIE and TURBITT 1982	17	90%	most	few	present	n.d.	n.d.	n.d.	n.d.
HAYNES et al. 1982a	11	80%	80%	20%	20%	n.d.	present	most	n.d.
HOLDEN et al. 1982a	5	61%	57%	14%	14%	n.d.	n.d.	n.d.	n.d.
MCMILLAN et al. 1982c	4	n.d.	n.d.	n.d.	n.d.	n.d.	present	n.d.	n.d.
SCHMITT et al. 1982	10	most	most	few	present	n.d.	n.d.	n.d.	n.d.
HAYNES et al. 1982b	4	most	most	5%	present	n.d.	50%	n.d.	n.d.
CHU et al. 1982d	91	60%	54%	8%	4%	3%	n.d.	n.d.	n.d.
WILLEMZE et al. 1983	21	40–90%	20–90%	5–25%	present	n.d.	n.d.	n.d.	n.d.
FELLER and STERRY (submitted)	25	most	80%	20–30%	present	n.d.	5–50%	20–80%	20–80%

OKT3, 4 or 8. This supports the view that all OKT6 positive dermal cells in fact are Langerhans cells; nevertheless, electron microscopic studies are needed to provide further clarification of this point.

Other interesting antibodies are those that react with all thymocytes but are lost in the periphery, like 3A1/Tü 14 or Leu 8. In our studies (STERRY et al. 1984) we found that the proportion of dermal cells positive for these antigens varies within wide ranges. These results may be interpreted as showing the possible existence of two malignant clones in mycosis fungoides that in individual patients would be derived either from Leu 8 positive or Leu 8 negative T lymphocytes (STERRY et al. 1984). Another explanation of this high variation would be that Leu 8 is gradually lost during the course of the disease as it is lost physiologically in T4-lymphocytes; Leu 8 would not then be suitable as clonal marker. This question can be answered by follow up studies to see whether Leu 8-positive patients turn to Leu 8-negative.

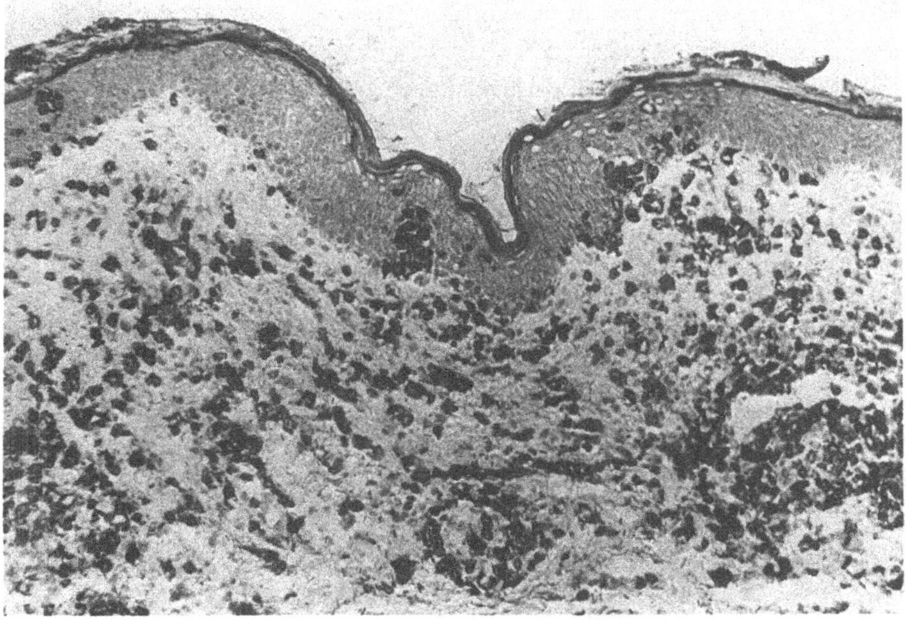

Fig. 14. Demonstration of a pan T antigen (Leu 4) in an early plaque of mycosis fungoides. Most of the infiltrating cells within the epidermis and the majority of the dermal lymphocytes are positive for pan T cell antigen. Immunoperoxidase. ×16

Phenotypes of immature lymphocytes have been observed by several investigators in the dermal infiltrate in mycosis fungoides. Up to 50% OKT10 positive cells were reported by McMillan et al. (1984) in three out of eight patients. Similarly, OKT9 is expressed by many epidermal and dermal lymphocytes (McMillan et al. 1982); both findings are in accordance with our own results. Even more important was the observation of Chu et al. (1982c) that in 15% of their patients a large percentage of the infiltrating cells simultaneously react with OKT4 and OKT8. The simultaneous expression of these two antigens is normally not found in adults but represents the phenotype of stage II intrathymic differentiation (Reinherz et al. 1980).

Activation antigens like the transferrin receptor (OKT9), or HLA-DR (OKT Ia1) and HLA-DS (Leu 10)-antigen are expressed on a variable proportion of the lymphocytes in the dermal infiltrate. According to our own results, the percentage of lymphocytes expressing HLA-DR and -DS varies between 10 and 70 with a tendency for DS to be expressed more frequently (Table 3).

Analysis of the dermal infiltrate with the monoclonal antibody Ki 67, which detects a nuclear antigen expressed during cell proliferation, gives data that are comparable with autoradiographic studies already published (Sterry et al. 1980a; Sterry et al. 1981a; Kummermehr and Burg 1982; Pierard et al. 1982); see also Table 4. In plaque lesions, 2–4% of the dermal infiltrate reacts with Ki 67.

Two monoclonal antibodies have been raised against the leukaemic helper-T-lymphocytes in cutaneous T cell lymphoma (Berger et al. 1982). These anti-

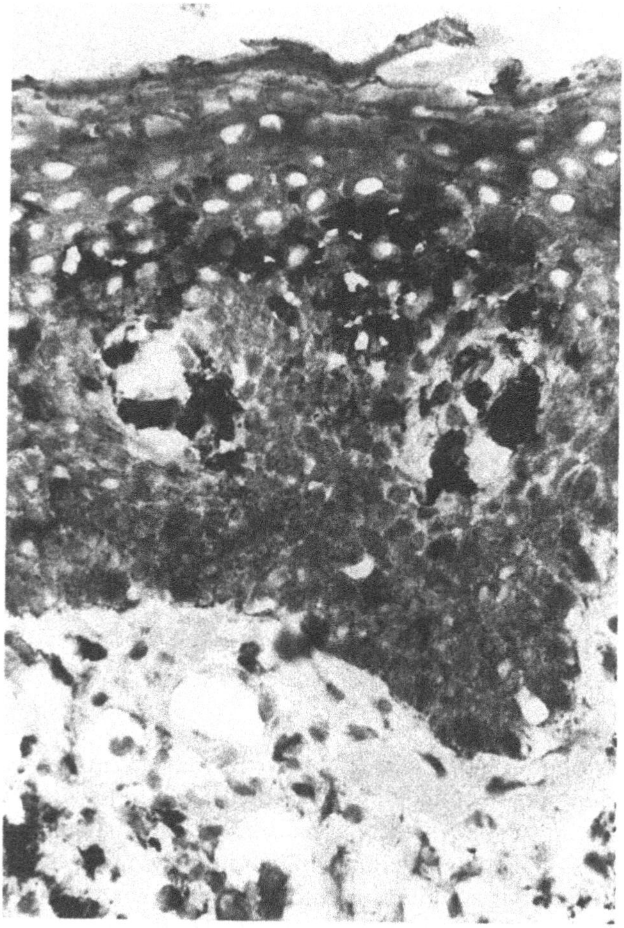

Fig. 15. Pautrier's microabscesses in early mycosis fungoides. Demonstration of T6 antigen reveals numerous Langerhans cells within the epidermis and the Pautrier's microabscesses. The negative cells within the abscesses represent lymphocytes (see Fig. 14) and keratinocytes. Immunoperoxidase. ×25

bodies termed BE1 and BE2 have been found to bind to lymphocytes from patients with cutaneous T cell lymphomas, some B-cell chronic lymphatic leukaemias, Epstein-Barr virus transformed B-cells, long term T cell lines, but not to normal lymphocytes. BE1 and BE2 could play an important role in early diagnosis of mycosis fungoides of myccosis fungoides, if these findings are confirmed.

In advanced cases in which histology shows an increase in lymphoblasts and immunoblasts, a differential loss of surface antigens by the T-cells has been described by several investigators (CHU et al. 1982d; WILLEMZE et al. 1982; HOLDEN et al. 1982b; SCHMITT et al. 1982). These blasts may be negative for Leu1 or Leu3a/OKT4 or both. The loss of the markers seems to herald a more aggressive course and indicates the terminal phase of the disease.

Our knowledge of the phenotype of the infiltrating lymphocytes in mycosis

Table 4. ^{3}H-thymidine labelling index in the dermal infiltrate of mycosis fungoides

Cutaneous lesion	Patient	Age	Sex	^{3}HI	
				Individual value	Mean value
Eczematous lesions (T1)	F.M.	71	m	1.6	1.2
	N.C.	35	m	0.8	
Plaques (T2)	J.K.	78	m	3.0	
	J.S.	71	m	1.7	
	E.W.	72	f	1.8	2.7
	I.E.	38	f	3.4	
	E.W.	65	f	3.5	
Tumors (T4)	M.B.	48	m	4.0	
	B.K.	39	m	3.9	3.6
	A.S.	71	f	2.8	

fungoides still is a framework; nevertheless it can be predicted that this technique will increase our understanding of this disease and its course. Probably, it will be possible to define phenotype constellations of diagnostic importance and perhaps of prognostic significance.

Enzyme-cytochemical methods have been used in the analysis of the dermal infiltrate in mycosis fungoides; the two enzymes that gave the most interesting results are *a*cid nonspecific alpha-*n*aphthyl*a*cetate *e*sterase (ANAE) and *d*i*a*mino-*p*eptidase IV/DAP IV or DPP IV). ANAE can be demonstrated specifically in T-lymphocytes of mouse lymph nodes (MÜLLER et al. 1975). Subsequently, ANAE was found to be a specific marker for T_M-lymphocytes (GROSSI et al. 1977). A major disadvantage of this technique is the fact that only large granular (dot-like) reaction products are specific for T_M-lymphocytes, whereas finely dispersed reaction products can be seen in T_G-lymphocytes and B-lymphocytes (GROSSI et al. 1978; STERRY et al. 1982). ANAE is present in most infiltrating lymphocytes in mycosis fungoides (STERRY et al. 1980c), thus confirming the T-cell nature of the infiltrate. Analysis of the reaction type reveals that in plaques 56% of the dermal lymphocytes show the typical dot-like reaction pattern specific for resting T_M-lymphocytes (Fig. 16a, b), whereas in tumours only 40% of the lymphocytes have a dot-like reaction product. The occurrence of a dot-like reaction is observed particularly around the dermal blood vessels, whereas this pattern is lost preferentially in the reticular dermis but also within the epidermis.

From these findings we conclude that T-lymphocytes leave the dermal blood vessels in resting state and are stimulated within the skin.

Beside lysosomal enzymes like ANAE, lymphocytes contain enzymes for protein degradation; among these is DAP IV, which can be demonstrated in about 50% of the peripheral blood lymphocytes (LOJDA 1977). Recently FELLER and PARWARESCH (1980a) demonstrated that DAP IV is almost selectively restricted to T_M-lymphocytes. This is true for normal and neoplastic T_M-lymphocytes (FELLER and PARWARESCH 1980b). We have shown that DAP IV can be demonstrated in the lymphocytes in mycosis fungoides (STERRY et al. 1982);

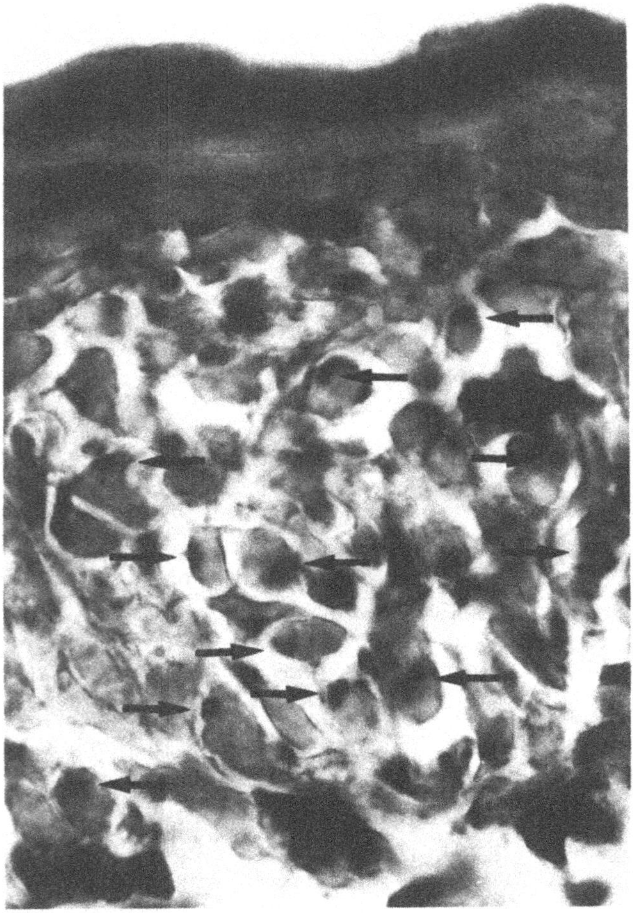

a

Fig. 16. **a** Pautrier's microabscess in an early plaque in mycosis fungoides; demonstration of ANAE. About half of the lymphocytes exhibit a dot-like reaction product (*arrows*); the remainder shows fine granular reaction products or is negative. Other cells exhibit a diffuse enzyme staining which is characteristic for cells of the monocyte-macrophage-series. **b** Dermal infiltrate of mycosis fungoides. Many lymphocytes show dot-like reaction of ANAE (*arrows*), while others show fine granules or are negative. Numerous macrophages can be identified by their diffuse staining

the percentages are similar to those obtained with dot-like ANAE (Table 5). It seems that DAP IV is lost earlier during the course of the disease than dot-like ANAE; patients with low values had longstanding disease. Within initial Pautrier's microabscesses, some lymphocytes may show DAP IV; in large microabscesses DAP IV is regularly lost. This observation is best explained by stimulation (Fig. 17a, b), because DAP IV is lost in T-lymphocytes after stimulation (STERRY et al., unpublished). The expression of HLA-DR and HLA DS as well of the transferrin receptor, which also indicates stimulation, is in good agreement with these enzyme-cytochemical findings.

Not only a change in the reaction pattern but also a complete loss of ANAE activity was observed in a patient with advanced cutaneous T cell lymphomas

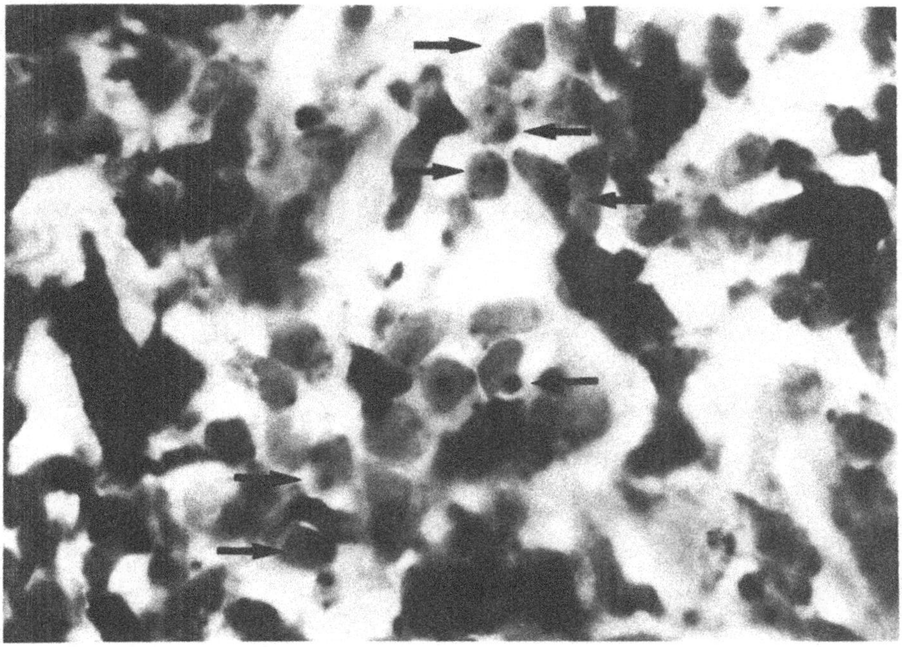

b

Table 5. Percentage of lymphocytes with dot-like ANAE-activity and DAP IV-activity in mycosis fungoides

Patient	Dot-like ANAE	DAP IV positive	Patient	Dot-like ANAE	DAP IV positive
1	61	4	7	76	67
2	81	52	8	19	19
3	44	27	9	27	30
4	72	70	10	78	11
5	38	31	11	10	9
6	17	3			

(HOLDEN et al. 1982); this most probably reflects de-differentiation and can be regarded an unfavourable prognostic sign like the appearance of immature phenotypes. We may speculate that in parallel to these events clonal markers appear in cytogenetic investigations.

3.2 Extracutaneous Manifestations

3.2.1 Lymph Nodes

Lymph node enlargement is observed in mycosis fungoides patients usually several years after onset of the skin lesions. When diagnosis is firmly established

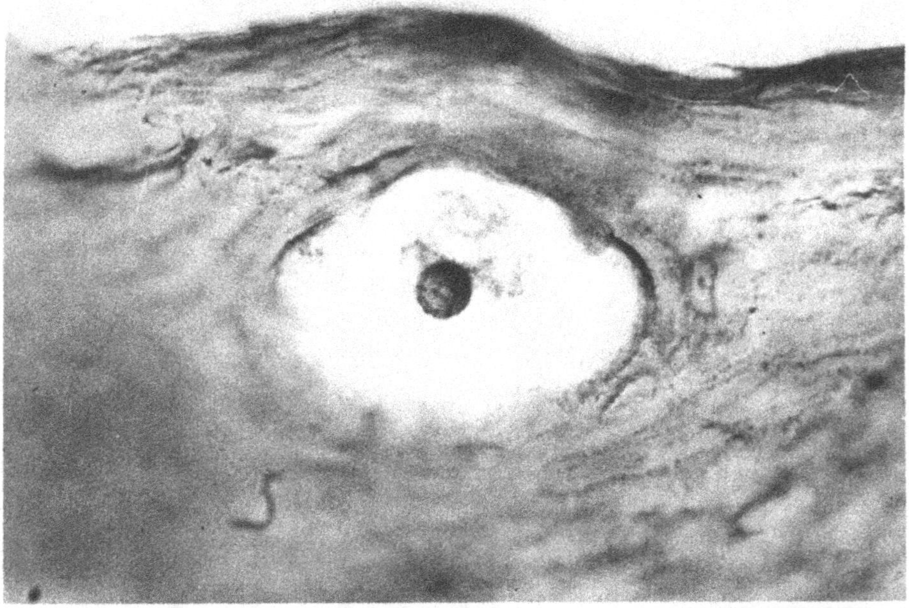

a

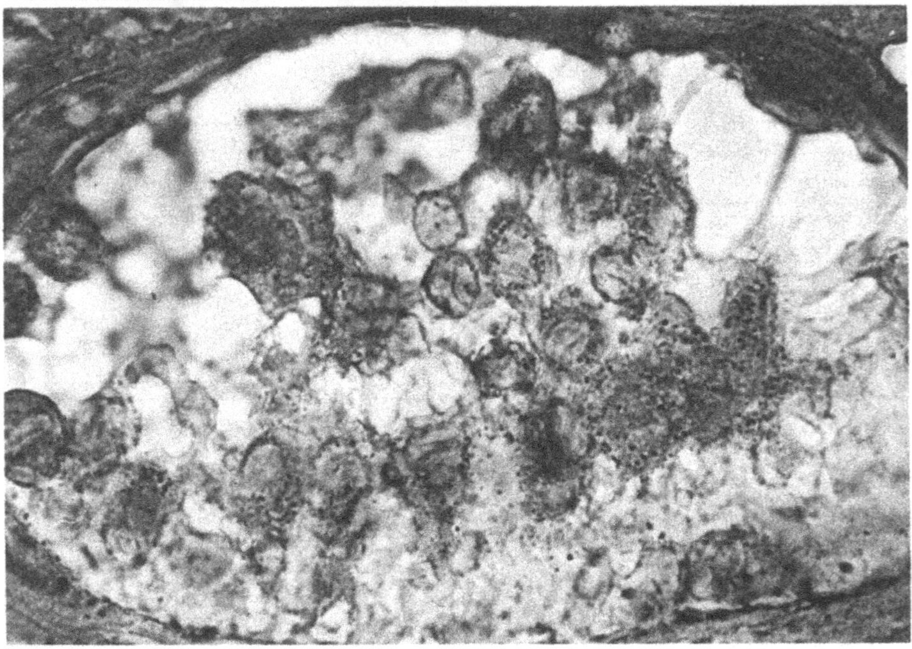

b

Fig. 17. a Early Pautrier's microabscess; demonstration of DAP IV. One lymphocyte within the early abscess shows reaction for DAP IV, and thus can be identified as T_M lymphocyte. **b** Large Pautrier's microabscess; DAP IV demonstration. All lymphocytes show a cerebriform nucleus; enzyme reaction is negative about 45% of the patients have palpable lymph nodes (Broder and Bunn 1980; Bunn et al. 1980).

Lymphadenopathy is least common in patients with limited plaques (17%) and most frequent in patients with cutaneous tumors (56%) and generalized erythroderma (79%) (Broder and Bunn 1980). Most frequently, inguinal and axillary lymph nodes are enlarged whereas nuchal, submandibular and supraclavicular lymph node regions are less frequently involved.

Excised lymph nodes seldom exceed two or three centimeters in diameter (Lennert 1978; Rappaport and Thomas 1974). Even at autopsy, lymph node conglomerates are an exception, in most cases the individual lymph nodes can be seperated easily from one another. The cut surface of fresh lymph nodes shows a graywhite tissue occasionally containing black stippling due to melanin deposits (Lennert 1978).

The involvement of lymph nodes by the specific mycosis fungoides infiltrate occurs gradually; during this process, several distinct stages may be separated according to Lennert (1978) and Scheffer, Meijer and van Vloten (1980). According to the results of these authors, we divide lymph node involvement in mycosis fungoides into five histological stages.

Dermatopathic Lymphadenopathy

Numerous pale large histiocytes are localized in the paracortical region and characterize the histological picture of dermatopathic lymphadenopathy (Pautrier and Worringer 1932). These changes are nonspecific and can be found in lymphadenopathy due to many benign dermatoses. Lymphocytes with cerebriform nuclei are present only in minimal numbers, so that by routine histology the diagnosis of mycosis fungoides cannot be established. However, cytogenetic (Huberman et al. 1979), electron microscopic (Scheffer et al. 1980), DNA-cytophotometric investigations and rosette-cytology (Huberman et al. 1979) have revealed that specific involvement is demonstrable in nearly every enlarged lymph node in mycosis fungoides.

Early Specific Involvement

Moderate amounts of small lymphocytes with cerebriform nuclei are found, intermingled mainly between the large pale histiocytes within the paracortical area. Additionally, those lymphocytes can be found within the marginal sinuses. Eosinophils may be present. If the diagnosis is suspected by the skin manifestations, routine histology with Giemsa-staining is sufficient for diagnosis.

Partial Effacement of the Lymph Node Architecture

Large clusters of small lymphocytes with cerebriform nuclei arise mainly within the paracortical area and sometimes below the marginal sinuses. There are almost always larger atypical lymphocytes with convoluted dark staining nuclei and basophilic cytoplasm, which correspond to so-called mycosis cells. Eosinophils may be numerous. In other areas of the lymph nodes, the features described for early specific involvement are present.

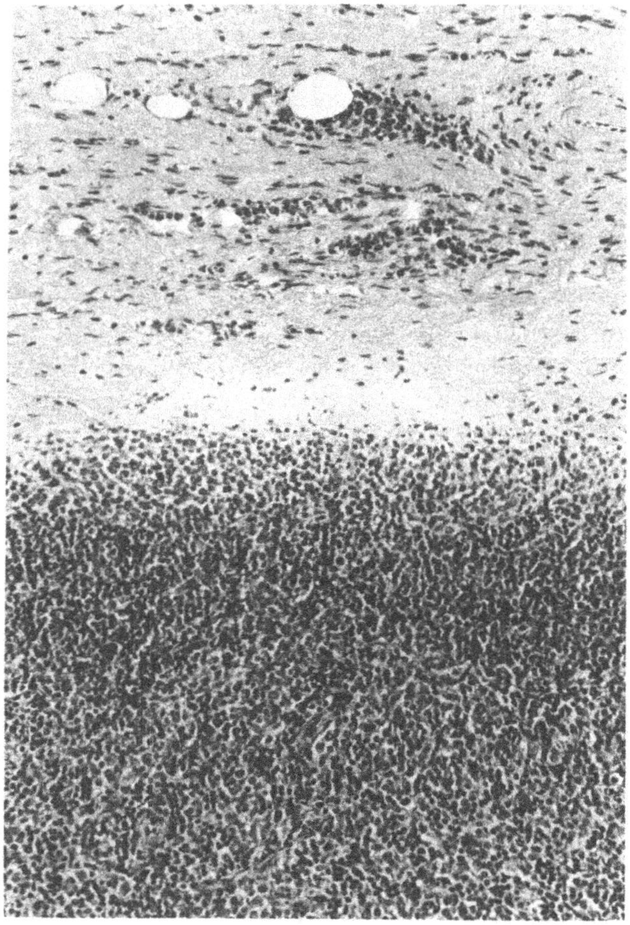

Fig. 18. Lymph node with complete effacement of the nodal architecture in mycosis fungoides. Note the infiltration of the lymph node capsule by small lymphocytes with hyperchromatic nuclei. ×16

Complete Effacement of Lymph Node Architecture

The whole lymph node is infiltrated by nodules of small lymphocytes with a cerebriform nucleus and by larger atypical mycosis cells. Lymph node histology is totally effaced. Within the nodules of such small lymphocytes numerous mitotic figures are seen (VARIOKOJIS et al. 1974). Focal areas of necrosis are frequent.

"Anaplastic" Stage

During the terminal stage of mycosis fungoides, high grade malignant lymphomas may develop (see chapter 3.2.5). In such cases, convoluted lymphoblasts or immunoblasts may be found in lymph nodes of mycosis fungoides patients.

The appearence of high grade malignant lymphomas is associated with a poor prognosis.

Subtle clues to diagnosis of mycosis fungoides lymph node involvement are the infiltration of the lymph node capsule (Fig. 18) and the absence of inflammatory changes within the lymph nodes like small germinal centers (LENNERT 1978).

3.2.2 Blood and Bone Marrow

There is considerable disagreement concerning the involvement of peripheral blood in mycosis fungoides. Whereas in the authors own patients with classical mycosis fungoides no increase in white blood count could be found, and an increase of convoluted cells above 5% was rare (3/43), many investigators from the United States describe a much higher proportion (MORAN et al. 1977; BRODER and BUNN 1980). This may be due to the fact that in United States there seems to be a greater variety of T-cell lymphomas with skin involvement which may be included in the concept of "cutaneous T cell lymphoma".

Despite these controversies blood involvement, with more than 10% of lymphocytes having a cerebriform nucleus, indicates a poor prognosis (see chapter 4). It must, however, kept in mind that in electron microscopic studies of normal peripheral blood nearly ten percent of the lymphocytes show highly convoluted nuclei (MEIJER et al. 1977).

Patients with disease limited to the skin show normal distribution of the various T-lymphocyte subsets, including E-rosettes (COOPERRIDER and ROENIGK 1978), T_M and T_G-cells (MUNSON et al. 1982), and helper- and suppressor phenotyping (CHU et al. 1983; WILLEMZE et al. 1983). The number of lymphocytes reacting with the tumour-associated antibodies BE1 and BE2 increases with duration of the disease (CHU et al. 1983a); these antibodies may therefore be of great importance in early diagnosis in mycosis fungoides.

With the appearance of tumours or internal involvement, abnormalities can be observed; these include quantitative changes due to increasing numbers of the neoplastic lymphocytes in the peripheral blood. More interesting, however, is the loss of antigens which leads to an increase of lymphocytes with OKT 3^--, 4^--, 8^--phenotype (WILLEMZE et al. 1983).

In contrast to many other malignant lymphomas, bone marrow involvement in classical mycosis fungoides is seen only in the preterminal phase; at autopsy 35 out of 97 patients had bone marrow infiltration (EPSTEIN et al. 1972; RAPPAPORT and THOMAS 1974). The distribution of the atypical lymphocytes is usually multifocal. Bone marrow involvement was not demonstrated in 17 patients in early stages (WORM et al. 1978).

3.2.3 Visceral Organs

Two larger studies concerning this topic have been published: in 1972 by EPSTEIN, LEVIN, CROFT and LUTZNER and in 1974 by RAPPAPORT and THOMAS;

Table 6. Visceral organs involved at autopsy in 66 patients. (Modified after EPSTEIN et al. 1972)

Organ	No. of patients	Organ	No. of patients
Lymph nodes	51	Kidney	23
Spleen	43	Tongue	16
Lung	37	Heart	15
Liver	35	Pancreas	15
Bone	23	Thyroid	1

the reader is referred to these papers for further details. Before this time it was believed by many pathologists and dermatologists that mycosis fungoides remained confined to the skin but could be complicated by lymphosarcomas (see CYR et al. 1966). Most frequently, spleen, lungs, liver, and kidneys are involved at autopsy (see Table 6).

Spleen. (RAPPAPORT and THOMAS 1974). A diffuse homogeneous appearance without destructive features is found most often; gross nodules are a rare observation. The histological picture shows great variability, as the white or the red pulp may be preferentially involved in different patients. Complete obliteration of the splenic architecture may also be found.

Lung (RAPPAPORT and THOMAS 1974). Involvement of the lung occurs more frequently than that of the liver (Table 6); histologically, preferential infiltration of the alveolar walls is observed. In contrast to Hodgkin's disease, contiguous extension of the disease from the tracheobrochial or bronchiopulmonary lymph nodes into the parenchyma is not observed.

Liver. Multiple nodules from one to several centimeters in diameter are frequently found at autopsy in livers with gross involvement (RAPPAPORT and THOMAS 1974). Interindividual differences were pronounced in the histological changes, varying from only periportal infiltration to nodular or diffuse infiltration of the liver parenchyma (RAPPAPORT and THOMAS 1974).

Liver biospies during staging laparoscopy have been published in two studies (GRIEM et al. 1975; HUBERMAN et al. 1980): 9 out of 57 patients showed histological involvement at time of diagnosis.

Kidney (RAPPAPORT and THOMAS 1974). 75% of kidneys with histological involvement showed macroscopically circumscribed tumors of variable size. On microscopic examination, there was interstitial infiltration of lymphocytes with preservation of both tubules and glomeruli. Sometimes, epitheliotropism to the tubular renal epithelium was observed, resembling epidermotropism in the skin.

Central nervous system. Involvement of meninges and brain is found in about 10% of cases at autopsy (EPSTEIN et al. 1972). Clinically, it may cause headache, back pain and dorsal column signs (BODENSTEINER and SKIKNE 1982). Additionally, seizures may complicate the course (WOLFF and LANDES 1984). Cranial and local radiotherapy and intrathecal methotrexate have induced a long lasting remission in one case (BODENSTEINER and SKIKNE 1982).

Other organs. Perforation of the bowel due to ulcerating tumours may complicate the course of mycosis fungoides (CAMISA and GOLDSTEIN 1981).

3.2.4 Clinical Immunology

Frank depression of the immune system in mycosis fungoides is seen mainly in patients with widespread disease and visceral involvement. In these and in patients with immunosuppression due to therapy, susceptibility to severe infections may be a clinical problem (see chapter 3.2.5.).

Intracutaneous testing of delayed type hypersensitivity and in vitro lymphocyte stimulation with T-cell mitogens have been studied by several investigators, however, with conflicting results (BLAYLOCK et al. 1966; MACKIE et al. 1976; NORDQVIST and KINNEY 1976; COOPERRIDER and ROENIGK 1978; DAVID et al. 1980; HARST-OOSTVEEN and VAN VLOTEN 1978). Summarizing all results, there is a tendency of decreasing in vitro and in vivo T-lymphocyte mediated functions with advancing disease.

Antibody-dependent cellular cytotoxicity is normal in patients with plaques (ASBELL et al. 1978), whereas natural killer cell mediated cytotoxicity was significantly lower in patients than in controls (NEILAN et al. 1983).

Lymphocytotoxic antibodies could be demonstrated in 11 out of 13 patients with mycosis fungoides in early stages (DOBORY et al. 1977; SCHOCKET et al. 1982). These lymphocytotoxic antibodies are directed against suppressor T-lymphocytes in most cases (7/9) and only rarely against helper T-lymphocytes (LEE et al. 1982). Another study has shown IgM-autoantibodies against T-lymphocytes that inhibit E-rosetting (YAMBE et al. 1981).

Serum IgE and IgA are elevated in the majority of mycosis fungoides patients (BREHM 1974; MACKIE et al. 1976; SCHLAEGER 1980). During remissions they return to normal values and increase several months before clinical signs of a relapse become evident.

Monocyte-mediated antibody-dependent cytotoxicity was found to be normal in one study (WIKLUND et al. 1979) and increased in another (KRAGBALLE et al. 1983). Granulocyte functions seems not to be altered in mycosis fungoides (HAMMINGA et al. 1982b).

3.2.5 Associated Disorders

Infections. Patients with mycosis fungoides are prone to viral infections, especially if extracutaneous involvement is present, or if immunosuppressive agents are given for therapy. Development of zoster is frequently observed, often with dissemination over the whole skin (VONDERHEID and VAN VOORST VADER 1980). Chronic herpes simplex (VONDERHEID et al. 1980) or dissemination of herpes simplex (GAHLEN-SCHULTE et al. 1982; GOLDGEIER et al. 1981; SEGAL et al. 1978) also may complicate mycosis fungoides, or had even been identified as the terminal event before systemic antiviral agents were available (EPSTEIN et al. 1972; SEGAL et al. 1978). 6 out of 86 patients autopsied by EPSTEIN et al. (1972) showed cytomegalovirus-infection. Widespread bacterial and mycotic infections have been found in 66% of 86 autopsied patients at post-mortem examination; most frequently, staphylococci, pseudomonas, yeasts and aspergillus were isolated (EPSTEIN et al. 1972).

Secondary malignancies. Four aetiological factors may be responsible for the frequent occurence of malignancies in mycosis fungoides. (1) Malignancies due to fortituous coincidence or due to a genetic susceptibility to cancer development, (2) malignancies due to immunodeficiency in the late stages, (3) malignancies due to the immunoregulatory functions of the mycosis fungoides lymphocytes, and (4) malignancies due to systemic or topical chemotherapy.

There are numerous reports on malignancies arising in patients with mycosis fungoides (reviewed by OLSEN et al. 1984); most frequently, carcinomas of various origin and leukaemias were observed. A history of cancer in a first-degree relative was reported in 30% of the mycosis fungoides patients; this strongly suggests a genetic predisposition to cancer in these families (GREEN et al. 1979).

Concurrent development of Hodgkin's disease and mycosis fungoides may be fortitious, although common aetiological factors have been suspected (LIPA et al. 1982; CAYA et al. 1984).

Kaposi's sarcoma develops in patients with immunodeficiency (see DAUL and DESHAZO 1983) or immunosuppression (GAUGE and JONES 1978). Its appearance in patients with mycosis fungoides has repeatedly been observed (see OLSEN et al. 1984), arising before, concurrently with or after the onset of mycosis fungoides. It then may be due to immune defects in late mycosis fungoides (see chapter 3.2.4) or immunesuppressive effects of therapy.

The same may be true in the development of high grade malignant lymphomas of T-immunoblastic or T-lymphoblastic type in late stages of mycosis fungoides (BÜCHNER and RUFLI 1979).

The malignant lymphocytes are phenotypically helper-T-cells (see chapter 5). Several observations of autoimmune haemolytic anemia (WHITE et al. 1984), monoclonal gammopathies (RUFFIEUX et al. 1984), mediterranean lymphoma (CASSUTO et al. 1981) or multiple myeloma (Bryant) in mycosis fungoides have been interpreted as the result of the chronic stimulation of the B-cell system.

In a series of 63 patients with cutaneous T cell lymphomas, seven developed a second malignancy; these patients had more chemotherapy than the others (OLSEN et al. 1984). All myelogenous and myelomonocytic leukaemias in mycosis fungoides patients occured after chemotherapy (OLSEN et al. 1984; WADELL et al. 1982). This is in concordance with similar observations in patients treated for Hodgkin's disease (COLEMAN et al. 1977).

4. Prognostic Signs and Staging Investigations

As has already been pointed out, the natural history of mycosis fungoides is that of initial cutanous manifestation and subsequent involvement of the whole organism. It is evident that prognosis beomes poorer during the natural course of the disease and therefore evaluation of the stage of disease in an individual patient will give us information on his prognosis. Moreover, patients with more advanced disease will not respond to therapies which are highly effective in early stages of mycosis fungoides. Therefore, careful examination of the patient will not only have prognostic implications, but also will influence the choice

Table 7. Staging of mycosis fungoides

Classi-fication	Description
T: Skin	
T_0	Clinically and/or histopathologically suggestive lesions
T_1	Limited plaques, papules, or eczematous patches covering 10% of the skin surface
T_2	Generalized plaques, papules, or erythematous patches covering 10% of the skin surface
T_3	Tumours
T_4	Generalized erythroderma
N: Lymph nodes	
N_0	No clinically abnormal peripheral lymph nodes, pathology negative for MF
N_1	Clinically abnormal peripheral lymph nodes, pathology negative for MF
N_2	No clinically abnormal peripheral lymph nodes, pathology positive for MF
N_3	Clinically abnormal peripheral lymph nodes, pathology positive for MF
B: Peripheral blood	
B_0	Atypical circulating cells not present (5%)
B_1	Atypical circulating cells present (>5%); record total WBC and total lymphocyte counts and number of atypical cells/100 lymphocytes
M: Visceral organs	
M_0	No visceral organ involvement
M_1	Visceral involvement (must have pathology confirmation and organ involved should be specified)

of therapy. Moreover, staging procedures are indispensible for control of therapeutic efficacy and follow up of treated patients. Among the numerous clinical manifestations of the disease there are some that have been shown to be of prognostic importance, and which will be discussed in this chapter.

In 1975 the Mycosis Fungoides Cooperative Study Group (LAMBERG et al. 1975) proposed a modification of the Tumour-Node-Metastasis (TNM)-system for mycosis fungoides (Table 7). According to this TNM-classification staging of the patients can be performed (Tables 7 and 8). This classification and staging system has been shown to be of prognistic significance (see below); it is logical and reproducable and has been adopted by the EORTC project group Cutaneous Lymphomas.

4.1 Skin Manifestations

Nearly all large retrospective and prospective studies, mainly performed in the United States of America, demonstrate that increasing skin involvement is asso-

Table 8. Staging classification of CTCL

Stage	Classification		
	T	N	M
IA	1	0	0
IB	2	0	0
IIA	1–2	1	0
IIB	3	0–1	0
III	4	0–1	0
IVA	1–4	2–3	0
IVB	1–4	0–3	1

ciated with worsening of prognosis, i.e. shortening of the mean survival time (BUNN et al. 1980; BRODER and BUNN 1980; COHEN et al. 1980; EPSTEIN et al. 1972; FUKS et al. 1973; GREEN et al. 1981; HAMMINGA et al. 1982a; KNOTH 1976; LAMBERG et al. 1979). Eczematous or plaque lesions involving less than 10% of the skin surface (T_1) without extracutaneous involvement indicates a very good prognosis: the mean five year survival rate is more than 90% (see BRODER and BUNN 1980). The prognosis decreases if more than 10% of the skin surface (T_2) is involved (5 year survival rate 70%), and becomes even poorer when tumours (T_3) or erythroderma (T_4) develop (five year survival 40%) (see BRODER and BUNN 1980) (Fig. 19a).

Examination of mycosis fungoides patients must therefore include an exact description of cutaneous findings; (Table 7); this is best performed using standardized photography or by schematic drawings.

Stages T_1 to T_4 must be confirmed histologically. If several variables are present simultaneously, the highest must be used for staging.

4.2 Lymph Nodes and Blood

Lymph nodes. Enlargement of lymph nodes is associated with pronounced impairment of prognosis: mean survival time is 10 years in patients with skin involvement only, in contrast to three years when lymph nodes are palpable (BRODER and BUNN 1980; EPSTEIN et al. 1972; GREEN et al. 1981; LAMBERG et al. 1979) (Fig. 19d).

Two other lymph node variables also influence prognosis: the number of enlarged lymph nodes and lymph node histology. Patients with only one lymph node have a better prognosis when compared with those with two to four enlarged lymph nodes; mean survival time decreases further when more than five lymph nodes are palpable (GREEN et al. 1981; LAMBERG et al. 1979). Lymph node histology gives important prognostic information (Fig. 19b); it must be stressed that nonpalpable lymph nodes that have been excised and that show specific involvement indicate a decrease of mean survival time when compared with enlarged lymph nodes with nonspecific pathological changes (see BRODER and BUNN 1980) (Fig. 19b).

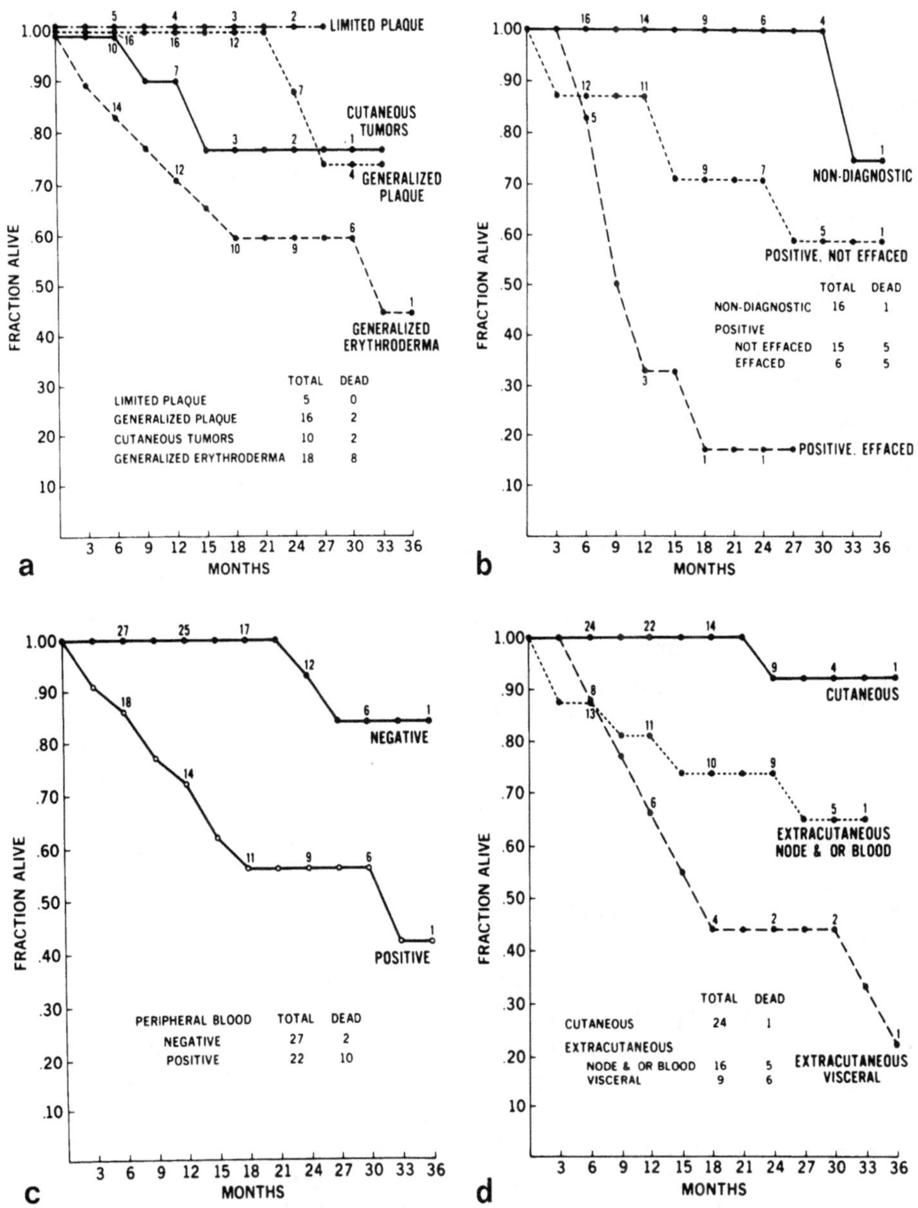

Fig. 19. a Actuarial survival of patients by skin stage. **b** Actuarial survival of patients with and without peripheral blood involvement by light microscopy. **c** Actuarial survival of patients on basis of lymph histology by light microscopy. **d** Actuarial survival of patients with disease confined to the skin, with extracutaneous disease confined to lymph nodes or peripheral blood, and with extracutaneous disease in visceral sites. (From BUNN et al. 1980; Annals of Internal Medicine *93*, 223–230, 1980; with kind permission)

The following investigations seem advisable for correct assessment of lymph node involvement in a given patient at the initial examination (Table 9): careful clinical palpation of axillary, inguinal, supraclavicular nuchal and submandibular lymph node groups. Excision of palpable lymph nodes with preference of other regions than the inguinal region. If there are no palpable lymph nodes,

Table 9. Staging investigations in mycosis fungoides (investigations for scientific purposes not included)

I. Diagnosis

A. Complete history and physical examination (see text)

B. Multiple skin biopsies including Epon-embedded and snap-frozen specimens

C. Laboratory investigations:
WBC, including percentage of atypical lymphocytes
Serum chemistry
Quantitative immunoglobulins

II. Extent of disease

A. Biopsy of enlarged lymph nodes (including snap-frozen material)

B. Biopsies from enlarged liver or spleen

C. chest-X-ray

excision of one lymph node from the axillary region by a skilled surgeon may be considered. Staging is performed according to Table 7. Lymphangiography and lymphadenopathy will not provide further informations and are not necessary during routine staging investigations. It has been argued that lymphadenography may reveal enlarged lymph nodes in the para-aortic and para-iliac regions (FUKS et al. 1974). However, isolated enlargement of these lymph nodes is rare and the prognostic significance uncertain. A more recent study showed that only 20 out of 31 patients with clinically enlarged lymph nodes had abnormal lymphadenography; all 13 patients without palpable lymph nodes had normal lymphadenography (HUBERMAN et al. 1979). These results were confirmed by CASTELLINO et al. (1979).

Blood. The Mycosis Fungoides Cooperative Group (BUNN et al. 1979) has added to their TNM-classification a B-(blood) category to indicate peripheral blood involvement; more than 5% atypical lymphocytes within peripheral blood smears stained by Pappenheim's technique are stated to be B I (see Table 7). Presence of lymphocytes with a cerebriform nucleus (Sézary cells; Lutzner cells) in peripheral blood smears is associated with an unfavourable prognosis: the mean survival time is only 12 months (BRODER and BUNN 1980; COHEN et al. 1980; EPSTEIN et al. 1972; GREEN et al. 1981; LAMBERG et al. 1979). This criterion has also been shown to be of prognostic importance in a prospective study (BUNN et al. 1980) (Fig. 19c). Moreover, patients with high percentages of circulating Sézary cells have a shorter survival time than those with lower percentages (VONDERHEID et al. 1979).

It must be repeated at this point, that in classical mycosis fungoides in Europe frank involvement of peripheral blood is unusual. Furthermore, it must be kept in mind that about 5% of peripheral blood lymphocytes in healthy persons show cerebriform nuclear contours in electron microscopic studies (MEIJER et al. 1977), so that this criterion probably needs further investigation.

For staging investigations total white blood cell and total lymphocyte counts and the number of atypical lymphocytes/100 lymphocytes should be recorded (see Table 6).

4.3 Visceral Organs

In general, involvement of viscera is associated with the very short survival time of approximately six months (COHEN et al. 1980; EPSTEIN et al. 1972) (Fig. 19d).

Spleen. The visceral organ most often involved in mycosis fungoides is the spleen (EPSTEIN et al. 1972) (Table 6). Splenomegaly represents a poor prognostic sign (COHEN et al. 1980; EPSTEIN et al. 1972). Szintigrams of the spleen are not helpful in early diagnosis of spleen enlargement (KLEIN 1976).

Liver. Specific infiltration of the periportal areas occurs many months before hepatomegaly becomes clinically evident, and is present in 15% of mycosis fungoides patients histological at the time of primary diagnosis (HUBERMAN et al. 1980). This percentage is even higher when liver biopsies are performed under sight during laparoscopy (HUBERMAN et al. 1980). Histological involvement of the liver without clinical enlargement, however, is not of prognostic importance; therefore, during routine staging procedures liver biopsies are not mandatory (Table 9).

If spleen or liver enlargement, have been found during the clinical examination, histological verification of specific involvement must be demanded (Table 9).

Bone marrow. Even in advanced mycosis fungoides the bone marrow usually is spared (KLEIN 1976; WORM et al. 1978). Bone marrow aspiration smears or biopsies are not therefore included in routine mycosis fungoides staging programs, and may be reserved for special cases (WORM et al. 1978). Involvement of viscera is recorded within the M-category.

After completion of the staging evaluations patients are categorized into the appropriate stage, as outlined in Table 8 (LAMBERG et al. 1979).

The recommended staging investigations are summarized in Table 9.

5. Cytogenetic Studies

There are several studies available concerning the DNA- content and chromosome analysis in mycosis fungoides lymphocytes. Using different techniques, the results obtained by the various study groups can be summarized as follows:

1. Early mycosis fungoides does not show any detectable DNA or chromosome aberrations.
2. Patients with more disseminated disease, usually beginning with generalized plaque lesions, show DNA abnormalities in most cases however, without clone formation.
3. Patients in the late stages of mycosis fungoides may have demonstrable clones, which can be observed in various organs simultaneously. Occurence of a clone in a given patient is associated with a change in histology (mainly "large cell" histology) and a poor prognosis.

Three different techniques for DNA- and chromosome analysis have been applied in mycosis fungoides: Feulgen DNA-cytophotometry, flow cytophotometry and chromosome-banding of metaphase-arrested lymphocytes.

Feulgen-DNA-cytophotometry can be regarded as abnormal if more than 5% of the cells within a dermal infiltrate show hyperdiploid DNA-distribution (VAN VLOTEN et al. 1974). All patients with proven mycosis fungoides (plaques and tumors) had abnormal DNA-histograms with more than 5% of the cells in the tetraploid and hypertetraploid region (VAN VLOTEN et al. 1974). 8 out of 15 patients which were suspected of having early mycosis fungoides had abnormal DNA-histograms; six from these eight developed mycosis fungoides or malignant reticulosis within one year (VAN VLOTEN et al. 1974).

In contrast, HAGEDORN and KIEFER (1977) were not able to isolate enough cells on imprints from large plaques parapsoriasis to perform DNA-measurements; moreover, they could not demonstrate DNA-abnormalities in two patients with plaques in mycosis fungoides, whereas in tumours the abnormal DNA distribution was confirmed (HAGEDORN and KIEFER 1977). Simultaneous enzyme cytochemistry confirmed that DNA-abnormalities were confined to the lymphocytes, whereas histiocytes were normal.

Feulgen-DNA-cytophotometry also seems to be of value in examination of enlarged lymph nodes with nonspecific histology; VAN VLOTEN et al. (1979) found abnormal DNA-histograms in 11 out of 22 of such lymph nodes. Abnormal histograms were associated with an unfavourable course.

A major limitation of Feulgen-DNA-cytophotometry is the fact that only a moderate number of cells can be analyzed. In contrast, with flow-DNA-cytophotometry larger numbers of cells can be measured. Using this technique, skin biopsies (LANGE WANTZIN et al. 1983) and lymph node and peripheral blood samples (BUNN et al. 1980) were investigated. The study from BUNN et al. suggested that in early mycosis fungoides no DNA abnormalities could be detected in lymph nodes or peripheral blood; with increasing duration discrete chromosomal abnormalities appear which could be identified by widened G_1 peaks; this corresponds to chromosome numbers from 41 to 48 in simultaneous cytogenetic studies. Late in the disease discrete aneuploid peaks appeared. These three stages were associated with decreasing prognosis. In contrast, LANGE-WANTZIN et al. (1983) observed discrete aneuploid peaks in 4 out of 6 patients with T_0 skin lesions. Further studies are needed to clarify these discrepancies.

The most sensitive of these techniques for DNA analysis is cytogenetic investigation by Giemsa-banding of metaphase chromosomes. Patients with extracutaneous dissemination always have demonstrable abnormal karyotypes (ERKMAN-BALIS and RAPPAPORT 1974). In these patients, individual lymphocytes of the same patient may show hyper-, hypodiploidia, chromosome translocations, trisomia or chromosome defects (BUNN et al. 1980; EDELSON et al. 1979; ERKMAN-BALIS and RAPPAPORT 1974; FUKUHARA et al. 1978; NOWELL et al. 1982; VAN VLOTEN et al. 1980; WHANG-PENG et al. 1982). Chromosome 1 is most frequently involved in structural abnormalities, while chromosomes 21 and 22 are most frequently involved in numerical abnormalities (WHANG-PENG et al. 1982).

Clone formation was seen only in patients with advanced clinical disease (EDELSON et al. 1979; WHANG-PENG et al. 1982). Clone formation is associated with change to "large cell" histology and poor prognosis (BUNN et al. 1982; WHANG-PENG et al. 1982). Evaluation of the data from the American literature is difficult, because Sézary syndrome, other T-cell lymphomas and mycosis fungoides are mixed up within the category of cutaneous T-cell lymphoma.

One finding of great importance for our understanding of the pathogenesis of mycosis fungoides is the fact that lymphocytes with DNA- abnormalities may occur in a high percentage in the peripheral blood without corresponding numbers of cerebriform lymphocytes (BUNN et al. 1980; VAN VLOTEN et al. 1980). This finding together with the observations of BERGER et al. (1982) that 20 to 40% of lymphocytes within the peripheral blood react with BE 1 and BE 2 without a similar number of lymphocytes with a cerebriform nucleus deserve further investigation. It can, however, concluded from these studies that in advanced mycosis fungoides there are lymphocytes within the peripheral blood that exhibit clear markers of the disease (i.e. DNA-abnormalities and tumour associated antigens) without showing a cerebriform nucleus, which is always regarded as constant marker of the malignant lymphocytes in mycosis fungoides.

6. Etiology and Pathogenesis

The aetiology of mycosis fungoides is still unknown. There are several studies that suggest that genetic, infectious, or chemical (including environmental) factors might be responsible for the development of the disease.

Genetic factors are suggested by the occurrence of familial mycosis fungoides; in the literature six families are documented, in which there were at least two members affected by mycosis fungoides. These reports include mycosis fungoides in siblings as well as in parents and their children (GREENE et al. 1979; SANDBANK and KATZENELLENBOGEN 1968; SHELLEY 1980; KAMERON 1933). Genetic factors are additionally suggested by the excessive frequency of HLA-antigens AW 31 and AW 32 (MACKIE et al. 1976).

C-type-virus-like particles have been demonstrated in skin biopsies and lymph nodes from patients with mycosis fungoides (VAN DER LOO et al. 1979). To date, these observations have not been confirmed, nor are there, at the moment, other hints for the viral aetiology of mycosis fungoides.

The relationship between occupational or environmental factors and mycosis fungoides has been stressed by several recent investigations. GREENE et al. (1979) found a high incidence of employment in a manufacturing occupation, especially petrochemical, textile, metal and machinery industries. The same study found elevated mycosis fungoides mortality rates in counties where petroleum, rubber, primary and fabricated metal, machinery and printing industries were located. COHEN et al. (1980) compared patients with age- and sex-matched controls and found a statistically significant correlation between industrial exposure and mycosis fungoides. Similar results were obtained by FISCHMANN et al. (1979), who reported exposure to potential carcinogenic agents in 91% of the patients. The most common chemicals were air pollutants (39%) pesticides (36%), solvents and vapors (30%) and detergents and desinfectants (14%). Development of mycosis fungoides was reported in a patient after use of thorotrast (a substance formerly used for contrasting in angiography until it became evident that thorotrast induced liver hemangiosarcomas); in this patient mycosis fungoides terminated in a high grade malignant lymphoma (HUNDEIKER et al. 1968). The occupational exposure to carcinogenic substances is a general problem which is not only importand for mycosis fungoides and which deserves further intensive investigations.

The fact that mycosis fungoides represents a fascinating disease entity is also documented by the numerous hypotheses concerning its pathogenesis that have been proposed. One of the classic models concerning the pathogenesis of mycosis fungoides is based on the clinical observation that many patients have a history of preexisting skin disorders, most often eczemas (STEIGLEDER 1974; STEIGLEDER 1976; SCHUPPLI 1976). In these theories, chronic antigen persistance leads to a continuous stimulation of the lymphocytes within the skin, which eventually leads to malignant transformation. If some of the lymphocytes are altered by viral infection, malignant transformations may occur even more readily (STEIGLEDER 1976). The demonstration of C-type virus-like partikels in Langerhans-cells in mycosis fungoides (VAN DER LOO et al. 1979) gave rise to the hypothesis that the initial event in mycosis fungoides might be viral infection of epidermal Langerhans cells (MACKIE 1981). These virus infected Langerhans cells would then continuously stimulate T-lymphocytes within the epidermis, until malignant degeneration of such chronically stimulated lymphocytes occurs. The view that Langerhans cells are of pathogenetic importance is also favored by ROWDEN and LEWIS (1976).

Normal epidermis generates a lot of soluble factors which influence immigrating lymphocytes. Among these are epidermal cell thymocyte activating factor (ETAF), that has been studied by LUGER et al. (1981) and by SAUDER et al. (1981), which is analagous to interleukin I, and a thymopoietin-like substance which can also be found in the epidermal keratinocytes (CHU et al. 1982). If these factors were produced abnormally, they could lead to pathological lymphocyte reactions, which finally might terminate in a malignant disease. Moreover, the enzyme terminal deoxynucleotidyltransferase (TdT) is expressed in human lymphocytes during co-cultivation with epidermal cells (RUBENFELD et al. 1981). TdT may act as a somatic mutagen, and may be responsable for be diversification of the T-cell antigen receptors. PATTERSON and EDELSON (1982) suggested that under abnormal circumstances the induction of TdT could lead to alterations of DNA and by this way to the generation of malignant T-cells.

The appearance of interdigitating reticulum cells, which are responsible for the homing of T-lymphocytes to the T-cell areas of lymph nodes within the skin could also serve as a possible explanation for the T-lymphocyte infiltrate in mycosis fungoides (GOOS 1976).

Another interesting aspect of the pathogenesis of mycosis fungoides represents the expression of class II major histocompatibility antigens on keratinocytes. TJERNLUND (1978) was the first to demonstrate that HLA-DR β-chains are expressed on the keratinocyte surface during the course of mycosis fungoides. As we have shown, HLA-SB-antigens are expressed as well (see chapter 3.1.2). These observations are important in two directions. First, the expression of class II HLA-antigens may lead to immunological reactions between lymphocytes and keratinocytes. This view would be supported by the report of PRICE and MIRKOVICH (1978). These authors cultured keratinocytes from diseased and uninvolved skin from patients with mycosis fungoides in the stages T1, T2 and T3. When lymphocytes from the same patients were added to this culture system lymphocytotoxicity with lysis of the keratinocytes from diseased skin was observed in patients with plaques and tumours. Recently it has been demonstrated that the T4-antigen on the T-lymphocyte surface is involved in the recognition of class II HLA antigens (BIDDISON et al. 1984). This constellation may be responsible for the degeneration of keratinocytes within Pautriers microabscesses, which are in close contact with Langerhans cells and lymphocytes (SCHMITT and THIVOLET 1980). Pathogenetically it is of great interest that class II HLA antigens are also expressed on keratinocytes in chronic graft versus host (gvh) disease (VOLC-PLATZER et al. 1984). In gvh-disease the donor lymphocytes attack the structures of the host; during this process class II histocompatibility antigens are expressed. It might be possible that the infiltrating lymphocytes in mycosis fungoides are an expression of an autoimmune phenomenon which, secondarily, leads to expression of class II histocompatibility antigens and subsequent degeneration of keratinocytes in Pautrier's microabscesses. Because lymphocyte chromosome abnormalities can be detected very early in disease (LANGE-WANTZIN et al. 1983) it may be speculated that lymphocytes are the primary cell-system disturbed in mycosis fungoides.

7. Therapy

7.1 PUVA-Therapy

PUVA-therapy of mycosis fungoides represents one of the most important treatment modalities. It was first used in the dermatology department of Wuppertal, West Germany, by MORTAZAWI and OBERSTE-LEHN (1972), using topical psoralen and UVA. Others supported their observation that topical PUVA-therapy induces remissions in mycosis fungoides and is equally effective in relapses (TRONNIER and LOEHNING 1974; WEBER 1975; FISCHER and SKOGH 1979).

Oral administration of psoralen together with subsequent UVA irradation undoubtedly improved the efficacy of therapy in mycosis fungoides (GILCHREST et al. 1976; HÖNIGSMANN et al. 1976; ROENIGK 1976) because clinically only slightly involved areas were also treated and psoralen reaches the dermis, in contrast to the effects of topical application. Several groups from all parts of the world confirmed and extended these findings (HJORTSHOJ and SCHMIDT 1977; HODGE et al. 1977; HÖNIGSMANN et al. 1984; HOFMANN et al. 1977; KONRAD et al. 1977; KONRAD et al. 1978; LOWE et al. 1979; OBERSTE-LEHN 1980; ROENIGK 1977; WARIN 1981; WOLFF 1978).

According to these studies PUVA-therapy is highly effective in stage IA, IB and probably IIA, regarding induction and duration of remissions. Eczematous and plaque lesions respond in nearly all patients.

Several follow up studies (GILCHREST 1979; HÖNIGSMANN et al. 1984; MOLIN et al. 1981a; ROENIGK 1977; WARIN 1981) indicate that most of the patients with early mycosis fungoides can be kept in remission for up to seven years.

According to the results of Hönigsmann et al. (1984) maintainance therapy is not necessary. There is agreement among all investigators that relapses respond as well to PUVA as the initial lesions; PUVA treatment may be repeated many times. Despite the good responses in early mycosis fungoides, in terms of duration of remissions PUVA-therapy must be regarded as less effective when tumours are present or lymph nodes and visceral organs are involved (Gilchrest 1979; Hönigsmann et al. 1984; Molin et al. 1981 b; Roenigk 1977; Warin 1981).

In these stages a progression of subcutaneous or visceral mycosis fungoides has been reported despite clearing of cutaneous lesions (Fischer et al. 1978; Molin et al. 1978).

Apart from the possible curative effect of PUVA treatment in early stages, another indication is stressed by many authors: adjunct therapy during systemic or topical chemotherapy, and therapy of relapses after all sorts of treatments. Its effectiveness may be enhanced by additional local application of meladinine.

Two mycosis fungoides-specific *side-effects* of PUVA-therapy should be mentioned. A clinical phenomenon that may cause irritation of the patient is worsening of lesions during the initial treatment period (Hönigsmann et al. 1984). Additionally, in appearantly uninvolved skin "new" patches may develop. This phenomenon of unmasking early lesions is transitory, but the patient should be prepared.

Patients with mycosis fungoides often show PUVA-erythema at low doses of UVA. This is due to increased UVA-sensitivity in mycosis fungoides (Volden and Thune 1977; Volden 1980). PUVA phototoxicity testing (Gschnait 1982) therefore is mandatory before starting this therapy.

During PUVA treatment new lesions may develop at sites not sufficiently reached by UVA irridiation (sanctuary sites, i.e. groins, perianal region, interdigital spaces, eyelides or the submammary region) (du Vivier and Vollum 1980). Such lesions may respond to additional therapy as local glucocorticoids or local nitrogen mustard application (du Vivier and Vollum 1980); sensitization to nitrogen mustard is, however, not prevented by concurrent PUVA treatment. Care must been taken to check the possibility that subcutaneous or visceral spread may occur despite clinical clearing of the skin lesions (Fischer et al. 1978; Molin et al. 1978; Tourbier and Schultze-Ehrenburg 1981).

At present there is no clear understanding of the action mechanism of PUVA in mycosis fungoides; however, its effects are mainly limited to those parts of the skin reached by UVA. Possible mechanisms are reduction of number and/or function of Langerhans cells (Stingl et al. 1981; Aberer et al. 1981), toxicity for T-lymphocytes (Lischka et al. 1977) or alteration of keratinocyte surface or mediator production (Sauder et al. 1983), just to mention a few. Depressed delayed type of hypersensitivity may recover during PUVA-therapy (Kubba et al. 1979).

7.2 Total Skin X-Ray and Electron Beam Irradiation Therapy

Total skin X-ray therapy has been used for treatment of mycosis fungoides since the turn of the century (Scholz 1902). Scholz reported that several patches

Table 10. Therapy studies with ERBT in mycosis fungoides. (After HERBST and MÜLLER 1984; with kind permission of the authors)

Author	Electron energy	Dose fractions	Duration of the study	No. of patients
TRUMP et al., Boston	2.5	1400 rad/10 weeks	1953	4
SMEDAL et al., Boston	2.5	600 or 800 rad within 8 or 10 days 600/750/900/1200 rad to 2000 rad	1951–1960	220
Lo et al., Burlington	3.5	800 rad/15 days	1964–1973	200
FUKS et al., Stanford	2.5	3000 rad/40 days	1957–1968	107
HOPPE et al., Stanford	2.5	3000–3600 rad/8–9 weeks	1966–1977	222
	4 (since 72)	1000 rad		18
		1000–2000 rad		46
		3000 rad		97
VAN VLOTEN et al., Leiden	4	2800–3500 rad/10 weeks	1975–1982	23
BUNN et al., NCI, Washington	3.2	2400–3000 rad/6–10 weeks	1975–1982	39
WALLNER et al., Philadelphia	3.8	2500–3000 rad/8 weeks	1975–1977	30
MEYLER et al., San Francisco	3.0	3000 rad/5 weeks	1971–1976	39
WILLIAMS et al., Manchester	3.0	2400 rad/18 days	1979	21
NISCE et al., New York	2.5/3.5	3000 rad/60 days	1973	21
HERBST, Erlangen	5/7	3600 rad/30 days	1979–1982	11

of mycosis fungoides showed ulceration after large doses of x-rays, healed afterwards and did not show any signs of recurrence. However, new patches and plaques appeared at nonirradiated sites in the same patient. Today, there are two main indications for x-ray therapy in mycosis fungoides. 1. Total skin radiation with teleroentgen or low voltage x-ray in patients with patches or plaques; 2. local irradiation of plaques or tumours resistant to other therapies.

Total skin teleroentgen therapy with 300 to 900 rad gives 100% remissions in patients with stage IA and IB, with almost no subjective side effects (WISKEMANN and BUCK 1978). After 1 year, 51% have relapsed, and after 4 years only 20.5% of these patients are still free of disease (WISKEMANN and BUCK 1978). Several techniques for total body x-ray irradiation have been described; details of the two most commonly used are given by LUKACS and BRAUN-FALCO (1973) and WISKEMANN and BUCK (1978).

Total-skin electron-beam radiation therapy (total skin EBRT) became possible after detection of the therapeutic effect of accelerated electrons for superficial neoplasia (TRUMP et al. 1940). After more than 10 years of experimental work at the High Voltage Research Laboratory (Cambridge, Massachusetts), in 1951 a large therapy-study was initiated, which was published in 1962 and comprised 220 patients with mycosis fungoides (SMEDAL et al. 1962). These authors used low megavolt (2.5 mV) electron therapy giving a total dose of 600 to 800 rad within 8 to 10 days. Initial remission was induced in nearly all patients; the survival rate within the different stages could not be evaluated properly because

Table 11. Comparison of x-ray and electron-beam radiation therapy of mycosis fungoides

	X-rays	Electrons
Tissue energy distribution	Moderate decrease of the dose in subcutaneous fat	Rapid dose decrease in subcutaneous fat
Therapeutic activity in mycosis fungoides	Good	Good
Technical difficulties	Low	High
Centers with technical equipment	Many	Few
Costs	Relatively low	High
Outpatient treatment possible	Yes	Yes

Table 12. Side effects and complications of total-skin x-ray and electron-beam irradiation therapy of mycosis fungoides

Cutaneous atrophy, radiation dermatitis, teleangiectasies
Hyper- and hypopigmentation
Hair loss, Loss of sweat glands, Nail shedding } more pronounced in EBRT
General cutaneous discomfort
Gynaecomastia
Overdosage in overlapping areas: prolonged bandlike dermatitis and pain
Underdosage in overlapping areas: bandlike relapses in overlapping areas (Fig. 20)
Underdosage in subcutaneous fat: relapses as subcutaneous mycosis fungoides (PROCTOR et al. 1978)
Induction of malignant skin tumors (WRIGHT and KENNEDY 1984)

of technical problems in follow up. Further refinement of total skin EBRT was achieved at Standford University. FUKS and BAGSHAW (1971) demonstrated that disease-free survival after the first treatment with electrons is stage-dependent; 80% of the patients with limited plaques and eczematous lesions (stage IA) showed complete remissions for up to 10 years; in patients with tumors, however, less than 10% of the patients remained in complete remissions for such a long period. The dose given as initial therapy was increased up to 3600 rad and administered within 2 to 3 months (MINNA et al. 1979). Several other groups confirmed these findings (see Table 10).

When conventional total skin x-ray therapy and total skin EBRT are compared, it becomes evident, that with corresponding doses both therapy modalities are comparable as to their therapeutic efficacy; both techniques have advan-

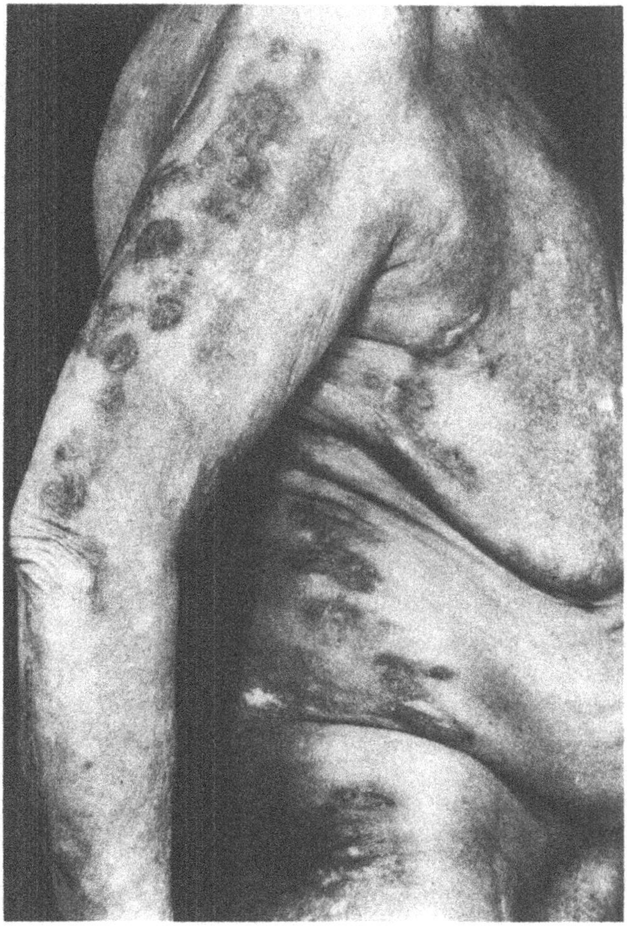

Fig. 20. Relapse of mycosis fungoides after EBRT treatment. The relapse is confined to those sites where underdosage due to tangential irradiation was present. Patient from the Department of Dermatology in Köln. (Prof. Dr. G.K. STEIGLEDER)

tages and disadvantages (Table 11), and choice of one or the other should be done according to the local facilities. Side effects of both techniques are summarized in Table 12.

7.3 Topical Chemotherapy

Topical application of mechlorethamine has been used since 30 years in mycosis fungoides (SIPOS 1956; HASERIK et al. 1959). Most experience with this therapy was gathered in United States, while it was used only sporadically by European dermatologists. Although mechlorethamine is principally effective in early mycosis fungoides, several problems concerning its application have prevented worldwide acceptance.

Like all alkylating agents, mechlorethamine forms strong covalent bonds with various nucleic acids, (CALABRESI and PARKS 1980). The antiproliferative effect seems not to be important in mycosis fungoides, as the proliferation rate is relatively low (see chapter 3.1.2). Mechlorethamine is a potent contact sensitizing agent, and immunological mechanisms probably mediate the action of mechlorethamine in mycosis fungoides (PRICE et al. 1977; VONDERHEID 1984).

In stages I A and I B, initial partial or complete remission is achieved in more than 80% of the patients; complete remissions with maintainance therapy for longer periods are achieved in 40–60% of patients in stage I A and B (MOLIN et al. 1979; VONDERHEID et al. 1979; HAMMINGA et al. 1982c; PRICE et al. 1977; PRICE et al. 1983; VONDERHEID 1984). In extracutaneous mycosis fungoides, topical mechlorethamine has no effect (PRICE et al. 1982; RICE et al. 1983). Most centers use the application method developed by VAN SCOTT and KALMANSON (1973) which permits treatment of the sensitization which occurs in half of the patients. The use of ointment-based mechlorethamine seems to reduce the rate of sensitization substantially (PRICE et al. 1982). Recently, the following time schedule has been proposed:

- daily applications until complete cleaning is achieved
- continuation of daily applications for further 6 months
- alternate-day applications for $2^1/_2$ years.
- discontinuation and control (VONDERHEID 1984)

Side effects of topical mechlorethamine therapy include contact allergy of delayed type (50% of the patients), immediate type (rare) and irritant contact dermatitis (cause for treatment discontinuation in 10% of the patients) (VONDERHEID 1984). Sensitization may also occur in the hospital staff. Additionally, lesions often heal with hyperpigmentation, and sometimes darkening of the whole skin is obseved (FLAXMAN et al. 1973). More serious is the development of squamous cell carcinomas and keratoakanthomas in sunexposed areas in 6,5% of the patients (DU VIVIER et al. 1978), or in other regions, frequently the genital area (LEE et al. 1982). Mechlorethamine therefore must be regarded as carcinogen or co-carcinogen. Systemic side effects have, up to now, not been observed (VONDERHEID 1984).

Other topical nitrosurea compounds are equally effective as mechlorethamine (ZACKHEIM and EPSTEIN 1975), but may exhibit systemic and local toxic effects. These compounds have not been followed in detail in the literature.

In conclusion, topical mechlorethamine is of equal effectiveness to other therapeutic regimens in early mycosis fungoides; however, several disadvantages like allergic and irritant contact dermatitis, tumour induction and the necessity of daily application have prevented worldwide acceptance.

7.4 Systemic Chemotherapy

Numerous cytostatic agents have been used in the therapy of mycosis fungoides; all of them given single or in combinations failed to induce stable remissions. This may in part be due to the fact that systemic chemotherapy has been used mainly in stages II B–IV B.

Table 13. Systemic chemotherapy in mycosis fungoides and Sézary's syndrome. (Modified after WINKLER and BUNN 1984)

Agent	No. of patients	% Response (partial and complete)
Bleomycin	32	62
Adriamycin	13	85
Doxorubicine	13	62
Streptonigrin	11	82
Mechlorethamine	86	64
Cyclophosphamide	86	67
BCNU	16	63
Methotrexate	91	68
High dose methotrexate	11	100
Azarabine	16	88
VP 16	15	67
Vinblastine	13	25
Vincristine	14	50
Deoxyformicine	7	57
Cisplatin	2	100
Prednisolone	50	50

Antibiotics: Using bleomycin alone, poor results with low response rates were obtained; moreover, many patients died during or after therapy from side effects (VAN VLOTEN and POLANO 1975; GROTH et al. 1979; SPIGEL and COLTMAN 1973; BAST et al. 1971; BERNADOU 1972; LEVI et al. 1977). The same holds true for combination regimens including bleomycin (GROTH et al. 1979). In contrast, adriamycin as a single agent in one series (LEVI et al. 1977) including 13 patients with advanced mycosis fungoides showed a remission rate of 85%. Therefore Adriamycin was included in many combination therapies.

Alkylating agents: Systemic administration of mechlorethamine leads to a remission rate of 78%, giving 3 mg/day in 41 patients (VAN SCOTT et al. 1975). 2 patients showed complete remission after cyclophosphamid therapy (KUBEC and KRTKOVA 1971).

Antimetabolites: Methotrexate (60–240 mg/m^2 i.v.) with subsequent administration of citrovorum factor induces complete remissions in 70% of stage II–III patients (MCDONALD and BERTINO 1978). A comparable effect is obtained with azarabine (MCDONALD and CALABRESI 1971). The effect of vepesid (VP 16, epipodophyllotoxin) seems to be more pronounced on lymph nodes involved by mycosis fungoides than on skin lesions (MOLIN et al. 1979).

Mitosis blocking agents (alkaloids): Vinblastin alone or vincristine alone only result in responses in less than half of the patients (LEVI and WIERNIK 1975).

Miscellaneous: Inhibition of adenosine desaminase by deoxycoformicin resulted in a complete remission in one patient with mycosis fungoides, lasting two months (KUFA et al. 1980). The rationale for the use of deoxycoformicin in mycosis fungoides is the high activity of adenosine desaminase in dermal lymphocytes (DAVIS and SIMPKINS 1979) as well as in the serum of mycosis fungoides patients (GLÜCK et al. 1983).

Details of remission rates are given in Table 13, which was modified after a recent review of WINKLER and BUNN (1984).

Combinations: Various combinations have been tested in mycosis fungoides; none of them has been fully convincing in terms of long-lasting complete remissions. A highly aggressive treatment with bleomycin and methotrexate gave 90% complete and partial remissions; however, 5 of the 10 patients died during continuation of therapy (GROTH et al. 1979); this regimen was therefore stopped by the Scandinavian Mycosis Fungoides Study Group. Vincristine and vinblastine (SERRI and BERNASCONI 1970), bleomycin, vinblastine and prednisolon (FOCAN et al. 1982), cyclophosphamide, vincristine and prednisolon (LEAVELL et al. 1976) and vepesid plus cyclophosphamid (MOLIN et al. 1979) was tested only in small series. Recently, BUNN et al. started a large study combining CAPO (cyclophosphamide, adriamycin, vepesid and vincristine) with total body electron beam radiation; results have not yet been published, however, in our hands even this aggressive therapy frequently shows relapses which are difficult to treat. Another complication of combined chemotherapy may be development of acute myeloblastic leukaemia (WADELL et al. 1982). For further details see the recent review of WINKLER and BUNN (1984).

7.5 Miscellaneous

7.5.1 Local Glucocorticoids

It has been shown in earlier investigations that local glucocorticoid ointments suppress eczematous and plaque lesions of mycosis fungoides; this effect depends on the strength of the applied glucocorticoid (FARBER et al. 1968). Relapses and rebound effects are frequently observed. However, this therapeutic possibility should be kept in mind especially in patients with resistant plaques or tumours, where intralesional glucocorticoids may be useful (MARMELZAT 1963).

7.5.2 Retinoids

Retinoids belong to the most interesting substances currently under investigation in mycosis fungoides. Etretinate and isotretinoin are both effective in usual doses in reduction of cutaneous manifestations of mycosis fungoides (CLAUDY et al. 1982; CLAUDY et al. 1983; KESSLER et al. 1983; SOUTEYRAND et al. 1981). Even more pronounced is the effect of these substances when they are added to PUVA therapy (HUNZIKER et al. 1983; IPPOLITO and GIACALONE 1982; SOUTEYRAND et al. 1981) or systemic polychemotherapy (ZACHARIAE et al. 1982).

Recently, MAHRLE et al. (1983) reported 3 complete and one partial remission, including one patient with tumours, after administration of arotinoid;

arotinoids are a highly potent new class of retinoids with an activity 100 to 1000 times stronger than etretinate and isotretinoin.

The effectiveness of retinoids in mycosis fungoides but not in Sézary's syndrome (MAHRLE et al. 1983; SOUTEYRAND et al. 1981) is particularly interesting with regard to the pathogenesis of these two disorders.

7.5.3 Transfer Factor

Transfer factor is a low molecular weight extract from human leukocytes with certain effects on the T-lymphocyte system (LAWRENCE 1969). Transfer factor was used as additional therapy in mycosis fungoides (ZACCHARIAE et al. 1975) and as such induced complete remission in one patient (ZACHARIAE et al. 1979).

7.5.4 TP-5

TP-5, the synthetic pentapeptide corresponding to the aminoacid residues 32 to 36 of thymopoietin, has recently been given in 6 patients with mycosis fungoides (PRZYBILLA et al. 1983). Partial remission was observed in two patients, no response in one patient, and disease progression in the other three patients.

7.5.5 Monoclonal Antibodies

Therapy of mycosis fungoides and Sézary's syndrome with monoclonal antibodies is currently under investigation in several laboratories, and at present it is difficult to give a satisfying overview on this field. BERNSTEIN et al. (1980) demonstrated in the mouse leukaemia model that monoclonal antibodies are principally effective in these disorders. Subsequently, MILLER and LEVY (1981) and OSEROFF et al. (1982) from the same group gave further evidence that monoclonal antibodies against T-lymphocytes are therapeutically active in mycosis fungoides. However, there are several technical problems to be overcome; the discussion of these is beyond the scope of this review.

7.5.6 Virustatic Agents

Recently, a remission of tumours in mycosis fungoides has been reported after administration of acyclovir (RESNICK et al. 1984). This observation must be confirmed before further conclusions can be drawn.

Acknowledgement: The excellent secretarial work of H. Guntzmann is gratefully acknowledged.

References

Aberer W, Schuler G, Stingl G, Hönigsmann H, Wolff K (1981) Ultraviolet light depletes surface markers of Langerhans cells. J Invest Dermatol 76:202–210

Ablin RJ, Morris AJ (1973) Thymus-specific antigens on thymic derived lymphocytes. Transplantation 15:415

Ackerman AB, Miller RC, Shapiro L (1966) Pustular mycosis fungoides. Arch Dermatol 93:221–225

Ackerman AB, Breza TS, Capland L (1974) Spongiotic simulants of mycosis fungoides. Arch Dermatol 109:218–220
Alibert JLM (1806) Description des maladies de la peau observées à l'Hopital St. Louis. Barrois l'aine' et Fils, Paris
Altmeyer P (1981) Disseminierte pagetoide Retikulose? Mycosis fungoides? Z Hautkr 56:63–74
Asbell SO, Gadol N, Saluk P, Vonderheid EC, Brady LW (1978) Antibody-dependent cellular cytotoxicity in patients with mycosis fungoides and Sézary syndrome. Int J Radiat Oncol Biol Phys 4:609–613
Bast C de, Moriame N, Wanet J, Ledoux M, Achten G, Kenis Y (1971) Bleomycin in mycosis fungoides and reticulum cell lymphoma. Arch Derm 104:508–512
Bazin E (1870) Lecons sur le traitment de maladies chroniques en general affections de la peau en particulier par l'emploi compare des eaux minerales de l'hydrotherapie et des moyens pharmaceutiques. Adrein Delahaye, Paris, p 425
Berger CL, Morrison S, Chu AC, Patterson J, Estabrook A, Takezak S, Sharon J, Warburton D, Irigoyen O, Edelson RL (1982) Diagnosis of cutaneous T cell lymphoma by use of monoclonal antibodies reactive with tumor-associated antigens. J Clin Invest 70:1205–1215
Bernardou A (1972) Bleomycin in the reticuloses. Br Med J 285–286
Bernstein ID, Tam MR, Nowinski RC (1980) Mouse leukemia: therapy with monoclonal antibodies against a thymus differentiation antigen. Science 207:68–71
Besnier E, Hallopeau H (1892) On the erythrodermia of mycosis fungoides. J Cutan Genitourin Dis 10:453
Biddison WE, Rao PE, Talle MA, Goldstein G, Shaw S (1984) Possible involvement of the T4 molecule in T cell recognition of class II HLA antigens. J Exp Med 159:783–797
Bluefarb SM (1955) Is mycosis fungoides an entity? Arch Dermatol 71:293–302
Bodensteiner DC, Skikne B (1982) Central nervous system involvement in mycosis fungoides. Diagnosis, treatment and literature review. Cancer 50:1181–1184
Bonneau H, Cosarini J-P (1967) Etude ultrastructurale d'un cas de mycosis fungoides. Bull Soc Fr Dermatol Syphil 74:612–617
Braathen LR, Førre Ø, Natvig J (1979) An antihuman T-lymphocyte antiserum: in situ identification of T cells in the skin of delayed-type hypersensitivity reaction, chronic photosensitivity dermatitis and mycosis fungoides. Clin Immun Immunopath 13:211–219
Braun-Falco O, Burg G, Schmoeckel C (1981) Recent advances in cutaneous lymphoma. Clin Exp Dermatol 6:89–109
Breathnach SM, McKee PH, Smith NP (1982) Hypopigmented mycosis fungoides: report of five cases with ultrastructural observations. Brit J Dermatol 106:643–649
Brehm G (1974) Verhalten vom Immunglobulin E bei ausgewählten Dermatosen. Arch Derm Forsch 248:329–337
Broder S, Bunn PA (1980) Cutaneous T-cell lymphomas. Semin Oncol 7:310–331
Brownlee TR, Murad TM (1970) Ultrastructure of mycosis fungoides. Cancer 26:686–698
Bryant E, Ronau SG, Iossifides IA (1982) Plasma cell myeloma in a patient with a cutaneous T-cell lymphoma. Cancer 50:2122–2125
Büchner S, Rufli T (1979) Manifestation eines malignen Lymphoms von hohem Malignitätsgrad im Spätstadium der Mycosis fungodes. Enzymzytochemische und immunzytologische Untersuchungen. Dermatologica 159:125–131
Bunn PA, Lamberg SI (1979) Report of the committee von staging and classification of cutaneous T-cell lymphomas. Cancer Treat Rep 63:725–728
Bunn PA, Huberman MS, Whang-Peng J, Schlechter GP, Guccion JG, Matthews MJ, Gazdar AF, Dunnick NR, Fischmann AB, Ihde DC, Cohen MH, Fossieck B, Minna JD (1980) Prospective staging evaluation of patients with cutaneous T-cell lymphomas. Ann Int Med 93:223–230
Bunn PA, Whang-Peng J, Carney DN, Schlam ML, Knutsen T, Gazdar AF (1980) DNA content analysis by flow cytometry and cytogenetic analysis in mycosis fungoides and Sézary syndrome. J Clin Invest 65:1440–1448
Burg G, Braun-Falco O (1975) T- and B-Lymphozyten in Hautveränderungen kutaner Lymphome. Dtsch med Wschr 100:2562–2564
Burg G, Rodt H, Grosse-Wilde H, Braun-Falco O (1978) Surface markers and mitogen response of cells harvested from cutaneous infiltrates in mycosis fungoides and Sézary's syndrome. J Invest Dermatol 70:257–259

Calabresi P, Parks RE (1980) Antiproliferative agents and drugs used for immunosuppression. In: The Pharmacological Basis of Therapeutics. Edited by Gilman AG, Goodmann LS, Gilman A. New York, Macmillan 1980, pp 1256–1313

Cameron OJ (1933) Mycosis fungoides in mother and in daughter. Arch Dermatol Syphilol 27:232–236

Camisa C, Goldstein A (1981) Mycosis fungoides. Small bowel involvement complicated by perforation and peritonitis. Arch Dermatol 117:234–237

Cassuto JP, Kövary PM, Campagni JP, Simoney J, Maiolini R, Schneider M (1981) Mycosis fungoides associated with mediterranean lymphoma. Arch Dermatol Res 270:17–23

Castellino RA, Hoppe RT, Blank N, Young ST, Fuks Z (1979) Experience with lymphography in patients with mycosis fungoides. Cancer Treat Rep 63:581–586

Caya JG, Choi H, Tieu TM, Wollenberg NJ, Almagro UA (1984) Hodgkin's disease followed by mycosis fungoides in the same patient. Cancer 53:463–467

Chu AC, MacDonald DM (1979) Identification in situ of T lymphocytes in dermal and epidermal infiltrates of mycosis fungoides. Br J Dermatol 100:177–189

Chu AC, Morgan EW, MacDonald DM (1980) Ultrastructural identification of T lymphocytes in tissue sections of mycosis fungoides. J Invest Dermatol 74:17–20

Chu AC, Berger CL, Kung P, Edelson RL (1982a) In situ identification of Langerhans' cells in the dermal infiltrate of cutaneous T-cell lymphoma. J Am Acad Dermatol 6:350–354

Chu AC, Berger CL, Lynfield Y, Esseessee I, Edelson RL (1982b) Pathogenesis of cutaneous T cell lymphoma. In: Lymphoproliferative disorders of the skin. Ed Goos M, Christophers E, pp 57–64, Springer Berlin-Heidelberg-New York

Chu AC, Patterson J, Berger C, Edelson R (1982c) T-cell subpopulations of cutaneous T-cell lymphoma (CTCL). J Invest Dermatol 78:334

Chu AC, Patterson J, Goldstein G, Berger C, Takezaki S, Edelson RL (1982d) Thymopoietin-like substance in human skin. J Invest Dermatol 78:330

Chu AC, Berger CL, Edelson RL, Spittle M, Russell C, Smith N (1983a) Circulating T cells in cutaneous T-cell lymphoma – a study using monoclonal antibodies against normal and malignant T cells. Br J Dermatol 108:219–246

Chu AC, Robinson D, Catovsky D, Smith N (1983b) The Sézary cell – a phenotypic study in different dermatoses. 10th SCUR Annual meeting and 4th International Dermatopathology Colloquium, Berlin, 15.–18.7.83. Booklet of Abstracts, pp 31–32

Civatte J, Kapetis E (1977) Problems in histological diagnosis of mycosis fungoides. Bull Cancer 64:187–190

Claudy A, Schmitt D, Alario A, Brochier J, Perrot H, Thivolet J (1977) Immunocytological characterization of the mycosis fungoides tumour cells. Bull Cancer 64:241–248

Claudy AL, Delomier Y, Hermier C (1982) Treatment of cutaneous T-cell lymphoma with a new aromatic retinoid (Ro 10-9359). Arch Dermatol Res 273:37–42

Claudy AL, Rouchouse B, Boucheron S, Le Petit JC (1983) Treatment of cutaneous T-cell lymphoma with etretinate. Br J Dermatol 109:49–59

Cohen SR, Stenn KS, Braverman IM, Beck GJ (1980) Mycosis fungoides: clinicopathologic relationships, survival, and therapy in 59 patients with observations on occupation as a new prognostic factor. Cancer 46:2654–2666

Coleman CN, Williams CJ, Flint A (1977) Hematologic neoplasia in patients treated for Hodgkin's disease. N Engl J Med 297:1249–1252

Cooperrider PA, Roenigk HH (1978) Selective immunological evaluation of mycosis fungoides. Arch Dermatol 114:207–212

Cyr DP, Geokas MC, Worsley GH (1966) Mycosis fungoides. Hematologic findings and terminal course. Arch Dermatol 94:558–572

Daul CB, De Shazo RD (1983) AIDS: an update and interpretation. Ann Allergy 51:351–361

David M, Shohat B, Hazar B, Feuerman EJ, Joshua H (1980) Identification of T- und B lymphocytes on skin sections from patients with lymphoproliferative disorders of the skin. J Invest Dermatol 75:491–494

David M, Shohat B, Trainin N, Feuerman E (1980) Cell-mediated immunity in patients with mycosis fungoides in clinical remission. Cancer 46:41–44

Davis BH, Simpkins H (1982) Mycosis fungoides and Sézary syndrome: malignant cells with T-cell enzymatic properties. Lab Invest 40:251

Dobozy A, Hunydi J, Husz S, Kenderessy AS, Simon N (1977) Autoimmune anti-T cell antibodies in the sera of patients with mycosis fungoides. Brit J Dermatol 97:543–546

Edelson RL (1979) Cutaneous T cell lymphoma. In: Moschella S (ed) Dermatology update, pp 195–207. Elsevier Press NewYork

Edelson RL (1980) Cutaneous T cell lymphoma: mycosis fungoides, Sézary syndrome, and other variants. J Am Acad Dermatol 2:89–106

Edelson RL, Kirkpatrick CH, Shevach EM, Schein PS, Smith RW, Green I, Lutzner M (1974) Preferential cutaneous infiltration by neoplastic thymus-derived lymphocytes. Ann Int Med 80:685–692

Edelson RL, Berger CL, Raafat J, Warburton D (1979) Karyotype studies of cutaneous T cell lymphoma: evidence for clonal origin. J Invest Dermatol 73:548–550

Epstein EH, Levin DL, Croft JD Jr, Lutzner MA (1972) Mycosis fungoides: survival, prognostic features, response to therapy and autopsy findings. Medicine 15:61–72

Erkman-Balis B, Rappaport H (1974) Cytogenetic studies in mycosis fungoides. Cancer 34:626–633

Farber EM, Zackheim HS, McClintock RP, Cox AJ (1968) Treatment of mycosis fungoides with various strengths of fluocinolone acetonide cream. Arch Dermatol 97:165–168

Fischer ER, Branimir LH, Wechsler HL (1972) Ultrastructural features of mycosis fungoides. Amer J Clin Path 58:99–110

Fischer T, Skogh M (1979) Treatment of parapsoriasis en plaques, mycosis fungoides, and Sézary's syndrom with trioxalen baths followed by ultraviolet light. Acta Dermatovenerol 59:171–173

Fischer T, van Vloten WA, Volden G (1978) Internal dissemination of mycosis fungoides despite successful local therapy. Acta Dermatovener 58:88–89

Fischmann AB, Bunn PA Jr, Guccion JG, Matthews MJ, Minna JD (1979) Exposure to chemicals, physical agents, and biologic agents in mycosis fungoides and the Sézary syndrome. Cancer Treat Rep 63:591–596

Flaxman BA, Zelazny G, van Scott EJ (1971) Nonspecificity of characteristic cells in mycosis fungoides. Arch Dermatol 104:141–147

Flaxman BA, Sosis AC, van Scott EJ (1973) Changes in melanosome distribution in caucasoid skin following topical application of nitrogen mustard. J Invest Dermatol 60:321–326

Focan C, Cryns-Lenain E, Bouhy F, Lapière C (1982) Clinical and histological staging as prognostic determinants in advanced cutaneous T cell lymphomas treated by sequential polychemotherapy with bleomycin, vinblastine and prednisone. Dermatologica 165:141–144

Fuks ZY, Bagshaw MA, Farber EM (1973) Prognostic signs and the management of the mycosis fungoides. Cancer 32:1385–1395

Fuks ZY, Castellino RA, Carmel JA, Farber EM, Bagshaw MA (1974) Lymphography in mycosis fungoides. Cancer 34:106–112

Fukuhara S, Rowley JD, Variakojis D (1978) Banding studies of chromosomes in a patient with mycosis fungoides. Cancer 42:2262–2268

Gahlen-Schulte S, Sterry W, Runne U (1982) Generalisierter Herpes simplex bei Mycosis fungoides (Ekzema herpeticum seu herpeticatum, Kaposi's varizelliforme Eruption). Z Hautkr 57:1757–1765

Gauge RW, Jones EW (1978) Kaposi's sarcoma and immunosuppressive therapy: an appraisal. Clin exp Dermatol 3:135–146

Gerdes J, Schwab U, Lemke H, Stein H (1983) Production of a mouse monoclonal antibody reactive with a human nuclear antigen associated with cell proliferation. Int J Cancer 31:13–20

Gerdes J, Dallenbach F, Lennert K, Lemke H, Stein H (in press a) Proliferation rate in malignant non Hodgkin's lymphomas as determined in situ with the monoclonal antibody Ki 67. Haematol Oncol

Gerdes J, Lemke H, Baisch H, Wacker H-H, Schwab U, Stein H (in press b) Cell cycle analysis of a cell proliferation associated nuclear antigen defined by the monoclonal antibody Ki 67. J Immunol

Gilchrest BA, Parrish JA, Tauenbaum L, Haynes HA, Fitzpatrick TB (1976) Oral methoxalen photochemotherapy of mycosis fungoides. Cancer 38:683–689

Glück S, Merck H, Sterry W, Goerz G, Schneider W (1983) Erhöhte Adenosin-Desaminase-Aktivität bei Patienten mit Mycosis fungoides. Hautarzt 34 (Suppl. VI):337–338

Goldgeier MH, Cohen SR, Braverman IM, Stenn KS (1981) An unusual and fatal case of disseminated cutaneous herpes simplex. J Am Acad Dermatol 4:176–180

Goos M (1976) T-cell specific microenvironment in mycosis fungoides. Arch Dermatol Res 255:215–218

Green SB, Byar DP, Lamberg SI (1981) Prognostic variables in mycosis fungoides. Cancer 47:2671–2677

Greene MH, Dalager NA, Lamberg SI, Argyropoulos CE, Fraumeni JF Jr (1979) Mycosis fungoides: epidemiologic observations. Cancer Treat Rep 63:597–606

Griem ML, Moran EM, Ferguson DS, Mettler FA, Griem SF (1975) Staging procedures in mycosis fungoides. Br J Cancer (Suppl.) 31:362–367

Grossi CE, Webb SR, Zicca A, Lydyard PM, Moretta L, Mingardi MC, Cooper MD (1978) Morphological and histochemical analysis of two human T-cell subpopulations bearing receptors for IgM and IgG. J exp Med 147:1405–1417

Groth O, Molin L, Thomsen K (1979) Tumor stage of mycosis fungoides treated with bleomycin and methotrexate: report from the scandinavian mycosis fungoides study group. Acta Dermatovener 59:59–63

Hagedorn M, Kiefer G (1977) DNA content of mycosis fungoides cells. Arch Derm Res 258:127–134

Hamminga L, Hermans J, Noordijk EM, Meijer CJLM, Scheffer E, van Vloten WA (1982a) Cutaneous T-cell lymphoma: clinicopathological relationships, therapy and survival in ninety-two patients. Br J Dermatol 107:145–156

Hamminga L, Leigh PC, Blussé van oud Alblas A, van Vloten WA, van Furth R (1982b) Functions of peripheral-blood monocytes and granulocytes in cutaneous T-cell lymphoma. Br J Dermatol 107:157–164

Hamminga B, Noordijk EM, van Vloten WA (1982c) Treatment of mycosis fungoides. Total-skin electron-beam irradiation vs topical mechlorethamine therapy. Arch Dermatol 118:150–153

Haserick JR, Richardson JR, Grant DJ (1959) Remission of lesions in mycosis fungoides following topical application of nitrogen mustard. Cleve Clin R 26:144–147

Haynes BF, Hensley LL, Jegasothy BV (1982a) Phenotypic characterization of skin infiltrating T-cells in cutaneous T-cell lymphoma: comparison with benign cutaneous T-cell infiltrates. Blood 60:463–473

Haynes BF, Hensley LL, Jegasothy BV (1982b) Differentiation of human T-lymphocytes: II Phenotypic differences in skin and blood malignant T-cells in cutaneous lymphoma. J Invest Dermatol 78:323–326

Heid E, Desvaux J, Brändle I, Grosshans E (1976) Der Verlauf der Parapsoriasis en plaques (Brocq'sche Krankheit). Z Hautkr 52:658–662

Herbst M, Müller R (1984) Ganz-Haut-Elektronentherapie der Mycosis fungoides und des Sézary-Syndroms. Hautarzt 35:16–21

Hjortshoj A, Schmidt H (1977) Photochemotherapy of mycosis fungoides. Danish Med Bull 24:40–42

Hodge L, Vella Briffa D, Warin AP, Gange RW, Bleeken S (1977) Photochemotherapy in mycosis fungoides. Br Med J 2:1257–1259

Hofmann C, Burg G, Plewig G, Braun-Falco O (1977) Photochemotherapie kutaner Lymphome. Orale und lokale 8-MOP-UVA-Therapie. Dtsch Med Wschr 102:675–679

Holden CA, Morgan EW, MacDonald DM (1982a) The cell population in the cutaneous infiltrate of mycosis fungoides: in situ studies using monoclonal antisera. Br J Dermatol 106: 385–392

Holden CA, Staughton RCD, Campbell MA, MacDonald DM (1982b) Differential loss of T-lymphocyte markers in advanced cutaneous T-cell lymphoma. J Amer Acad Dermatol 6:507–513

Hönigsmann H, Konrad K, Gschnait F, Wolff K (1976) Photochemotherapy of mycosis fungoides VIIth International Congress of Photobiology, Rome, Italy, 29. Aug.–3. Sept. 1976, Book of Abstracts, p 222

Hubermann MS, Bunn PA Jr, Matthews MJ, Ihde DC, Gazdar AF, Cohen MH, Minna JD (1980) Hepatic involvement in the cutaneous T-cell lymphomas. Cancer 45:1683–1688

Hundeiker M, Berger H, Petres J (1968) Mycosis fungoides nach Thorotrastanwendung mit Entwicklung zur Retikulumzellsarkomatose. Arch klin exp Forsch 232:56–65

Hunziker T, Zala A, Krebs A (1983) Retinoid-orale Photochemotherapie (RePUVA) als Kombinationsbehandlung bei Mycosis fungoides. Dermatologica 166:165–168

Ippolito F, Giacalone B (1982) Sur un cas de mycosis fungoide avec manifestations tumorales traité avec Ro 10-9359 (Tigason). Ann Dermatol Venerol 109:65–72

Kerl H (1981) Das Sézary Syndrom. Zbl Haut Geschlkr 144:359–380

Kerl H, Hödl S, Smolle J, Konrad K (1984) Klassifikation und Prognose kutaner T-Zell-Lymphome. Z Hautkr (in press)

Klein D (1976) Staging procedures in mycosis fungoides. Proc Am Soc Clin Oncol 17:277

Knoth W (1976) Reticulosen. Hautarzt Suppl I:295

Kragballe K, Herlin T, Ellegaard J (1983) Stimulation of monocyte-mediated, antibody-dependent cytotoxicity in mycosis fungoides. Arch Dermatol 119:203–206

Kresbach H (1981) Kutane maligne Lymphome. Ältere Vorstellungen und neuere Konzepte. Münch med Wschr 35:1291–1296

Kubba RK, Bailin PL, Roenigk HH (1979) Immunological evaluation in mycosis fungoides: Before and after PUVA therapy. Arch Dermatol 116:178–181

Kubec K, Krtkova J (1971) Clinical experiences with cyclophosphamide in the treatment of two cases of mycosis fungoides. Cesk Dermatol 46:166–169

Kufe D, Major P, Agarwal R, Reinherz E, Frei E (1980) Phase I-phase II trial of deoxycoformycin (DCF) in T cell malignancies. Proc Am Assoc Cancer Res 21:328

Kummermehr J, Burg G (1982) Autoradiographic pattern of cell proliferation in cutaneous malignant lymphoma. In: Lymphoproliferative diseases of the skin. Eds. Goos M, Christophers E, pp 71–78 Springer Berlin-Heidelberg-New York

Lamberg SI, Diamond EL, Lorincz AL, Caro WA, Rappaport H, Variakojis D, Block JB, Fuks ZY, van Scott EJ (1975) Mycosis fungoides cooperative study. Arch Dermatol 111:457–459

Lamberg SI, Green SB, Byar DP, Block JB, Clendenning WE, Epstein EN, Fuks ZY, Golitz LE, Lorincz AL, Michel B (1979) Status report of 376 mycosis fungoides patients at 4 years – Mycosis fungoides cooperative group. Cancer Treat Rep 63:701–707

Lange Wantzin G, Larsen JK, Christensen IJ, Bruun Rasmussen B, Thomsen K (1983) Aneuploidy in cutaneous T-cell lymphoma. Acta Derm Venerol 63:283–289

Lawrence H (1969) Transfer factor. Advance Immunol 11:195–201

Leavell UW, DeSimone P (1976) Combined chemotherapy (COP) in treatment of mycosis fungoides: report of four cases. South Med J 69:915–917

Lee LA, Fritz KA, Golitz L, Weston WL (1982) Second cutaneous malignancies in patients with mycosis fungoides treated with topical nitrogen mustard. J Am Acad Dermatol 7:592–598

Lee LA, Ryan SR, Huff JG, Schocket AL (1982) Lymphocytotoxic antibodies in mycosis fungoides are predominantly antisuppressor cell. J Invest Dermatol 78:337

Lefeber WR, Robinson JK, Clendenning WE, Dunn JL, Colton T (1981) Attempts to enhance light microscopic diagnosis of cutaneous T cell lymphoma (mycosis fungoides). Arch Dermatol 117:408–411

Lennert K (1978) Malignant lymphomas other than Hodgkin's disease. Spriner Verlag Berlin-Heidelberg-New York, pp 165–185

Lever WH, Schaumburg-Lever G (1983) Histopathology of the skin. 6th edition. J.P. Lippincott Co, Philadelphia

Levi JA, Wiernik PH (1975) Management of mycosis fungoides: Current status and future prospects. Medicine 54:73–88

Lipa M, Kunynetz R, Pawlowski D, Kerbel G, Haberman H (1982) The occurence of mycosis fungoides in two patients with preexisting Hodgkin's disease. Arch Dermatol 118:563–567

Lischka G, Bohnert E, Bachtold G, Jung EG (1977) Effects of 8-methoxypsoralen (8-MOP) and UVA on human lymphocytes. J Invest Dermatol 68:245

Lowe NJ, Cripps DJ, Dufton PA, Vickers FH (1979) Photochemotherapy for mycosis fungoides. A clinical and histological study. Arch Dermatol 115:50–53

Luger TA, Stadler BM, Katz SI, Oppenheim JJ (1981) Epidermal cell (keratinocyte)-derived thymocyte-activating factor (ETAF). J Immunol 127:1493–1502

Lutzner MA, Hobbs JW, Horwvath P (1971) Ultrastructure of abnormal cells in Sézary syndrome, mycosis fungoides, and parapsoriasis en plaques. Arch Dermatol 103:375–386

Lutzner M, Edelson R, Schein P, Green I, Kirkpatrick C, Ahmed A (1975) Cutaneous T-cell lymphomas: the Sézary syndrome, mycosis fungoides and related disorders. Ann Int Med 83:534–552

MacKie RM (1981) Initial event in mycosis fungoides of the skin is viral infection of epidermal Langerhans cells. Lancet 2:283–285

MacKie RM, Turbitt ML (1982) The use of a double-label immunoperoxidase monoclonal antibody technique in the investigation of patients with mycosis fungoides. Br J Dermatol 106:379–384

MacKie R, Dick HM, De Sousa MB (1976a) HLA and mycosis fungoides. Lancet 1 (7970), 1179

MacKie R, Sless FR, Cochran R, De Sousa M (1976b) Lymphocyte abnormalities in mycosis fungoides. Br J Dermatol 94:173–178
Mahrle G, Thiele B, Ippen H (1983) Chemotherapie kutaner T-Zell-Lymphome mit Arotinoid. Dtsch med Wschr 108:1753–1757
Marmelzat WL (1963) Mycosis fungoides: local injections of triamcinolone. Calif Med 98:139–141
McMillan EM, Beeman K, Wasik R, Everett MA (1982a) Demonstration of OKT6-reactive cells in mycosis fungoides. J Am Acad Dermatol 6:880–887
McMillan EM, Wasik R, Beeman K, Everett MA (1982b) In situ immunologic phenotyping of mycosis fungoides. J Am Acad Dermatol 6:888–892
McMillan EM, Wasik R, Jackson I, Peters S, Everett MA (1982c) OKT6-reactive cells in mycosis fungoides. J Cut Pathol 9:55–60
McNutt NS, Crain WR (1981) Quantitative electron microscopic comparison of lymphocyte nuclear contours im mycosis fungoides and in benign infiltrates in skin. Cancer 47:698–709
Meijer CJ, van Leeuwen AW, van der Loo EM, van der Putte LB, van Vloten WA (1977) Cerebriform (Sézary-like) mononuclear cells in healthy individuals: a morphologically distinct population of T cells. Relationship with mycosis fungoides and Sézary's syndrome. Virch Arch Cell Pathol 25:95–104
Meijer CJ, van der Loo E, van Vloten WA, Cornelisse J (1978) Early diagnosis of mycosis fungoides and Sézary's syndrome by computer assisted morphometric analysis of lymphoid cells. J Invest Dermatol 70:234
Meijer CJ, van der Loo EM, van Vloten WA, van der Velde EA, Scheffer E, Cornelisse CJ (1980) Early diagnosis of mycosis fungoides and Sézary's syndrome by morphometric analysis of lymphoid cells in the skin. Cancer 45:2864–2871
Miller RA, Levy R (1981) Response of cutaneous T cell lymphoma to therapy with hybridoma monoclonal antibody. Lancet I:226–230
Molin L, Skogh M, Volden G (1978) Successful PUVA-treatment in the tumour stage of mycosis fungoides associated with the appearance of lesions in organs other than the skin. Acta Dermatovener 58:189–190
Molin L, Thomsen K, Volden G (1979) Mycosis fungoides plaque stage treated with topical nitrogen mustard with and without attempts at tolerance induction: report from the scandinavian mycosis fungoides study group. Acta Dermatol 59:64–68
Molin L, Thomsen K, Volden G, Groth O (1980) Photochemotherapy (PUVA) in the pretumour stage of mycosis fungoides: a report from the scandinavian mycosis fungoides study group. Acta Dermatovenerol 61:47–51
Molin L, Thomsen K, Volden G, Groth O (1981) Photochemotherapy (PUVA) in the tumour stage of mycoses fungoides: a report from the scandinavian fungoides study group. Acta Dermatovenerol 61:52–54
Moran EM, Walther JR, Arouson IK, Variakojis D (1977) Clinical significance of circulating Sézary cells in mycosis fungoides. Proc Am Soc Clin Oncol 18:276
Mortazawi SAM, Oberste-Lehn H (1973) Lichtsensibilisatoren und ihre therapeutischen Fähigkeiten. Erste vorläufige Mitteilung. Z Hautkr 48:1–9
Munson D, Bunn PA, Schechter GP (1982) Fc-Receptor-defined T-lymphocyte subpopulations in patients with cutaneous T-cell lymphoma. J Invest Dermatol 79:317–321
Neilau BA, Vonderheid EC, O'Neill KJ (1983) Natural cell-mediated cytotoxicity in cutaneous T-cell lymphomas. J Invest Dermatol 81:176–178
Nordqvist CB, Kinney PJ (1976) T and B cells and cell mediated immunity in mycosis fungoides. Cancer 37:714–721
Nowell PC, Finan JB, Vonderheid EC (1982) Clonal characteristics of cutaneous T cell lymphomas: cytogenetic evidence from blood, lymph nodes, and skin. J Invest Derm 78:69–75
Oberste-Lehn H (1980) Photochemotherapie der T-Zellen-Lymphome. Z Hautkr 55:1335–1339
Olsen EA, Delzell E, Jegasothy BV (1984) Second malignancies in cutaneous T cell lymphoma. J Am Acad Dermatol 10:197–204
Oseroff AR, Miller RA, Stratte PJ, Levy R (1982) Monoclonal anti-T cell antibody in the therapy of mycosis fungoides. J Invest Dermatol 78:337
Patterson JAK, Edelson RL (1983) Interaction of T-lymphocytes with the epidermis: immunopathological studies. J Cut Pathol 10:540–549
Pautrier LM, Woringer F (1932) Note préliminaire sur un tableau histologique particulier de lésions

ganglionnaires accompagnant des éruptions dermatologiques généralisées prurigineuses, de types cliniques différents. Bull Soc Francaise Dermatol Syphilol 39:947–967

Payne CM, Nagle RB, Lynch PJ (1984) Quantitative electron microscopy in the diagnosis of mycosis fungoides. A simple analysis of lymphocytic nuclear convolutions. Arch Dermatol 120:63–75

Pierard GE, Franchimont C, de la Brassinne TLE, Lapiere CM (1982) Proliferation rate of cutaneous T cell lymphomas in the skin – relationship with histologic pattern and cytology. In: Lymphoproliferative diseases of the skin. Eds. Goos M, Christophers E, pp 65–70. Springer Verlag Berlin-Heidelberg-New York

Price NM, Mirkovich AM (1978) Lymphocytotoxicity in mycosis fungoides. Br J Derm 98:97–102

Price NM, Constantine VS, Hoppe RT, Fuks ZY, Farber EM (1977) Topical mechlorethamine therapy for mycosis fungoides. Br J Dermatol 97:547–555

Price NM, Fuks ZY, Hoffman TE (1977) Hyperkeratotic and verrucous features of mycosis fungoides. Arch Dermatol 113:57–60

Price NM, Deneau DG, Hoppe RT (1982) The treatment of mycosis fungoides with ointment-based mechlorethamine. Arch Dermatol 118:234–237

Price NM, Hoppe RT, Deneau DG (1983) Ointment-based mechlorethamine treatment for mycosis fungoides. Cancer 52:2214–2219

Przybilla B, Burg G, Schmoeckel C, Braun-Falco O (1983) Treatment of cutaneous T-cell lymphomas with TP-5. Acta Dermatol Venerol 63:524–529

Rappaport H, Thomas LB (1974) Mycosis fungoides: the pathology of extracutaneous involvement. Cancer 34:1198–1229

Reinherz EL, Kung PC, Goldstein RH, Levey RH, Schlossman SF (1980) Discrete stages of human intrathymus differentiation: analysis of normal thymocytes and leukemic lymphoblasts of T-cell lineage. Proc Natl Acad Sci USA 77:1588–1592

Resnick L, Schleider-Kushner N, Horwitz SN, Frost P (1984) Remission of tumor-stage mycosis fungoides following intravenously administered acyclovir. JAMA 251:1571–1573

Robb-Smith AHT (1944) The reticular tissue and the skin. Br J Dermatol 56:151–165

Roenigk HH (1977) Photochemotherapy of mycosis fungoides. Arch Dermatol 113:1047

Roenigk HH Jr, Castrovinci AJ (1971) Mycosis fungoides bullosa. Arch Dermatol 104:402–406

Rosas-Uribe A, Variakojis D, Molnar Z, Rappaport H (1974) Mycosis fungoides: an ultrastructural study. Cancer 34:634–645

Rowden G, Lewis MG (1976) Langerhans cells: involvement in the pathogenesis of mycosis fungoides. Br J Dermatol 95:665–672

Ruffieux C, Stalder M, Tran-Thang C (1984) Mycosis fungoides et gammopathie monoclonale. Association fortuite ou causale. Dermatologica 168:170–174

Russel Jones R, Chu AC (1981) Pagetoid reticulosis and solitary mycosis fungoides. Distinct clinicopathological entities. J Cut Path 8:40–51

Samman PD (1972) The natural history of parapsoriasis en plaques (chronic superficial dermatitis) and prereticulotic poikiloderma. Br J Dermatol 87:405–411

Sanchez JL, Ackerman AB (1979) The patch stage of mycosis fungoides. Criteria for histologic diagnosis. Am J Dermatopathol 1:5–26

Sandbank M, Katzenellenbogen I (1968) Mycosis fungoides of prolonged duration in siblings. Arch Dermatol 98:620–627

Sauder DN, Carter C, Katz SI, Oppenheim JJ (1981) Epidermal cell production of thymocyte activating factor. Clin Research 29:285 A

Sauder DN, Noonan FP, DeFabo EC, Katz SI (1983) Ultraviolet radiation inhibits alloantigen presentation by epidermal cells: partial reversal by the soluble epidermal cell product, epidermal cell-derived thymocyte-activating factor (ETAF). J Invest Dermatol 80:485–489

Scheffer E, Meijer CJLM, van Vloten WA (1980) Dermatopathic lymphadenopathy and lymph node involvement in mycosis fungoides. Cancer 45:137–148

Schein PS, MacDonald JS, Edelson R (1976) Cutaneous T-cell lymphoma. Cancer 38:1859–1861

Schlaeger M (1980) Immunglobulin E bei kutanen Lymphomen und bei der Parapsoriasis en plaques (Brocq). Dermatologica 161:1–7

Schmitt D, Thivolet J (1980) Lymphocyte-epidermis interactions in malignant epidermotropic lymphoma: I. Ultrastructural aspects. Acta Dermatovener 60:1–11

Schmitt D, Alario A, Touraine JL, Claudy AL, Perrot H, Thivolet J (1977) Specific surface antigen of human B and T lymphocytes: the use in the ultrastructural identification of cells extracted from cutaneous infiltrations. J Cut Pathol 4:211–235

Schmitt D, Souteyrand P, Brochier J, Czernieliwski J, Thivolet J (1982) Phenotype of cells involved in mycosis fungoides and Sézary syndrome (blood and skin lesions): Immunomorphological study with monoclonal antibodies. Acta Dermatovenerol 62:193–199

Schmoeckel C, Burg G, Braun-Falco O (1979) Quantitative analysis of lymphoid cells in mycosis fungoides, Sézary's syndrome and parapsoriasis en plaques. Arch Dermatol Res 264:17–28

Schocket AL, Huff JC, Carr RI, Norris DA (1982) Humoral immunity in stage I mycosis fungoides: an increased incidence of lymphocytotoxic antibodies. Br J Dermatol 107:285–291

Schuppli R (1976) Is mycosis fungoides an "Immunoma"? Dermatologica 153:1–6

Segal RJ, Watson W (1978) Kaposi's varicelliforme eruption in mycosis fungoides. Arch Dermatol 114:1067–1069

Shelley WB (1980) Familial mycosis fungoides revisited. Arch Dermatol 116:1177–1178

Sipos K (1965) Painting treatment of nitrogen mustard in mycosis fungoides. Dermatologica 130: 3–11

Smith RW, Terry WD, Buell DN, Sell KW (1973) An antigenic marker for human thymic lymphocytes. J Immunol 110:884

Souteyrand P, Thivolet J, Fulton R (1981) Treatment of parapsoriasis en plaques and mycosis fungoides with an oral aromatic retinoid (Ro 10-9359). In: Retinoids. Advances in basic research and therapy. Edited by Orfanos CE, Braun-Falco O, Farber EM, Grupper Ch, Polano MR, Schuppli R, pp 313–316. Springer-Verlag, Berlin-Heidelberg-New York

Steigleder GK (1974) Die lymphoretikuläre Reaktion. Eine neue Theorie zur Entstehung der Lymphoblastome (Immunoblastome). Z Hautkr 49:987–995

Steigleder GK (1976) Benign and malignant proliferative response. Acta Dermatovener 56:33–41

Steigleder GK (1978) Zur Pathogenese der kutanen malignen Lymphome und Pseudolymphome der Haut. Hautarzt Suppl III 29:31–33

Sterry W, Feller AC (1984) Immunohistochemical phenotyping of cutaneous T-cell lymphomas. Arch Dermatol Res 276:258

Sterry W, Pullmann H, Steigleder GK, Meisterernst E (1980a) Autoradiographic and enzyme cytochemical investigations in cutaneous lymphomas. Cell Tiss Kin 13:210

Sterry W, Steigleder GK, Nikolai B (1980b) Elevated colchicine sensitivity of dermal lymphocytes in mycosis fungoides. Acta Dermatovener 60:257–259

Sterry W, Steigleder GK, Pullmann H (1980c) In situ identification and enumeration of T lymphocytes in cutaneous T cell lymphomas by demonstration of granular activity of acid non-specific esterase. Br J Dermatol 103:67–72

Sterry W, Pullmann H, Steigleder GK (1981a) Proliferation kinetics of the dermal infiltrate in cutaneous malignant lymphomas. Arch Dermatol Res 270:285–290

Sterry W, Schulze HJ, Steigleder GK (1981b) Altered lymphocyte surface in mycosis fungoides. Arch Dermatol Res 270:249

Sterry W, Schulze HJ, Steigleder GK (1981c) Veränderte Zelloberfläche der dermalen Lymphozyten bei Mycosis fungoides. – Eine rasterelektronenmikroskopische Untersuchung. Z Hautkr 56:498–508

Sterry W, Steigleder GK, Goos M, Meisterernst E (1982) In situ identification and enumeration of helper T lymphocytes in cutaneous malignant lymphomas by dipeptidyl-peptidase IV (DPP IV). J Cut Pathol 9:119–120

Sterry W, Jansen M, Haneberg F, Steigleder GK (1983) Saure Esterase und Dipeptidyl-Peptidase IV als Marker immunologischer Lymphozytenpopulationen. Acta histochemica 28:181–190

Stingl G, Knapp W (1977) Characterization of neoplastic mononuclear cells on tissue sections. Haematol Blood Transfus 20:189–196

Stingl G, Gazze-Stingl LA, Aberer W, Wolff K (1981) Antigen presentation by murine epidermal Langerhans cells and its alteration by ultraviolet B light. J Immunol 127:1707–1713

Symmers D (1932) Mycosis fungoides as a clinical and pathological nonexistent. Arch Dermatol Syphil 25:1–5

Thomas JA, Janossy G, Graham-Brown RAC, Kung PC, Goldstein G (1982) The relationship between T-lymphocyte subsets and Ia-like antigen-positive nonlymphoid cells in early stages of cutaneous T-cell lymphoma. J Invest Dermatol 78:169–176

Tjernlund UM (1978) Epidermal expression of HLA-DR antigens in mycosis fungoides. Arch Derm Res 261:81–86

Touraine JL, Touraine F, Kiszkiss DF, Choi YS, Good RA (1974) Heterologous specific antiserum for identification of human T lymphocytes. Clin Exp Immunol 16:503–520

Tourbier H, Schultz-Ehrenburg U (1981) Etagenwechsel by Mycosis fungoides unter systemischer PUVA-Therapie. Z Hautkr 56:923–929

Tronnier H, Loehning R (1974) About the current status of the methoxalen UV-A therapy in dermatology. Castellania 2:267–271

United States Bureau of the Census (1963) In: US Census of population, 1960. Washington DC US Government Printing Office, Vol 1

van Leeuwen AWFM, Meijer CJLM, De Man JCH (1975) T-cell membrane characteristics of mycosis cells in the skin and lymph node. J Invest Dermatol 65:367–369

van Scott EJ, Kalmanson JD (1973) Complete remission of mycosis fungoides lymphoma induced by topical nitrogen mustard (HN2): Control of delayed hypersensitivity to HN2 by desensitization and by induction of specific immunologic tolerance. Cancer 32:18–30

van Vloten WA, van Duijn P, Schaberg A (1974) Cytodiagnostic use of Feulgen-DNA measurements in cell imprints from the skin of patientes with mycosis fungoides. Br J Dermatol 91:365–371

van Vloten WA, Scheffer E, Meijer CJLM (1978) DNA cytophotometry of lymph nodes from patients with mycosis fungoides and Sézary's syndrome. J Invest Dermatol 70:234

van Vloten WA, Scheffer E, Meijer CJLM (1979) DNA-cytophotometry of lymph node imprints from patients with mycosis fungoides. J Invest Dermatol 73:275–279

van Vloten WA, Pet EA, Geraedts JPM (1980) Chromosome studies in mycosis fungoides. Br J Dermatol 102:507–513

van der Harst-Oostveen CJGR, van Vloten WA (1978) Delayed-type hypersensitivity in patients with mycosis fungoides. Dermatologica 157:129–135

van der Loo EM, van Muijen GNP, van Vloten WA (1979) C-type virus-like particles specifically localized in Langerhans cells and related cells of skin and lymph nodes of patients with mycosis fungoides and Sézary syndrome. Virchows Arch B (Cell Pathol) 31:193–203

van der Loo EM, van Vloten WA, Cornelisse CJ, Scheffer E, Meijer CJLM (1981) The relevance of morphometry in the differential diagnosis of cutaneous T cell lymphomas. Br J Dermatol 104:257–269

van der Putte SCJ, van der Meer (1981) Mycosis fungoides: a morphological study. Clin exp Dermatol 6:57–76

Variakojis D, Rosas-Uribe A, Rappaport H (1974) Mycosis fungoides – pathologic findings in staging laparotomies. Cancer 33:1589–1600

Vidal E, Brocq L (1885) Étude sur le mycosis fungoide. Le France Medical 2:946, 957, 969, 983, 993, 1005, 1019, 1085

Viver A du, Vollum DI (1980) Photochemotherapy and topical nitrogen mustard in the treatment of mycosis fungoides. Br J Dermatol 102:319–322

Vivier A du, Vonderheid EC, van Scott EJ, Urbach F (1978) Mycosis fungoides, nitrogen mustard and skin cancer. Br J Dermatol 99:61–63

Volc-Platzer B, Majdic O, Wolff K, Knapp W, Stingl (1984) Ia antigens on keratinocytes in diseased skin. Arch Dermatol Res 276:258–259

Volden G (1980) A study of the photosensitive factor in relation to skin lesions of mycosis fungoides patients. Dermatologica 161:89–92

Volden G, Thune PO (1977) Light sensitivity in mycosis fungoides. Br J Dermatol 97:279–284

Vonderheid EC (1984) Topical mechlorethamine chemotherapy. Considerations on its use in mycosis fungoides. Int J Dermatol 23:180–186

Vonderheid EC, van Voorst Vader PC (1980) Herpes Zoster-Varicella in cutaneous T-cell lymphomas. Arch Dermatol 116:408–412

Vonderheid EC, van Scott EJ, Wallner PE, Johnson WC (1979) A ten year experience with topical mechlorethamine for mycosis fungoides: comparison with patients treated by total-skin electron-beam radiation therapy. Cancer Treat Rep 63:681–689

Vonderheid EC, Milstein HJ, Thompson KR, Wu BC (1980) Chronic herpes simplex infection in cutaneous T-cell lymphomas. Arch Dermatol 116:1018–1022

Wadell CC, Zubler MA, Gore WS (1982) Acute myeloblastic leukemia following chemotherapy for mycosis fungoides. Arch Dermatol 118:179–182

Warin AP (1981) Photochemotherapy in the treatment of psoriasis and mycosis fungoides. Clin Exp Dermatol 6:651–657

Weber G (1975) Blacklight-Meladinine: eine neue Dimension in der Dermatotherapie. Dtsch Ärzteblatt 72:1407–1410

Whang-Peng J, Bunn PA, Knutsen T, Matthews MJ, Schechter G, Minna JD (1982) Clinical implications of cytogenetic studies in cutaneous T-cell lymphoma (CTCL). Cancer 50:1539–1553

White SI, Marsden JR, Marks JM, Proctor S (1984) Autoimmune haematolytic anaemia occuring in a patient with mycosis fungoides. Br J Dermatol 110:495–497

Wiklund D, Norris DA, Morris RJ, Sanderson RJ, Weston WL (1979) Monocyte function and subpopulation in mycosis fungoides. Clin Res 27:139A

Willemze R, de Graff-Reitsma CB, Cnossen J, van Vloten WA, Meijer CJLM (1983) Characterization of T-cell lymphomas and benign inflammatory dermatoses. J Invest Dermatol 80:60–66

Winkler CF, Bunn PA (1984) Combination chemotherapy in cutaneous lymphomas. In: Progress in diseases of the skin. Vol. 2. Ed. Fleischmajer R. Grune and Stratton. Orlando – San Diego – San Francisco – New York – London – Toronto – Montreal – Sydney – Tokyo – Sao Paulo, pp 185–215

Wiskemann A (1980) Röntgentherapie der Haut. In: Dermatologie in Praxis und Klinik. Hrsg.: Korting GW, Thieme Verlag, Stuttgart, Bd 1, pp 734–749

Wolf AF, Landes E (1984) Mycosis fungoides mit Beteiligung des Zentralnervensystems. Hautarzt 35:22–26

Worm AM, Hastrup N, Hou-Jensen K, Thomsen K (1978) Bone marrow involvement in mycosis fungoides demonstrated by needle biopsy. J Cutan Pathol 5:31–34

Yamamura T, Aozasa K, Sano S (1984) The cutaneous lymphomas with convoluted nuclei. J Am Acad Dermatol 10:796–803

Yambe H, Ishii Y, Kikuchi K, Jimbow K (1981) E-rosette inhibitory factor in sera from patients with mycosis fungoides. J Invest Dermatol 76:376–380

Yeckley JA, Weston WL, Thorne EG (1975) Production of Sézary-like cells from normal human lymphocytes. Arch Dermatol 111:29–32

Zachariae H, Grunnet E, Ellegaard J, Thestrup-Pedersen K (1975) Transfer factor as an additional therapeutic agent in mycosis fungoides. Acta Allergol 30:272

Zachariae H, Grunnet E, Thestrup-Pedersen K (1979) Transfer factor in mycosis fungoides: a case report on a patient "cured". Acta Dermatovenerol 59:375–378

Zachariae H, Grunnet E, Thestrup-Pedersen K, Molin L, Schmidt H, Starfelt F, Thomsen K (1982) Oral retinoid in combination with bleomycin, cyclophosphamid, prednisone and transfer factor in mycosis fungoides. Acta Dermatovenerol 62:162–164

Zackheim HS, Epstein EH (1975) Treatment of mycosis fungoides with topical nitrosourea compounds. Arch Dermatol 111:1564–1570

Bullous Dermatoses

A.C. Chu

1. Introduction

The clinical manifestation of blistering may be the end result of a large number of different pathogenetic mechanisms. The bullous dermatoses thus represent a heterogeneous group of disorders which may result from infection, inflammation, trauma or genetic factors. The main reason for grouping these diseases are:

1. the clinical presence in all these diseases of blisters, and
2. the fact that similar specialised techniques are often used to identify and investigate the bullous diseases regardless of pathogenesis.

Frequently, the clinical appearance of the eruption is distinctive enough to allow the clinician to make a diagnosis, Even if this is not the case, the clinical appearance of individual bullae may give valuable clues as to the correct diagnosis. If the blister is tense, this suggests a subepidermal bulla, while if it is flaccid and easily ruptured, this suggests an intraepidermal blister. The age of the patient, distribution of the eruption, presence or absence of itching, associated inflammation in the skin, all help the clinician and pathologist towards a diagnosis.

Histopathology not only demonstrates the site and possible underlying mechanism of bulla formation, but even subtle differences will allow the pathologist to differentiate similar dermatoses. In certain bullous diseases, however, additional techniques are often used to augment histopathology in establishing a definitive diagnosis.

In the immunologically induced dermatoses, immunohistochemistry is extremely valuable and will allow the differentiation of clinically and histologically similar dermatoses. In the dermatoses associated with increased skin fragility, electron microscopy is useful in correctly categorising the abnormality in the skin. This is of particular importance in the group of genodermatoses, epidermolysis bullosa, as the different variants can only be correctly identified by characterising the defect in the skin by electron microscopy.

In this chapter we will examine the mechanisms of blister formation in the skin and will discuss some of the additional tests used in the diagnosis and investigation of the bullous dermatoses. The more important bullous diseases will be described to illustrate these points, but an exhaustive list of all the bullous skin disorders is beyond the scope of this book.

2. Mechanisms of Bullous Formation in the Skin

Anatomically, bullae may form at four sites: subcorneal, suprabasal, subepidermal and intradermal.

2.1 Intradermal

This type of blister formation is observed in bullous amyloidosis. The underlying mechanism is increased skin fragility due to the accumulation of an abnormal protein in the dermis, through which a cleavage plane develops.

2.2 Subepidermal

Subepidermal bullae may form as a result of damage to the papillary dermis, basal lamina or the basal keratinocyte.

2.2.1 Papillary Dermis

In many dermatoses, inflammation in the upper dermis leads to oedema of the papillary tips. If intense, a subepidermal blister develops in which the basal lamina is situated in the root of the blister.

2.2.2 Dermoepidermal Junction

Damage to the dermoepidermal junction may result from decreased tensile strength in this region of the skin due to an inherited abnormality or may result from inflammation centred on the dermoepidermal junction. In some disorders, the basal lamina is found in the roof, in some the floor and in some, both roof and floor, of the blister.

2.2.3 Basal Cell

Damage to the basal cell layer, may result from inflammation, giving rise to liquifractive degeneration of the basal cell layer, from abnormal fragility of the basal cells or from direct physical damage to the basal keratinocytes. Blisters caused by this mechanism have the basal lamina situated in the floor of the blister.

2.3 Intraepidermal

2.3.1 Inter- and Intracellular Oedema

Inflammation in the skin may result in inter and intracellular oedema, and when intense, spongiotic vesicles may form as a result of reticular degeneration of the keratinocytes and disruption of the desmosomal attachments of the cells. This type of blister formation is characteristic of eczema, but may also be seen in erythema multiforme.

2.3.2 Acantholysis

Acantholysis describes a process in which the keratinocytes become detached from each other because of damage to or an abnormality of the intercellular substance. As the keratinocytes detach, they become rounded up to form acantholytic cells. Acantholysis is often seen in bullous dermatoses in which the bulla formation is not primarily due to acantholysis, and in such cases is a secondary phenomenon, possible as the result of proteolytic enzymes released by the inflammatory process.

2.3.3 Viral Blisters

Certain viral infections of the skin – herpes simplex, herpes zoster, varicella – are characterised by the formation of vesicles or bullae in the skin. These blisters develop by balloon degeneration and reticular degeneration of the infected keratinocytes.

2.3.4 Direct Damage to Keratinocytes

This is the underlying mechanism of bulla formation due to physical causes, such as friction blisters. Keratinocytes in the stratum malpighii show necrotic change, resulting in the formation of an intraepidermal cleft.

2.3.5 Subcorneal

In some conditions, attack of the epidermis is centred on the subcorneal region. The reasons for this selective attack on the granular cells is unclear. Subcorneal blisters, may form as a result of acantholysis (pemphigus foliaceus), cytolysis of granular cells (subcorneal pustular dermatosis) or oedema in this area (toxic epidermal necrolysis).

3. Immunofluorescence Techniques and Bullous Dermatoses

Immunohistochemistry is an important additional technique in the diagnosis and investigation of the bullous dermatoses. Many bullous diseases are mediated by an immunological assault on the epidermis or basal lamina. In such diseases, immunohistochemistry will identify and localise the immunoreactants in the skin and can substantiate or establish a diagnosis of a specific dermatosis. In some dermatoses, e.g. dermatitis herpetiformis, immunohistochemistry may be the only way of making a definitive diagnosis, as both clinical and histological features may be non specific.

In some dermatoses, circulating antibodies are present which specifically bind to structures in the skin. These can be of great diagnostic value, and in pemphigus vulgaris and bullous pemphigoid, may also be of prognostic importance.

Immunohistochemistry may also be used in diseases where the anatomical situation of the cleft is diagnostically or prognostically important e.g. in the epidermolysis bullosa group of disorders, and the use of immunohistochemistry with specific marker antibodies may obviate the need for standard transmission electronmicroscopy.

The basic techniques used in immunohistochemistry will be briefly described, and the immunohistochemical characteristics of the individual dermatoses will be described with the dermatosis in question.

3.1 Specimen Collection

The site from which the skin biopsy is taken for immunohistochemistry is of paramount importance. As a generalisation, the biopsy should be taken from the margin of a fresh blister, including both normal and lesional skin. The age of the blister is of obvious importance from a histopathological view point, as regeneration of the epidermis may turn a subepidermal blister into an intraepidermal cleft, and the cell population present in the infiltrate may change with age, and become less diagnostic.

In some dermatoses, e.g. dermatitis herpetiformis, the immunoreactants in the skin are often removed by the inflammatory reaction. Perilesional or uninvolved skin is thus needed for immunohistochemistry in these diseases.

In a recent study, Wojnarowska et al. (1982) have shown that in bullous pemphigoid and pemphigus vulgaris, the immunoreactants are found as frequently in normal uninvolved skin, as in perilesional and lesional skin. These authors recommend that in these dermatoses normal skin is examined by immunohistochemistry.

Table 1. Stock solutions can be stored indefinitely, but buffer and fixatives should be prepared fresh each week

Buffer	
1 M potassium citrate buffer (pH 7.0)	2.5 mls
0.1 M magnesium sulphate	5.0 mls
0.1 M methylmaleimide	5.0 mls
Distilled water	87.5 mls
Adjust pH to 7.0 with 1 M potassium hydroxide.	
Fixative	
Buffer	100 mls
ammonium sulphate	55 gms

Following biopsy, the specimen can either be stored in transport medium (Table 1) for up to 7 days or can be snap frozen and stored at −80° C until needed. Specimens stored in transport medium should be washed carefully in two changes of wash buffer before being frozen. Failure to do this results in an unacceptable diminution in the staining obtained and may lead to false negative results (Skeete and Black 1977).

In indirect immunohistochemistry, the blood of the patient is examined for the presence of cirulating antibodies directed against skin components. Venous blood should be allowed to clot, and the serum removed after centrifugation. The serum can be frozen and stored at −20° C until used. Whole blood should never be frozen.

3.2 Direct Immunofluorescence

In direct immunofluorescence, the patient's skin is examined for the presence of immunoreactants. 4–5 μm cryostat sections of the skin are cut onto glass slides and stained with antibodies against human IgA, IgG, IgM, C_3 and fibrin. For more specialised studies, anti C_{1q}, C_2, C_4, properdin and factor B antibodies can also be used.

3.2.1 Staining Procedure

Sections are fan dried for 10 min and then washed in phosphate buffered saline (PBS) for 20 min. After fan drying for a further 10 min, the sections are incubated with the anti-immunoreactants at suitable dilutions for 30 min in a humidity chamber. The sections are then washed for 30 min in PBS and after air drying for 10 min are incubated with the fluorescein conjugated anti-immunoglobulin for 30 min in a humidity chamber. After a final wash in PBS for 30 min, the sections are counterstained for one minute in Evans blue stain, washed in tap water and mounted in buffered glycerol under a cover slip before examination under the fluorescence microscope. The immunoreactants are visualised by their bright green fluorescence.

3.3 Indirect Immunofluorescence

In this technique, circulating antibodies against structures in the skin are identified using a substrate of normal skin, monkey oesophagus, or guinea pig lip. In several studies, monkey oesophagus has been found to be the best substrate, but normal human skin is more accessible and is generally adequate.

3.3.1 Staining Procedure

4–5 μm cryostat sections of the substrate are cut and dried for 10 min. After a 20 min wash in PBS, the sections are air dried for 10 min, and incubated with the patient's serum diluted 1:4 or 1:16 in PBS for 30 min in a humidity chamber. In pemphigus vulgaris, where the titre of the circulating antibody is of prognostic value, doubling dilutions to 1:320 are used. After a 30 min wash in PBS and fan dry for 10 min, the sections are incubated with a fluorescein conjugated anti human anti serum for 30 min in a humidity chamber. After a final wash, the sections are counterstained with Evans Blue stain and examined under the fluorescence microscope.

3.4 Indirect C_3 Technique

This method detects circulating antibody which will activate complement. This is of most value in herpes gestationis, where the circulating HG factor is of diagnostic importance and is often not detected by indirect immunofluorescence.

3.4.1 Staining Procedure

Two 4–5 μm cryostat sections of normal human skin are fan dried and washed in PBS for 20 min, then fan dried for 10 min. The sections are first incubated with the patient's serum neat or diluted 1:4 in PBS for 30 min in a humidity chamber. The sections are washed in PBS for 30 min, fan dried for 10 min and then incubated with a source of complement (normal human serum diluted 1 in 5 in complement diluting buffer) for 30 min in a humidity chamber, washed in PBS for 30 min and fan dried for 10 min. The sections are finally incubated with a fluorescein conjugated anti C_3 for 30 min in a humidity chamber. After a final wash in PBS, the sections are mounted in buffered glycerol and examined with a fluorescence microscope.

3.5 Localisation of the Cleft

In certain diseases, i.e. the epidermolysis bullosa group of diseases, the localisation of the cleft in the skin is of major diagnostic and prognostic importance. The standard method of ascertaining this is by standard transmission electron microscopy. Immunohistochemistry will however, differentiate the three major subgroups, when electron microscopy is not available.

This technique makes use of the fact that the lamina lucida and lamina dense contain different antigenic determinants. The major marker for the lamina lucida is the bullous pemphigoid antigen and for the lamina densa is type 4 collagen. Using a high titre serum from patients with bullous pemphigoid and a commercially available anti-type 4 collagen, the position of the lamina lucida and lamina densa in the blister cavity can be ascertained. In intraepidermal blisters, both type 4 collagen and bullous pemphigoid antigen will be situated in the floor of the blister. In bullous pemphigoid and junctional epidermolysis bullosa, where the cleft is through the lamina lucida, the bullous pemphigoid antigen will be in both floor and roof of the blister while type 4 collagen will be restricted to the floor. In subepidermal blistering diseases, i.e. dystrophic epidermolysis bullosa both bullous pemphigoid antigen and type 4 collagen will be found in the roof of the blister.

4. Dermoepidermal Junction – Ultrastructure

The dermoepidermal junction is a complex structure involving the basal keratinocytes, the basement membrane and upper dermis.

Ultrastructurally, the dermoepidermal junction can be divided into four parts:

1. Basal keratinocyte plasma membrane
2. Lamina lucida
3. Basal lamina
4. Subbasal lamina fibrous elements.

The basal keratinocyte plasma membrane is about 8 nm thick and is trilaminate. On the cytoplasmic side are the hemidesmosomes which are 20–40 nm thick and act as anchoring points for the tonofilaments of the basal cells. The lamina lucida is 30 nm thick and is seen under the electron microscope as an amorphous pale zone. Within the lamina lucida and adjacent to the hemidesmosones are electron dense subbasal dense plaques, through which anchoring filaments connect the plasma membrane to the basal lamina.

The basal lamina is an electron dense fibrillar and amorphous layer 30–50 nm thick. It is a continuous layer, but reduplication is often seen, resulting from basal cell division and upward migration.

There are three types of subbasal lamina fibrous elements, the anchoring fibrils, microfibril bundles and collagen fibres. The anchoring fibrils and microfibril bundles are attached to the basal lamina. The anchoring fibrils have a unique periodicity compared to other human collagens.

The microfibril bundles are arranged perpendically and obliquely to the basal lamina and pass through to the deep dermis. These fibril bundles are thought to be composed of elastic tissue.

The collagen bundles are not attached to the basal lamina, and the collagen fibrils seen close to the basal lamina are not grouped into bundles.

All the structures making up the dermoepidermal junction are necessary to maintain the integrity of this zone. Genetic abnormalities of structures of the dermoepidermal junction manifest themselves as reduced cohesion between the dermis and epidermis and increased fragility of the skin resulting in blister formation. Many inflammatory disease also involve an attack on structures in the basement membrane zone and may result in clinical blister formation.

5. Bullous Pemphigoid

Bullous pemphigoid is a benign chronic blistering disease which predominantly affects people in the sixth, seventh or eight decades. The bullae may arise in clinically normal skin or in areas of macular erythema or urticated plaques. Blistering is usually accompanied by pruritus which may be severe. Individual bullae are tense and may attain a considerable size (up to 10 cm) before rupturing to leave denuded areas of skin. These denuded areas tend to heal, unlike pemphigus, where the tendency is for further extension.

Sites of predeliction for the eruption are axillae, groins, upper inner thighs, abdomen and flexor forearms. 33% of patients also have oral mucosa involvement, which usually presents as intact blisters. There is no racial or sexual predominance.

5.1 Histology

The histological appearance of bullous pemphigoid parallels the clinical activity or age of the lesion biopsied. In blisters arising from normal appearing skin, the inflammatory infiltrate may be insignificant, while in a blister arising from an erythematous site, the inflammatory cell infiltrate may be intense. Also, reepithelialisation of the blister cavity occurs early, starting as early as 48 h. Thus an older blister may show an intraepidermal or subcorneal, rather than subepidermal cleft. Early biopsy, preferably from a lesion on an erythematous base is therefore preferable.

Within the dermis, the earliest change which can be detected either in normal looking skin away from bullous or erythematous lesions, or in perilesional skin, is a perivascular infiltration of mononuclear cells which is predominantly lymphocytic (Dvorak et al. 1982). As the lesions progress from clinically normal skin to macular erythema, urticated erythema and bullous formation, the extent and composition of the dermal infiltrate alters. In the erythematous macule and plaque, the predominant cell in the perivascular infiltrate is the eosinophil, with a few basophils, neutrophils and macrophages. With clinical blister formation, more marked lymphocytic and eosinophilic infiltration occurs. At the periphery of some bullae, microabscesses composed predominantly of eosinophils are seen in the papillary tips, similar to, but less extensive than those seen in dermatitis herpetiformis.

Electron microscopic studies have shown that eosinophils in normal appearing skin and macular lesions are morphologically normal. However, in the ery-

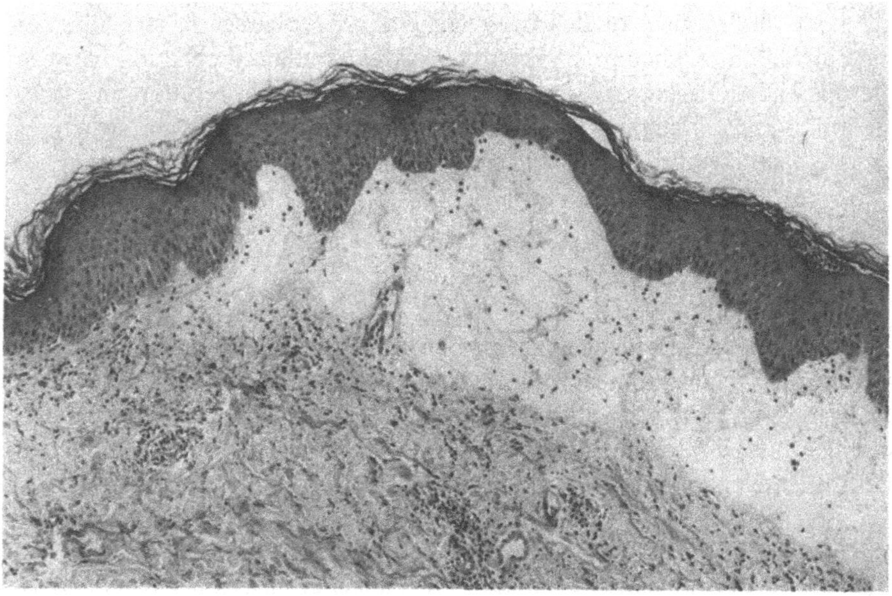

Fig. 1. Bullous pemphigoid. A well developed subepidermal bulla. The perivascular infiltrate is composed predominantly of eosinophils and eosinophils are seen scattered throughout the loose fibrin network within the blister cavity

thematous plaques and bullous lesions, numerous free eosinophils granules are found throughout the dermis (DVORAK et al. 1982). Some of the granules appear normal, but many show loss of density of either the central crystal or the entire granule. Release of eosinophils granules appears to be the result of karyorrhexis and karyolysis with release of membrane bound granules.

Mast cells in bullous pemphigoid show a progressive change with the clinical stage of the disease. In early lesions, only few mast cells are found high in the papillary dermis and these appear to be normal. In plaque lesions, however, many mast cells are found in the upper reticular dermis, many of which show excentric nuclei, tail like cytoplasmic projections, suggesting active movement of the cells, and hypogranulation.

Vascular changes are restricted to the venules. In early lesions, the lymphocytic infiltration is accompanied by endothelial cell hypertrophy and focal luminal obliteration. As the lesion progresses, more marked hypertrophy is seen with focal endothelial cell necrosis and apparent sloughing of endothelial cells. On electron microscopy, a conspicuous feature of the endothelial cells is the presence of numerous Weibel Palade bodies. In plaque and bullous lesions, basement membrane thickening of veins is seen, which has been shown, ultrastructurally to result from basal lamina reduplication.

Interstitial fibrin deposition is first evident in macular lesions, but becomes more intense in the upper reticular dermis below plaque and bullous lesions. Fibrin is absent from venules and perivascular spaces. With well developed blisters, a fibrin network with eosinophils scattered throughout is present in the floor of the blister (Fig. 1).

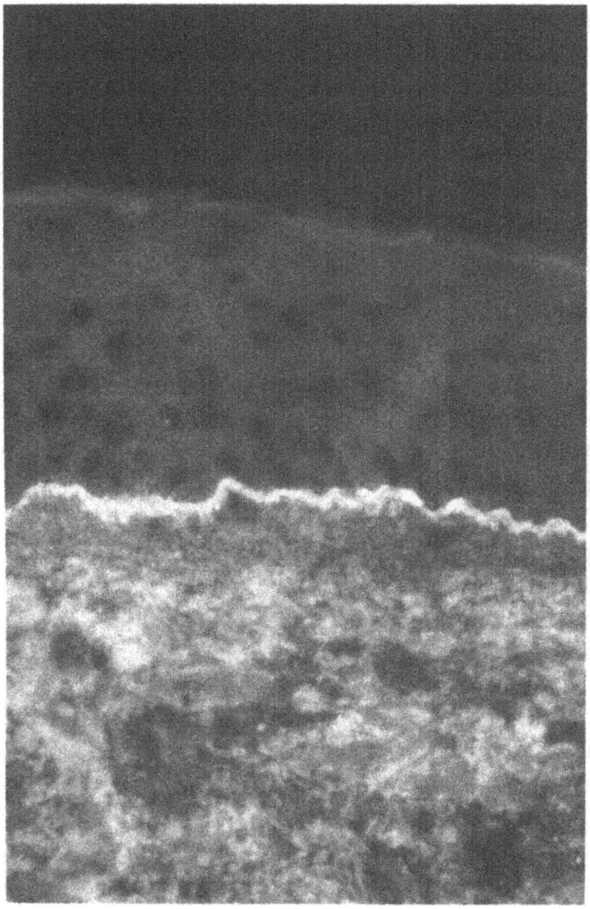

Fig. 2. Bullous pemphigoid. Direct immunofluorescence shows a linear band of IgG along the basement membrane zone

Bullae arise from areas of oedema of the papillary dermis. As the oedema becomes more intense, vacuoles develop which eventually coalesce to form a subepidermal cleft. Electron microscopic studies have shown that blister formation is preceded by the fragmentation of the basal lamina (SCHAUMBURG-LEVER et al. 1972). Re-epitheliatisation of the blister floor occurs rapidly from the margins of the blister.

5.2 Immunohistochemistry

The characteristic finding in lesional skin of bullous pemphigoid is the linear deposition of C_3 and IgG at the basement membrane zone (BEUTNER et al. 1970). Occasionally other immunoglobulins are also found, IgM and IgA, and occasionally properdin and factor B, suggesting that complement activation may be mediated via the classical or alternative pathways (Fig. 2).

In 60–70% of patients, circulating IgG against the basement membrane zone is found. In one study using an indirect C_3 test, 58% patients were found to have circulating IgG using a standard indirect immunofluorescence technique, while 76% were found to have circulating IgG using an indirect C_3 test (HODGE et al. 1978). This demonstrates the greater sensitivity of the C_3 test in detecting circulating IgG and also the higher prevalence of circulating anti basement membrane zone IgG in patients with bullous pemphigoid.

5.3 Pathogenesis

Bullous pemphigoid is an autoimmune disease, in which tissue damage is mediated by a circulating, complement fixing IgG directed against the basement membrane zone of the skin. The antigen against which this antibody is directed, is produced by the basal keratinocytes and is found predominantly in the lamina lucida. A 31,000 mw protein has been characterised by DIAZ et al. (1977) as the putative bullous pemphigoid antigen. This protein is found in the lamina lucida and also in the saliva and urine of normal individuals. It has been found to block bullous pemphigoid antibody binding in normal human skin.

Keratinocytes have been shown to produce the bullous pemphigoid antigen in tissue culture. This protein also seems to be an integral part of the basal keratinocyte cytoplasmic membrane, as it is retained by basal keratinocytes following trypsin separation of individual epidermal cells and can be demonstrated as a polar cap by binding of bullous pemphigoid anti serum.

A possible mechanism for the tissue damage seen in bullous pemphigoid, is the binding of IgG to the bullous pemphigoid antigen in the lamina lucida, with complement fixation, resulting in the influx of inflammatory cells and damage to the basal lamina.

Within the blister fluid of bullous pemphigoid, at least three chemoattractant factors have been characterised. Neutrophil and eosinophil chemotaxis has been attributed to the C_{5a} fraction of the fifth complement component (DIAZ-PEREZ and JORDAN 1976) and to a mast cell derived chemoattractant. Activation of mast cells by C_{3a} and the subsequent degranulation of mast cells seen in early bullous pemphigoid, is thought to lead to release of ECF-A (eosinophil chemotactic factor) by the mast cells (WINTROBE et al. 1977).

A further chemoattractant factor has more recently been characterised by CENTER et al. (1983). This factor, which is chemoattractant for lymphocytes shows many of the characteristics of the human lymphocyte chemoattractant lymphokine (CENTER et al. 1982). It is a 56,000 μm cationic protein with an isoelectric point of 8.6–9.0. It is heat resistant but sensitive to trypsin and neurominidase. This factor may be responsible for the early lymphocytic infiltration which precedes the influx of eosinophils.

Despite the great weight of evidence in favour of an immunological, complement mediated mechanism for the damage seen in bullous pemphigoid, no direct evidence for this has been reported. Of particular note is that passive transfer experiments have as yet failed to demonstrate this mechanism in vivo. SAMS and GLEICH (1971) infused large amounts of bullous pemphigoid antibody into monkeys. Although the bullous pemphigoid antibody could be shown to be bound to the basement membrane zone for several days, none of the animals developed clinical disease.

5.4 Bullous Pemphigoid and Carcinoma

Numerous anecdotal reports have appeared in the literature, of the association between bullous pemphigoid and underlying systemic malignancy. In a study of 134 patients with bullous pemphigoid, HODGE et al. (1981) found a significant difference between those patients with and without circulating bullous pemphigoid antibody in relation to malignancy. 93 patients were shown to have circulating anti-basement membrane antibody and 4% of these were found to have an associated systemic carcinoma. In the 35 patients who showed no circulating antibody, however, 23% had an associated carcinoma. This study, therefore, suggests that all seronegative bullous pemphigoid patients should be investigated for possible underlying neoplasm.

6. Cicatricial Pemphigoid (Benign Mucus Membrane Pemphigoid)

This is a chronic bullous dermatosis primarily involving the mucous membranes. It affects predominantly middle aged and elderly patients with a pedeliction for oral and ocular mucous membranes. On occasions, cutaneous lesions may also be present.

An unusual varient of this disease was described by BRUNSTING and PERRY in 1957, in which localised cutaneous bullous lesions occurred, predominantly on the head and neck, with relative sparing of the mucosal surfaces.

Conjunctival involvement leads to severe scarring and eventually to blindness in about 20% of patients.

6.1 Histology

Histologically, cicatricial pemphigoid is indistinguishable from bullous pemphigoid. With more chronic lesions, significant scarring is present in the upper dermis. Ultrastructurally, the basal lamina may show evidence of replication (SUSI and SHKLAR 1971) or may be largely destroyed.

6.2 Immunohistochemistry

On direct immunofluorescence, IgG and C_3 are found in 80–97% of patients with cicatricial pemphigoid in a linear fashion along the basement membrane zone. Only 10–36% of patients, however, have circulating anti basement membrane zone IgG as detected by indirect immunofluorescence, even using oral mucosa as the substrate.

On immunoelectronmicroscopy, the immunoreactants are deposited in the lamina lucida, similar to bullous pemphigoid, herpes gestationis and linear IgA dermatosis. Studies using suction blister techniques, however, have shown that the localisation of immunoreactants in suction blisters is different in cicatricial and bullous pemphigoid. In bullous pemphigoid, the immunoreactants are localised to the roof of the blister, while in cicatricial pemphigoid, the immunoreactants are localised to the floor of the blister. This suggests that different antigens may be involved in the two diseases, which may explain the different clinical presentations of the diseases (FINE et al. 1984).

7. Herpes Gestationis

Herpes gestationis is an uncommon, pruritic bullous eruption of pregnancy. The incidence is between 1:3000–4000 pregnancies (RUSSELL and THORNE 1957) and the onset is usually in the 20th–28th week of pregnancy but it may occur in the first trimester or in the puerperium. Frequently there is an exacerbation of the eruption post partum, and the eruption may recur with the first menstrual cycle post partum or with starting the contraceptive pill. Its duration following delivery is usually more than three weeks and in the majority the bullous lesions subside after eight weeks. It may however run a protracted course and one patient has been documented in which the eruption has lasted for over 10 years (HOLMES et al. 1982).

The eruption starts as pruritic urticated papules and plaques which progress to vesicles, target lesions and polycyclic erythema followed after a mean of four weeks by bullous formation (HOLMES et al. 1982). Characteristically the eruption starts around the umbilicus and then spreads to the trunk and limbs. Occasionally the face, palms, soles and oral mucosa are involved.

7.1 Histology

The earliest change seen on electron microscopy is damage to basal keratinocytes (HARRINGTON and BLEEHEN 1979). This is seen even in clinically uninvolved skin. In early urticated lesions, there is a perivascular infiltrate of lymphocytes, histiocytes and eosinophils in the superficial and deep dermal plexuses.

Eosinophils may be present in large number, occasionally comprising 50% of the dermal infiltrate (HOLMES et al. 1982). As the lesion evolves, there is progressive oedema of the dermal papillary tips, with overlying spongiosis and focal necrosis of basal keratinocytes. The necrotic basal keratinocytes occasionally resemble the colloid bodies seen in lichen planus and lupus erythematosus. Eosinophils may be seen collecting at the tips of oedematus dermal papillae forming eosinophilic microabscesses (HERTZ et al. 1976). Eosinophils and lymphocytes collect in spongiotic foci, and eosinophils may show fragmentation of their nuclei (SCHAUMBURG-LEVER et al. 1973). Bullae arise from areas of basal cell necrosis and are subepidermal.

On electron microscopy, there is marked degeneration and necrotic change in basal keratinocytes with intracellular oedema and vacuolar degeneration (HARRINGTON and BLEEHEN 1979). The plasma membrane of basal cells becomes discontinuous and the contents of the cells are seen to protrude through these gaps. The basal lamina remains predominantly intact but may show small gaps through which pseudopods of basal keratinocytes protrude.

7.2 Immunohistochemistry

The characteristic finding in herpes gestationis is the linear deposition of C_3 at the basement membrane zone (KATZ et al. 1976). In 25–30% of patients, IgG may also be detected. Occasionally properdin and factor B of the alterative pathway and C_{1q} and C_4 of the classical pathway of complement activation, may be found.

Indirect immunofluorescence demonstrates circulating IgG against basement membrane zone in about 20% patients, but using the more sensitive indirect C_3 test, 90% patients show a circulating HG factor which is a complement fixing IgG directed against the basement membrane zone.

C_3 deposition may be present in the skin of patients up to 1 year after clinical resolution of the eruption.

Immunoelectron microscopy has shown that the C_3 and IgG are deposited in the lamina lucida and at the plasma membrane of basal keratinocytes, in the same pattern as that seen in bullous pemphigoid (YAOITA et al. 1976).

7.3 Pathogenesis

Herpes gestationis probably represents an autoimmune disease, with the deposition of the HG factor at the basement membrane zone which fixes complement and mediates the damage to basal keratinocytes. Although properdin and factor B are occasionally found in herpes gestationis skin, testing in vitro with a C_2 deficient human serum as a source of complement has shown that the HG factor fixes complement by the classical pathway.

In patients with herpes gestationis, there is a high incidence of anti-thyroid auto antibodies and of clinical Graves disease (HOLMES et al. 1982). There is also a high incidence of HLA B8 and HLA DR3 in these patients suggesting some genetic predisposition to the disease.

8. Dermatitis Herpetiformis

Dermatitis herpetiformis is an intensely pruritic papulovesicular dermatosis. Although it may occur at any age, the peak incidence is in the 2nd and 3rd decades. The eruption consists of erythematous papules, urticated plaques, vesicles which are usually heavily excorated, and on rare occasions, bullae. The distribution of the eruption is on extensor surfaces, affecting the elbows, knees,

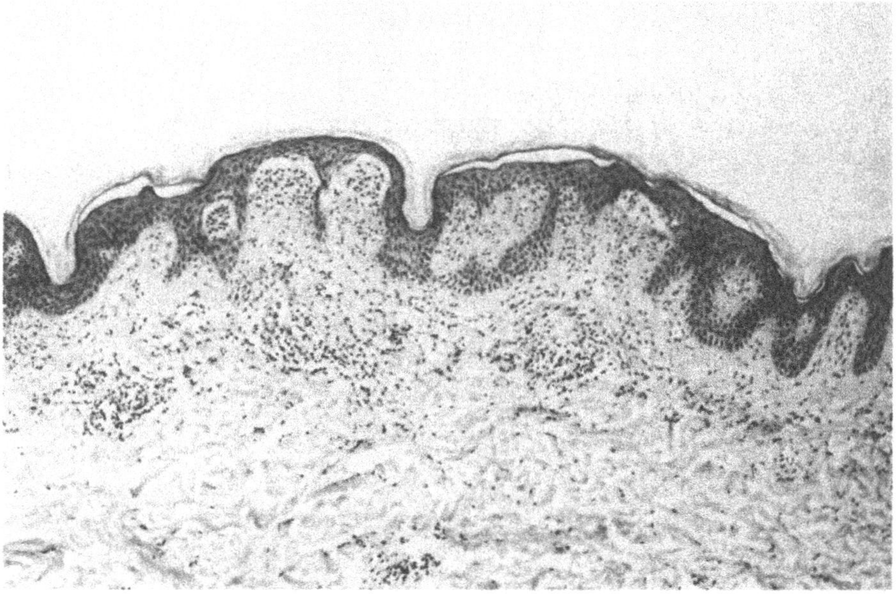

Fig. 3. Dermatitis herpetiformis. Neutrophilic microabscesses are present in the dermal papillae which show early vesicle formation

buttocks, nuchal region, scalp, sacrum and shoulders. The oral mucosa is not affected (Tolman et al. 1959). Males are affected twice as frequently as females. The eruption tends to be life long with brief spontaneous remissions. Response to suphones (dapsone) is dramatic, with rapid relief of symptoms.

The majority of patients with dermatitis herpetiformis have an associated asymptomatic gluten sensitive enteropathy. The relationship between the skin and gastrointestinal abnormalities will be further discussed under pathogenesis.

Characteristic histological changes are best seen in early urticated lesions or in perivesicular areas. In many patients, histological examination may be unhelpful and multiple biopsies are necessary before the diagnosis can be established.

8.1 Histology

Chronologically, the first abnormality found in dermatits herpetiformis is the presence of a perivascular mononuclear cell infiltrate in the upper dermis. Reitamo et al. (1981) showed that the majority of these cells, in the earliest lesions were B cells, but T cells become more numerous with the evolution of the lesion. At this stage, fibrin and fibronectin can be shown to be deposited in the dermal papillae, asociated with oedema of the papillae.

As the lesion evolves, the upper dermis and immediate subepidermal zones become the centre of the inflammatory process. Characteristically, polymorphs and eosinophils form tightly packed collections or microabscesses in the tips of dermal papillae. Neutrophils usually predominate, but eosinophils may be

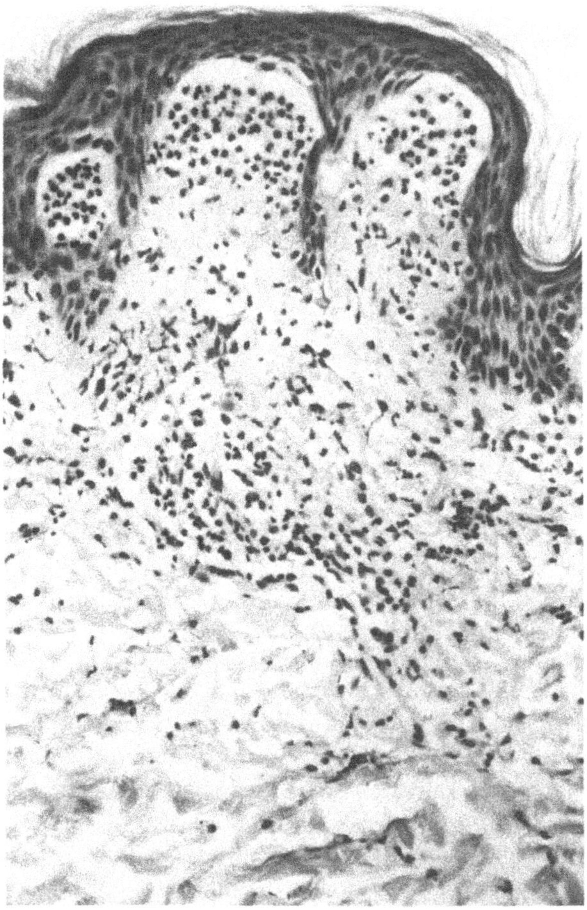

Fig. 4. Dermatitis herpetiformis. The upper dermal infiltrate is predominantly of neutrophils with a few eosinophils. Leucocytoclasis is a prominant feature

present in equal numbers or may even predominate (Fig. 3). Scattered throughout the dermal papillae are polymorphs, with a few eosinophils and some histiocytes and lymphocytes.

Leucocytoclasis is seen in the majority of cases. This is diffusely distributed throughout the papillary dermis associated with the fibrin deposition (CONNOR and WILSON JONES 1972) (Fig. 4).

Papillary and subpapillary capillaries and venules may show some endothelial cell swelling, and this may be associated with loss of red blood cells into the papillary dermis. Fibrin deposition is not generally associated with blood vessels, and leukocytotasis shows no spatial concentration around blood vessels. CONNOR and WILSON JONES (1972), have, however, reported one case of dermatitis herpetiformis in which fibrinoid necrosis of small blood vessels was observed.

Within the epidermis, spongiosis and slight acanthosis may be seen. Focal basal cell degeneration associated with an underlying papillary tip microabscess or early vesicle formation is seen in most cases.

The blister in dermatitis herpetiformis starts as oedema and subsequent separation of the epidermis and dermis overlying a papillary microabscess. Frequently the bullae are multilocular, but the locules coalesce to form a single cleft. PAS stain shows basement membrane disruption overlying the papillary microabscesses.

Ultrastructurally, the earliest changes in blister formation is the formation of vacuoles beneath an intact basal lamina, (RICHES et al. 1973). More vacuoles form and the basal lamina is disrupted and basal keratinocytes damaged.

Acantholysis is a recognised feature of dermatitis herpetiformis, but is not a primary cause of blister formation. The acantholytic cells are seen either as single cells or in clumps, and are only seen in vesicles or bullae in which polymorphs are also present within the blister cavity, and the basal cell layer is disrupted.

8.2 Immunohistochemistry

The pathopneumonic change in dermatitis herpetiformis is the depostion of IgA within the skin (FRY and SEAH 1974). In 80% of patients the IgA is distributed in a granular fashion in the dermal papillae (Fig. 5). In 12–18%, the distribution is as a linear, continuous or more rarely granular band along the basement membrane zone. Longitudinal studies have shown that the IgA deposition does not change its pattern in individual patients (HALL et al. 1981).

The IgA is frequently associated with deposition of C_3 and also properdin, factor B, and C_5, suggesting complement fixation via the alternative pathway. IgA deposition is found in perilesional and clinically normal skin. Immunoreactants, however, are frquently absent from skin showing active blister formation. The site of biopsy is thus extremely important in dermatitis herpetiformis.

The IgA is polyclonal and does not contain the secretory piece of IgA. Deposition of IgA and C3 is unchanged by treatment with sulphones, but may be reduced following a gluten free diet (FRY et al. 1973).

Circulating IgA against the basal membrane zone is seen in 2% of patients with granular papillary IgA deposition and in 30% of patients with linear IgA deposition (YAOITA and KATZ 1977).

17–22% patients with dermatitis herpetiformis also show circulating IgG anti-reticulin antibodies (SEAH et al. 1971). Some authors have implicated these antibodies in the pathogenesis of dermatitis herpetiformis, but IgG deposition in the skin in this disease is very uncommon.

Immunelectron microscopic studies have shown in the granular papillary pattern IgA dermatitis herpetiformis, that IgA is deposited as aggregates associated with microfibrillar bundles and with micro fibrillar components of the elastic tissue (STINGL et al. 1976). In the linear pattern, deposition of IgA may be associated with the anchoring fibrils in the dermis or occasionally in the lamina lucida (YAOITA and KATZ 1976).

8.3 Pathogenesis

Granular IgA – dermatitis herpetiformis, is associated with a gluten enteropathy in almost all patients (MARKS et al. 1966). In most this is asymptomatic, and

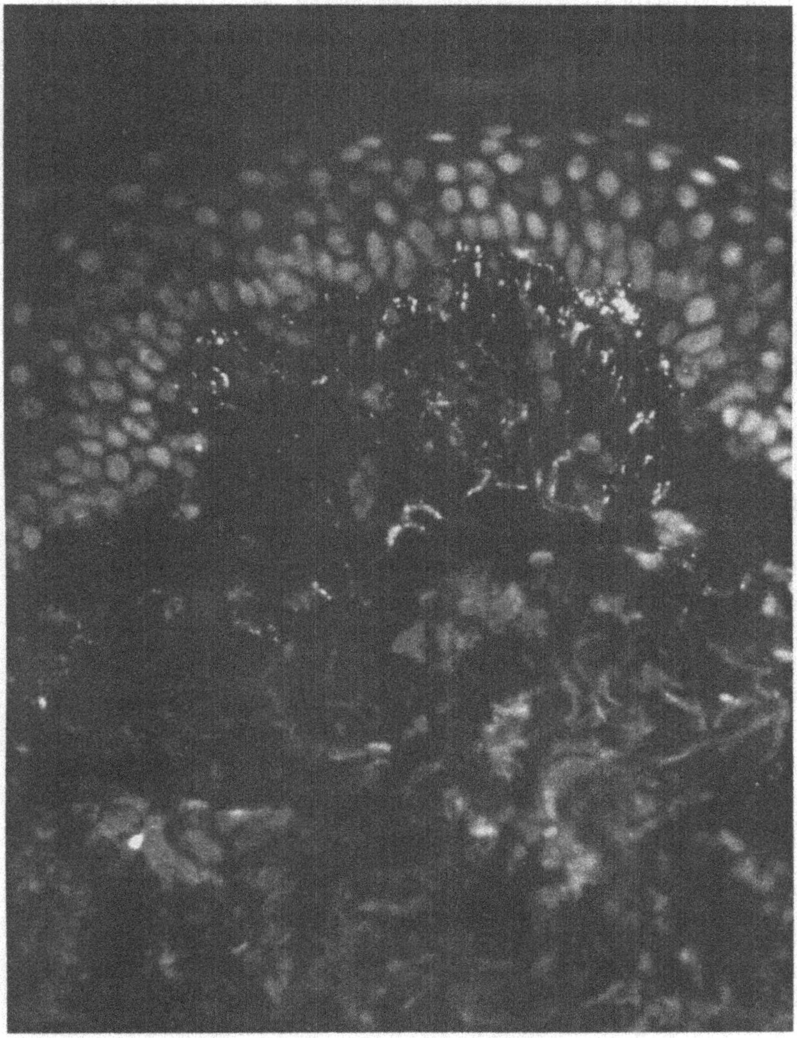

Fig. 5. Dermatitis herpetiformis. Direct immunofluorescence shows granular deposits of IgA in the dermal papillae. Counterstaining with Evans blue allows the visualisation of keratinocyte nuclei in the epidermis

in some patients, histological changes of villous atrophy of jejunal mucosa may only become evident following a gluten load (WEINSTEIN 1974).

In view of this association, many groups have postulated a casual relationships between gluten and dermatitis herpetiformis.

IgA secretion in the gastro-intestinal tract is increased in dermatitis herpetiformis (STINGL et al. 1976) and IgA immune complexes have been demonstrated in 30% of patients with dermatitis herpetiformis (ZONE et al. 1980). There is however, no correlation between the levels of immune complexes and disease activity or treatment. A gluten free diet, has however been shown to reduce the need for suphone therapy in patients with dermatitis herpetiformis. FRY et al. (1973) treated 20 patients with a strict gluten free diet, 50% were able to discontinue sulphone therapy and 30% were able to reduce the dose of dapsone by 75%. Gluten avoidance for 5–12 months was necessary to achieve these results.

17–20% of patients with dermatitis herpetiformis have circulating anti-reticulin antibodies. SEAH et al. (1971) have shown that circulating anti-reticulin antibody can be absorbed from serum by gluten or gluten fraction III, suggesting a cross reaction with gluten. It has thus been suggested that in dermatitis herpetiformis, circulating gluten anti-gluten IgA complexes are trapped in the skin by reticulin bound anti-reticulin antibody which cross reacts with gluten. IgA could then fix complement via the alternative pathway (PROVOST and TOMASI 1974). This mechanism would explain the immunoelectron microscope findings of the close association between the IgA depositions and microfibrillar bundles, and elastic tissue.

This mechanism does however have many factors against it. The incidence of IgA immune complexes in dermatitis herpetiformis is only 30%. The incidence of circulating anti-reticulin antibodies is also low and IgG is are rarely seen deposited in the skin in dermatitis herpetiformis suggesting that the antireticular antibodies are not deposited in the skin. Also IgA and C_3 persist for some months in the skin of patients in clinical remission on dapsone.

A strong association between dermatitis herpetiformis and HLA B8 has been demonstrated. LAWLEY et al. (1980) showed HLA B8 to be present in 88% of patients with granular papillary IgA dermatitis herpetiformis, compared to a control population and linear IgA dermatitis herpetiformis where the incidence is 20–30%. There is also a significantly higher incidence of HLA DW3 and HLA DRW3 in patients with granular IgA dermatitis herpetiformis.

8.4 Linear IgA Dermatosis (Linear IgA Dermatitis Herpetiformis)

This dermatosis is clinically indistinguishable from granular IgA dermatitis herpetiformis, but differs in many parameters from granular IgA dermatitis herpetiformis.

Linear IgA dermatitis herpetiformis is not associated with a gluten enteropathy, and there is no increased incidence of HLA B8 or HLA DW3/DRW3 in these patients. On immunohistochemistry, the deposition of IgA in the skin is always in a linear fashion at the basement membrane zone, generally as a continuous band but occasionally as a granular deposition (Fig. 6).

On immunoelectron microscopy, the IgA is deposited on the anchoring fibrils in the dermis, or the in lamina lucida, similar to the distribution of IgG in bullous pemphigoid (YAOITA and KATZ 1976).

Histologically, linear continous and granular IgA dermatitis herpetiformis are indistinguishable. BLENKINSOPP et al. (1983), however, showed that acantholysis and fibrin deposition at the papillary tips was more commonly seen in granular papillary IgA – dermatitis herpetiformis, than in linear IgA dermatitis herpetiformis. These differences, were however very subtle, and would not allow the differentiation of the two groups of dermatitis herpetiformis without immunofluorescence techniques.

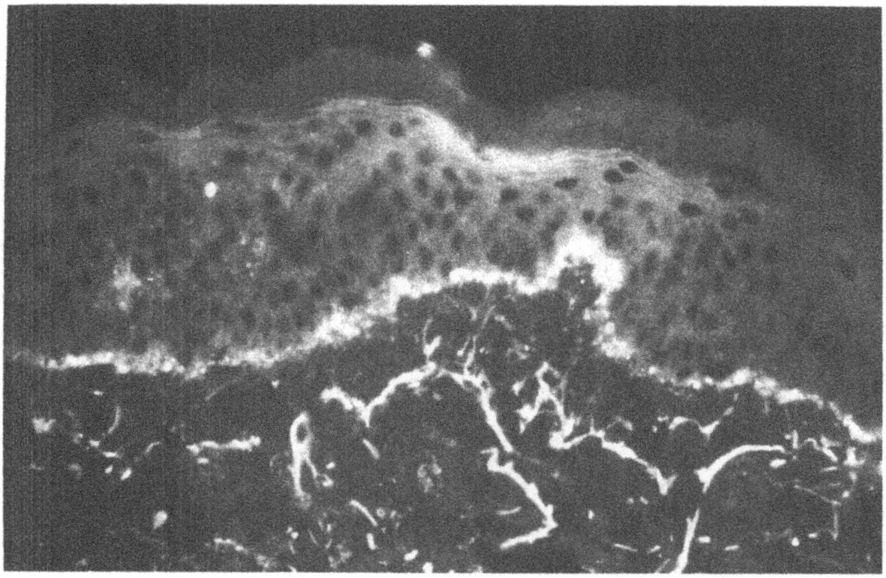

Fig. 6. Linear IgA dermatosis. Direct immunofluorescence shows the linear deposition of IgA in a granular fashion along the basement membrane zone

9. Chronic Bullous Disease of Childhood

This is an acquired, self limiting, blistering disease which represents a form of linear IgA disease occuring in children. The mean age of onset of the disease is 5 years, and the eruption usually spontaneously resolves after two to three years. The eruption consists of large tense clear or haemorrhagic bullae on normal or erythematous skin. In association with the bullae, grouped vesicles similar to those seen in dermatitis herpetiformis are occasionally seen. Sites of predeliction are the lower trunk, buttocks, thighs and genitalia.

Pruritis is a variable feature and may be severe. Unlike dermatitis herpetiformis, but in common with linear IgA disease, there is no associated gastrointestinal involvement (Castillo 1983).

9.1 Histology

The characteristic finding in these disease is of a subepidermal blister filled with neutrophils, eosinophils or both. Papillary microabscesses of neutrophils may be present and help to establish a diagnosis (Van der Meer et al. 1977). Often, however, papillary microabscesses are absent and a predominance of eosinophils in the dermal and epidermal infiltrates may give a histological picture indistinguishable from bullous pemphigoid. In such cases, immunofluorescence is invaluable in making the correct diagnosis (Marsden et al. 1980).

9.2 Immunofluorescence

Direct immunofluorescence shows a linear deposition of IgA at the basement membrane zone (Chorzelski, Jablonska 1979). More than one biopsy may be needed to demonstrate the IgA deposition.

Indirect immunofluorescence shows circulating IgA which binds to the basement membrane zone, in up to 60% of cases (Marsden et al. 1980). Immunoelectronmicroscopy shows that the IgA in this disease is deposited in the lamina lucida, in the same pattern as that seen in linear IgA disease and in the same pattern as IgG is deposited in bullous pemphigoid.

10. Pemphigus Vulgaris

Pemphigus is a chronic mucocutaneous blistering disease, which before the advent of corticosteroid therapy, was usually fatal. Two main types of pemphigus each with a variant, are recognised, on the basis of the position of the blister within the epidermis. Pemphigus vulgaris and its variant pemphigus vegetans exhibit suprabasilar cletting, while pemphigus foliaceus and its variant, pemphigus erythematosus show an upper epidermal cleft which is subcorneal and either within the granular or upper malpighian layers.

Pemphigus is predominantly a disease of middle age, but no age group is exempt. There is no sex preponderance. Early reportes suggested an increased incidence in those of Jewish or Mediterranean extraction but subsequent studies have not substantiated this. There is, however, an association between pemphigus vulgaris and HLA A10, HLA B13 and HLA DR W4 haplotype (Singer et al. 1981).

The characteristic skin lesion in pemphigus vulgaris is a flaccid, easily ruptured vesicle or an erosion which shows a tendency to increase in size rather than to heal. The earliest lesion is a vesicle or bulla which is clear and tense and may arise from normal, erythematous or urticated skin. The initial lesion may remain localised for weeks or months before further lesions appear. As the lesion ages, the fluid becomes tubid, the blister more flaccid and this eventually ruptures to leave a denuded area. Coalescence of several denuded areas or extension of individual lesions may result in large erosions. The individual lesions heal with little scaring, but leave areas of hypo- or hyperpigmentation. Pruritus is an uncommon symptom, but patients often complain of pain or burning of eroded areas.

95% patients have oral mucus membrane involvement and in 25% this is the primary site. Blisters are unusual in the mouth, but painful erosions are the typical clinical manifestation.

An unusual but not uncommon presentation of pemphigus vulgaris is as a paronychia.

In all patients, a positive Nikoloky's sign can be elicited. This is induced by digital friction to normal or perilesional skin, which induces cleft formation and sliding of the epidermis over the basal cell layer.

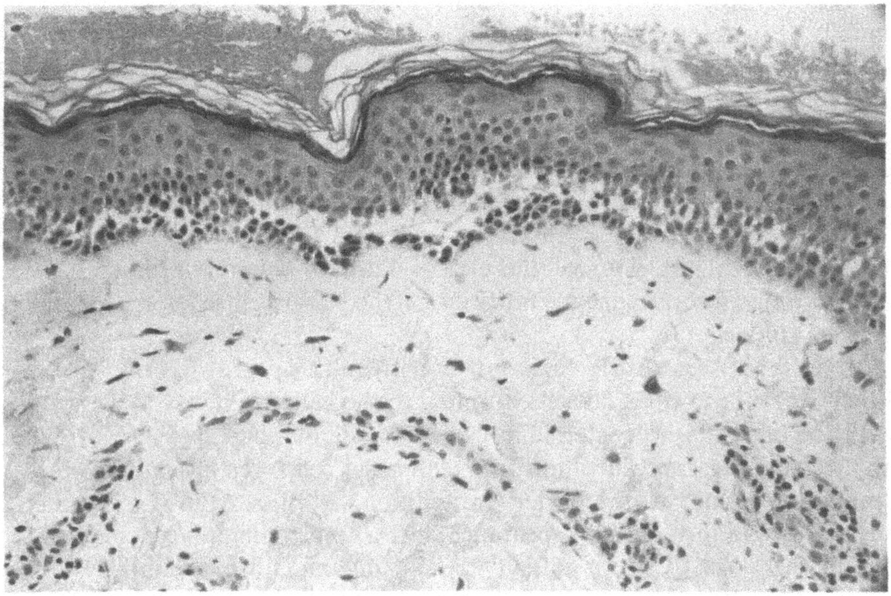

Fig. 7. Pemphigus vulgaris. A suprabasalar acantholytic cleft is seen, with intercellular oedema and separation of keratinocytes at the margins of the blister. Within the dermis there is only a very sparse cellular infiltrate

Skin eruptions which are clinicopathologically and immunohistochemically identical to pemphigus vulgaris and pemphigus foliaceus may be induced by the drugs D penicillamine, rifampicin, cataprine and practolol.

10.1 Histology

Pemphigus vulgaris is characterised histologically by suprabasal, acantholytic vesicles. With acantholysis, the epidermal cells lose cohesion between each other, become separated and rounded up and lie singly or in clumps within the blister cavity. Individual acantholytic cells are round and have homogenous cytoplasm and hyperchromatic nuclei. The presence of acantholytic cells is used diagnostically in the Tzank test, in which a fresh blister is deroofed and a smear made of the scrapings from the floor. Staining with haematoxylin and eosin or gemisa allows the identification of acantholytic cells.

Skin, mucus membranes and outer root sheaths of hair follicles are similarly affected.

The earliest change seen in pemphigus vulgaris is intercellular oedema and separation of the cells in the lower epidermis (Fig. 7). Ultrastructurally, this is seen to be the result of dissolution of the intercellular cement between the cells in the lower epidermis with detachment of desmosomes (Hashimoto, Lever 1967). As the lesion progresses, desmosomes are lost, tonofilaments retract to a perinuclear position and the epidermal cells develop interdigitating cytoplasmic processes.

Occasionally, the epidermis shows marked spongiosis and infiltration with eosinophils, a pattern described as eosinophilic spongiosis by Emmerson and Wilson Jones (1968). This is an early sign of pemphigus and precedes frank acantholysis. It is not however, specific for pemphigus vulgaris as it may be observed in other types of pemphigus such as pemphigus vegetans and foliaceus, and an identical histological picture may be observed in dermatitis herpetiformis, herpes gestationis and in the vesicular stage of incontinentia pigmenti (Knight et al. 1976).

In early lesions, the floor of the cleft is lined by a monolayer of basal cells. Anchoring fibres retain the integrity of the basal cell layer by binding to the basal lamina.

Other changes seen in the epidermis are irregular up growths of papillae lined by a single layer of basal cells, forming the so called villi, and downward proliferation of strands of epidermal cells between dermal papillae.

As the lesion ages, regeneration from the basal cell layer gives the picture of a mulilayered floor to the blister. In addition, down growth of epidermal strands may give a histological appearance similar to pemphigus vegetans.

Within the dermis there is initially a mild inflammatory cell infiltrate of eosinophils and plasma cells which becomes more marked as the lesion ages.

11. Pemphigus Vegetans

Clinically, pemphigus vegetans represents the vegetating, less aggressive form of pemphigus vulgaris. Two types are recognised on clinical grounds. The first is the Neumann variant in which the initial lesion is a clear blister. This form of the disease has a tendency to develop into classical pemphigus vulgaris. The second variant is the Hallopeau type, in which the initial lesion is a pustule, and this variant has a very benign clinical cause.

In both variants, the sites of predeliction are the intertriginous areas, in which papules, plaques and verrucoid masses develop.

11.1 Histology

In the earliest lesion suprabasilar clefts containing acantholytic cells may be observed, with acanthosis, papillomatosis and epidermal microabscesses composed of eosinophils (Lever 1965).

In the Hallopean type, the acantholytic clefts are filled with eosinophils and degenerated acantholytic cells. This is associated with a pronounced infiltration of the epidermis with eosinophils and associated spongiosis (Fig. 8).

As the lesion ages, the histological picture is dominated by papillomatosis, acanthosis and hyperkeratosis and the eosinophilic infiltrate and microabscess formation are lost. At this stage the histology become totally non specific and diagnosis relies upon immunofluorescence findings.

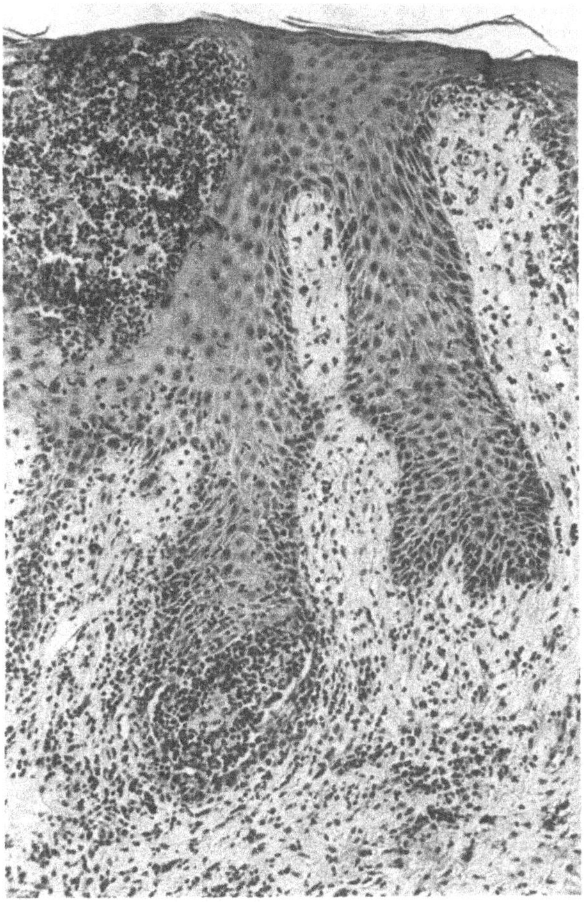

Fig. 8. Pemphigus vegetans. An acantholytic blister is present in the lower epidermis. The blister cavity is filled with eosinophils and eosinophils are seen infiltrating the spongiotic epidermis. A large eosinophilic microabscess is seen high in the epidermis

12. Pemphigus Foliaceus

In this form of pemphigus, the acantholytic process predominantly affects the upper epidermis and granular cell layer. Clinically it can be divided into a generalised form presenting as an exfoliative dermatitis, or as a localised form with scattered lesions over the scalp, malar area of face and upper trunk.

The initial lesion is a very superficial flaccid vesicle or bulla which quickly ruptures and becomes crusted. The eruption can start on normal skin or on an erythematous, urticated base. Crusting is the dominant clinical feature. An endemic form of pemphigus foliaceus, Fogo selvagem – is recognised in some parts of Brazil. This is clinically, histologically and immunologically identical to pemphigus foliaceus.

12.1 Histology

Histology of the skin in pemphigus foliaceus may be totally unrewarding, as the statum corneum may be lost during processing, and acantholysis is often not a striking feature (Fig. 9).

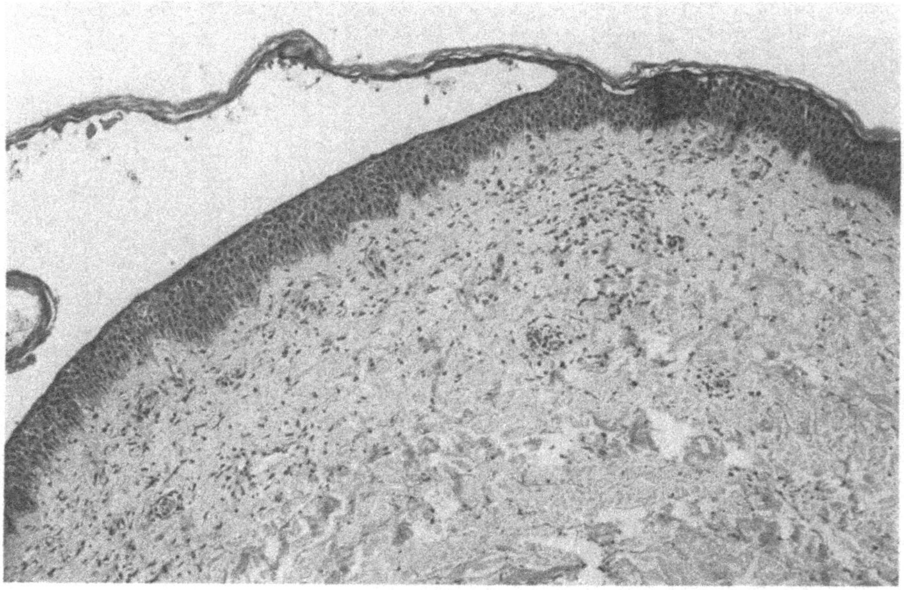

Fig. 9. Pemphigus foliaceus. An intraepidermal cleft is seen below the stratum granulosum, in which a few acantholytic cells are seen free in the blister cavity or partially attached to the roof of the blister

One of the earliest signs in pemphigus foliaceus is the finding of small nests of eosinophils high in the epidermis. This is followed by the formation of an acantholytic cleft high in the epidermis below the stratum corneum. The acantholytic cells are usually too well differentiated to round up and appear as deeply basophilic cells, similar to the grains seen in Darier's disease.

In older lesions, acanthosis, mild papillomatosis, hyperkeratosis and parakeratosis may be observed. The hyperkeratosis often involves hair follicles producing hyperkeratotic plugs and is associated with hypergranulosis.

Within the dermis, only mild changes are seen which consist of an inflammatory cell infiltrate predominantly of eosinophils.

13. Pemphigus Erythematosus – Senear Usher

In this variant of pemphigus foliaceus, the clinical and immunopathological features of pemphigus foliaceus and lupus erythematosus are often combined.

The lesions occur over the scalp, face and upper trunk, and usually involve the butterfly area of the face. Facial lesions clinically resemble lupus erythematosis or seborrhoeic dermatitis. On the trunk, thin walled blisters are always seen, which rapidly rupture and heal to leave hyperpigmented macules.

Histology is identical to pemphigus foliaceus. Immunofluorescence studies, however, often show the features of pemphigus together with a linear basement membrane zone immunoglobulin deposition and the presence of anti nuclear antibodies, characteristic of lupus erythematosus (JABLONSKA et al. 1977).

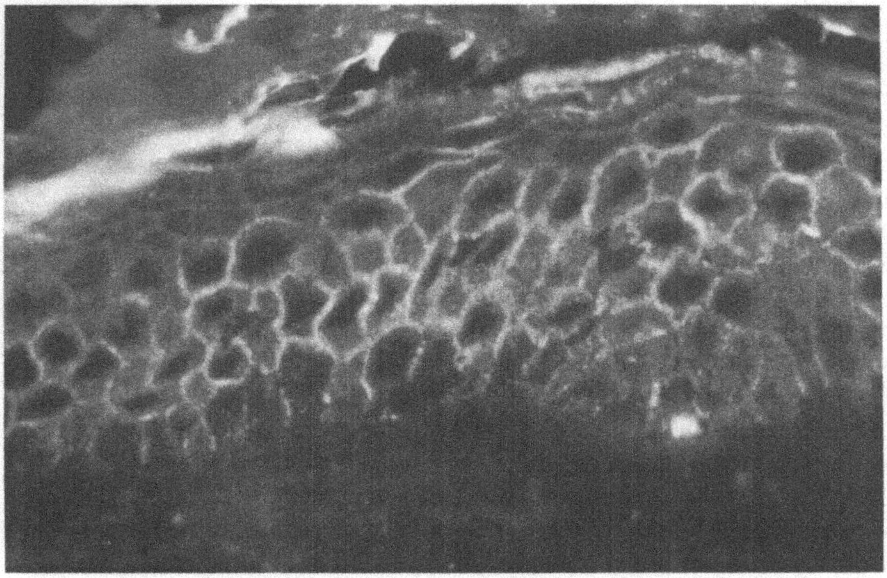

Fig. 10. Pemphigus vulgaris. Direct immunofluorescence shows deposition of IgG in the intercellular spaces, giving the crazy paving appearence

13.1 Immunohistochemistry

The pathopneumonic finding in all forms of pemphigus, is of immunoglobulin bound to the intercellular substance of the epidermis. The immunoglobulin is usually IgG but occasionally IgM and IgA may be found. C_{1q}, C_4 and C_3 deposition has been reported (BEUTNER and JORDAN 1964) (Fig. 10).

The staining is found throughout the epidermis, and is found in lesional, perilesional and clinically normal skin.

In the majority of patients there is a circulating IgG against the intercellular substance. Several reports have suggested that the titre of this circulating antibody correlates well with the clinical activity of the disease, and the antibody titre is used regularly in some hospitals to monitor the response of the disease to therapy (JUDD and LEVER 1979). In a study at St. John's Hospital for Diseases of the Skin, in which 19 patients were followed for prolonged periods, however, only in 47% was there a good correlation between disease activity and antibody titre, in 32% a fair correlation and in 21% a poor correlation.

Circulating antibodies against the intercellular substance are not restricted to pemphigus. They are observed in anti A and B blood group sera, and can be absorbed out by AB substances. They are also found in penicillin morbilliform drug eruptions, trichophyton fungal infections, bullous pemphigoid, cicatricial pemphigoid and thermal burns. These circulating antibodies are always of low titre.

Using the indirect C_3 technique, it has been shown that the circulating pemphigus antibody does not fix complement in vitro.

13.2 Pathogenesis

Pemphigus is an autoimmune disease in which the damage to the epidermis is mediated by circulating autoantibodies directed to the intercellular substance of the epidermis.

Schiltz and Michel (1976) have demonstrated that pemphigus antibody will induce acantholysis in organ culture in the absence of complement. The antigen is not species specific and human pemphigus antibody will induce acantholysis in mouse or rabbit as well as human skin organ cultures. In organ culture and tissue culture systems, acantholysis induced by pemphigus antibody can be inhibited by the use of soya bean trypsin inhibitor which inhibits serine proteinases, and also by β_2 macroglobulin which is a broad spectrum proteinase inhibitor (Singer et al. 1981). It has thus been suggested, that the tissue damage seen in pemphigus is due to the activation by the antibody, of soluble hydrolytic enzymes which dissolve the intercellular cement and split the desmosomes.

Schiltz et al. (1978), in one study was able to demonstrate that after incubation with pemphigus antibody for five days, epidermal cells release a soluble substance which is not an immunoglobulin, which will induce acantholysis in fresh explants. This soluble factor, they suggest, is an enzyme released by the keratinocyte, but needs further biochemical investigation.

14. Benign Familial Chronic Pemphigus (Hailey and Hailey Disease)

Benign familial chronic pemphigus is a genodermatosis passed as a dominant trait with variable penetrance. It never manifests itself before puberty and has a peak incidence between 15 and 30 years of age. There is no sex proponderence, but the disease is much more common in caucasians (Michel 1982).

The eruption consists of plaques of vesicles and bullae which rupture to leave an exudative base on which a crust develops. As the skin dries, deep painful fissures develop. The eruption is well localised and sharply marginated. With central resolution and peripheral extension, annular and serpiginous lesions develop. Nikolsky's sign may be positive, demonstrating the underlying pathological mechanism of acantholysis.

Atypical forms of benign familial chronic pemphigus have been described (Lyles et al. 1958) in which the primary lesions are hyperkeratotic, verrucous, papulovesicular or vesiculopustular.

Sites of prediliction are the flexural and intertriginous areas, including the nape and sides of the neck, axillae, groins, scrotum, perineum and vulva. The disease tends to run a chronic course, with periods of remission and exacerbation. Lesions heal without scarring but leave areas of hyperpigmentation.

14.1 Histology

The histology of benign familial chronic pemphigus, varies with the age of the lesion biopsied. In early lesions, the basal cell layer remains intact, but intercellular oedema and loss of intercellular bridges in the malphigian layer leads to partial or complete separation of cells giving rise to the so called "delapidated brick wall" appearence in the lower epidermis. Lacunae develop in which fully acantholytic cells may be observed. These cells have well defined nuclei and well preserved cytoplasm (Fig. 11).

In older lesions, there is downward proliferation of the rete ridges which elongate as cords of basal cells into the dermis. Villi lined by a single layer of basal cells, extend from papillae into the blister cavity.

The upper layers of the epidermis remain well preserved and dyskeratosis is rarely present. Cells resembling the corps ronds and grains of Darier's disease are only occasionally observed. PIERARD (1968) in an ultrastructural study, suggested that in Hailey and Hailey disease, true corps ronds or grains are not found but cells resembling them are shrunken acantholytic cells or parakeratotic scale. The dermal inflammatory response is variable, and increases with more clinically active lesions.

Electron microscopic studies have shown that basal keratinocytes lose adhesion on their lateral and superior margins, but remain attached to the basement membrane by hemidesmosomes. The cells show a characteristic abnormal thickening of tonofilaments in the perinuclear and juxtanuclear positions. In the malphigian layer, there is widening of intercellular spaces and partially separated cells show abnormal microvillous processes, which may be clubbed, elongated or narrowed (GOTTLIEB and LUTZNER 1970).

14.2 Pathogenesis

Benign familial chronic pemphigus is an abnormal skin response to a number of different stimuli in a genetically predisposed individual. Skin lesions are induced naturally, and can be induced experimentally, by friction, mild trauma, cold injury, thermal burns, ultraviolet irradiation, chemical irritants and contact allergic reactions. Bacteria and yeasts may also induce clinical lesions (CHORZELSKI 1962).

Evidence for the role of bacteria and yeasts in the pathogenesis of benign familial chronic pemphigus was reviewed by MONTES et al. in 1970. Evidence in favour of their involvement includes:

1. isolation of bacteria from intact bullae
2. finding bacteria in skin lesions on histological examination
3. clearing or improvement of the clinical lesions following antibiotic therapy
4. experimental production of skin lesions by cutaneous innoculation of Staphylococcus aureus.

The common organisms isolated from lesions of benign familial chronic pemphigus are Staphylococcus aureus, β haemolytic streptococci, Proteus mirabilis, Pseudomonas aeuroginosa and Candida albicans.

Immunofluorescence studies show no immunoreactants in the skin in benign familial chronic pemphigus, which helps to differentiate this disease from pemphigus vulgaris, and also suggests that immunological mechanisms are not involved in this disease.

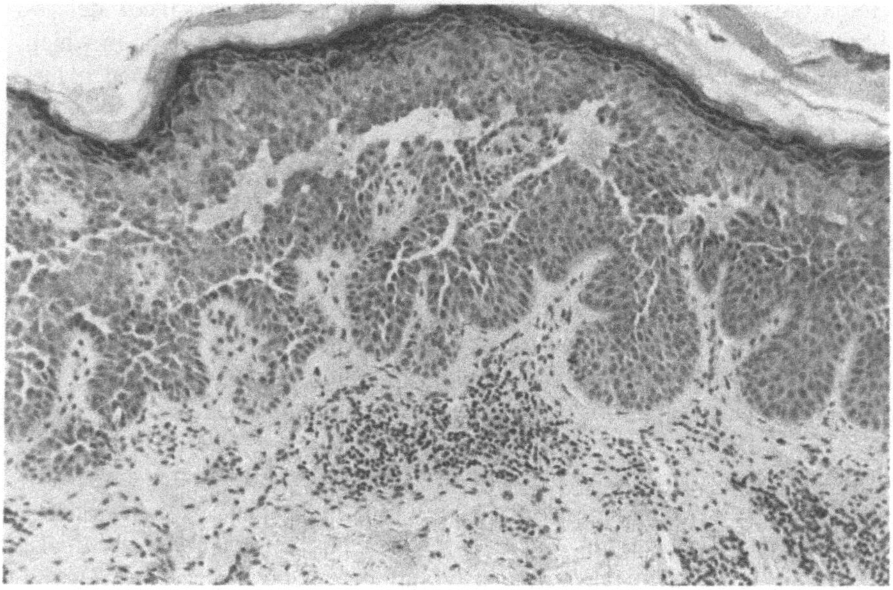

Fig. 11. Hailey-Hailey disease. Within the epidermis are the typical intraepidermal lacunae, and the "delapidated brick wall" appearence of the partially separated keratinocytes in the lower epidermis

15. Darier-White Disease (Keratosis Follicularis)

Darier-White disease is a genetic disorder of keratinisation, inherited as an autosomal dominant trait. Clinical manifestations of the disease are rare before 5 years of age, but usually start in the first or second decades.

The eruption consists of recurrent skin coloured papules which develop a yellowish to tan coloured scaly crust over the surface. When the crust is removed, a porelike opening is revealed. The name keratosis follicularis is misleading, as the lesions are not follicular. Sites of predilection are the seborrhoeic areas of the body, including the back, chest, nasolabial folds, ears, forehead, scalp and groins.

On the palms and soles, small punctate keratoses are present. Nail involvement is seen as V-shaped scalloping of the nails and subungual thickening. Mucosal surfaces are involved including the oral and rectal mucosa and oesophagus. In the mouth, a characteristic small, cobble stone-like change is seen. Asymptomatic corneal abnormalities are commonly found (Blackman et al. 1980).

Individual keratotic papules may coalesce to form warty hypertrophic masses, and in the intertriginous areas, the lesions beome vegetative and foul-smelling.

Bullous forms of Darier-White disease are uncommon, but have been reported (Hori et al. 1982).

The eruption is usually worse in the summer and seems to be aggravated by sunlight (Rand and Baden 1983).

15.1 Histology

The pathological changes seen in Darier-White disease can be divided into two parts:

1. Acantholysis leading to intraepidermal lacunae.
2. Dyskeratosis with the development of two characteristic forms of dyskeratotic cells – corps ronds and grains.

The lacunae are suprabasilar, extend throughout the malpighian layer, and are more extensive in clinically vesicular and bullous lesions than in keratotic papules. Within the lacunae, acantholytic cells and occasionally corps ronds and grains are found.

Corps ronds are found predominantly in the granular cell layer, and are characterised by their large pyknotic nuclei, surrounded by dense eosinophilic cytoplasm and an outer glistening membrane. These cells are found either singly or in small groups. Grains are found predominantly in the stratum corneum and are small cells with elongated nuclei and scanty cytoplasm. Many authors believe that grains develop from corps ronds.

Irregular upward proliferations of papillae results in papillomatosis and is associated with hyperkeratosis and parakeratosis. The dermis is relatively spared with only a sparse lymphocytic infiltrate in the upper dermis and no abnormality of collagen, elastic tissue or dermal blood vessels (Caufield and Wilgram 1963).

The primary abnormality in Darier-White disease appears to be a defect in synthesis, organisation or maturation of tonofilament – desmosome complexes. Electron microscopic studies have however supported conflicting ideas on the mechanism of acantholysis and dyskeratosis in Darrier-White disease. Caufield and Wilgram (1963) demonstrated the separation of tonofilaments from desmosomes and suggested that aggregation of these with keratokyaline granules led to the formation of corps ronds. Mann and Haye (1970) however, demonstrated that tonofilaments remain attached to desmosomal attachment plaques during splitting of desmosomes and subsequent separation of cells. The tonofilaments then retract perinuclearly and aggregate to form dense bands within corps ronds.

Gottlieb and Lutzner (1973) highlighted the vacuolation of basal cells and prickle cells and suggested that this was the primary abnormality triggered by the mutant gene. Vacuolated keratinocytes with increased tonofilament aggregates represent precursors of corps ronds and further vacuolation of the cells gives rise to grains.

15.2 Pathogenesis

Marks et al. in 1978, demonstrated no abnormality in the humoral immunity in patients with Darier-White disease, but showed reduced cell mediated immunity as demonstrated by function T cell studies. Jegasothy and Humeniuk (1981) supported these findings by demonstrating cutaneous anergy in the majority of their patients with Darier-White disease, and a selective reduced response to the T cell mitogen concanalavin A but normal response to phytohaemagglutenin and poke weed mitogen.

Immunofluorescence studies on involved skin in Darier-White disease show no immunoreactants in the skin.

The immune system does seem to be involved in Darier-White disease, but seems to be secondarily affected rather than playing a part in the primary skin condition.

16. Transient Acantholytic Dermatosis (Grover's Disease)

This is a relatively new clinicopathological entity; first described by GROVER in 1970. It is a self limiting, usually pruritic eruption, which generally affects white males over the age of 50. Clinically, the eruption is not distinctive, and usually presents as a fairly sparse eruption of keratotic or erythematovesicular papules, over the upper chest, back and to a lesser extent, arms and legs. Bullous transient acantholytic dermatosis has been reported, (WAISMANN et al. 1976) but this is a rare occurrence. A diagnosis of acne, seborrhoeic dermatitis, miliaria rubra or follicutitis is usually made. As the name suggests, in the majority of patients the disease is transient lasting for only 2–3 months and then spontaneously regresses. In some patients, however, it may persist for up to six years (SIMON et al. 1976).

16.1 Histology

Four patterns of epidermal change have been reported in transient acantholytic dermatosis by CHALET et al. (1977). This is a somewhat artificial division of the histopathological changes seen in this disease, as in any one lesion, more than one of these patterns may be observed. The patterns do, however, correlate fairly well with the clinical appearance of the lesion, and the hyperkeratotic papules usually show the Darier-like pattern, while the erythematovesicular papules usually show more the pemphigus vulgaris-like pattern.

Darier-like. In this pattern, there is focal suprabasilar clefting with acantholytic cells and dyskeratotic cells scattered throughout all levels of the epidermis, and usually associated with overlying parakeratosis.

Pemphigus vulgaris-like. In this pattern, focal suprabasal clefts are associated with only little overlying acantholysis and no dyskeratosis.

Hailey-Hailey-like. In this pattern, the focal suprabasal clefts are associated with marked acantholysis extending throughout the malpigian layer, but with little or no dyskeratosis.

Spongiotic. In this pattern, there is once again focal suprabasal clefting, but acantholytic cells are found within spongiotic vesicles. Often, slight intracellular oedema is seen associated with the spongiosis and acantholysis. This pattern of change is rarely seen on its own and is usually seen associated with the pemphigus vulgaris-like pattern.

Within the dermis, there is a mild lymphohistiocytic infiltrate around the superficial dermal plexus. In some patients, a moderate number of eosinophils are present within the infiltrate, and in these patients, it is usually associated with spongiosis of the epidermis.

16.2 Pathogenesis

There is no good evidence for a genetic cause of this dermatosis and the late onset and transient nature would be against this. Immunofluorescence studies show no significant abnormalities (Bystryn J-C 1979; Heehan and Quirk 1980) to suggest an immunological cause.

Transient acantholytic dermatosis has, however, often been associated with drying of the skin, by excessive washing, irritant contact, prolonged sun exposure and asteototic change due to environmental factors, which have led some authors to suggest a primary irritant cause of the disease.

17. Erythema Multiforme

Erythema multiforme is an acute, self limiting disease affecting the skin and mucous membranes. A large number of different aetiological agents have been implicated in the disease, but its pathogenesis remains unclear. The clinically distinctive lesions of erythema multiforme is the iris or target lesion, but as the name suggests, many morphologically different lesions may be present including erythematous macules, papules, iris lesions and bullae. The distribution of erythema multiforme is typically acral and mucosal surfaces may be involved. In some cases, the disease is restricted to mucosal surfaces.

17.1 Histology

The histology of erythema multiforme depends on the clinical character of the lesion biopsied. In the macular lesions, the major change is seen in the dermis, while in bullous lesions the maximal changes occur in the epidermis. Several authors, have tried to divide the histological changes of erythema multiforme into three patterns, the predominantly dermal, mixed dermal and epidermal and predominantly epidermal (Orfanos et al. 1984). This artificial splitting of the histological picture is of little diagnostic value, as all three patterns may be seen in a single iris lesion, and in any given patient, all clinical lesions may be present and these will show the full range of histological change.

In the dermis, the inflammatory process is centred on the superficial dermal plexus with an accumulation of mononuclear cells either forming a sleeve-like infiltrate around the vessels, or in more florid cases, filling the papillary dermis. The infiltrate may occasionally extend to the reticular dermis, but this is unrelated to the clinical stage or severity of the disease. Eosinophils may be present in significant numbers in the dermal infiltrate and Bedi and Pinkus (1976) reported this in 37% of the erythema multiforme lesions they examined. In

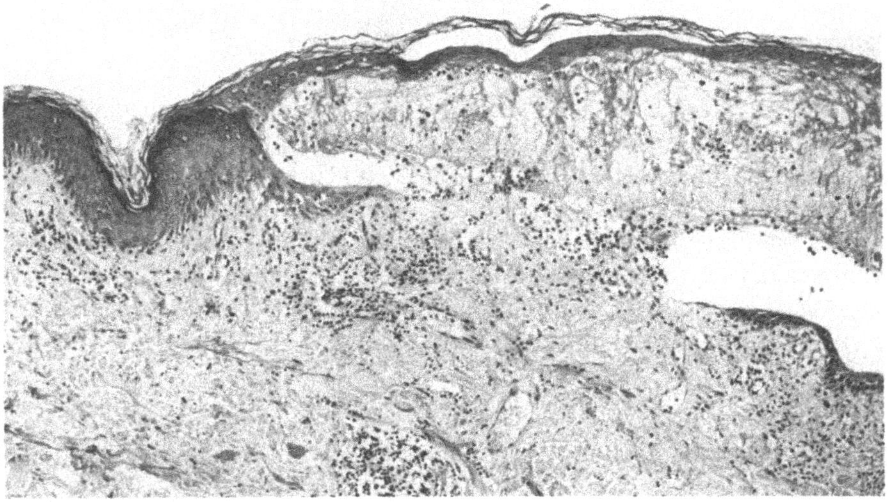

Fig. 12. Erythema multiforme. This shows the epidermal pattern, with generalised necrosis of the epidermis. Regeneration from the margins of the blister is already occuring

their study, eosinophils were conspicuously absent from iris lesions. In macular lesions, the blood vessels appear normal but in more advanced lesions show vasodilation, endothelial cell swelling and fluid exudation. In some iris and bullous lesions, red blood cell extravisation may be observed.

At no stage is there evidence of immune complex vasculitis with destruction of vessel walls, fibrinoid change or leucocytoclasis. Variable numbers of neutrophils may be present in older lesions, but represent secondary inflammatory cells.

Within the epidermis, focal or generalised necrosis may occur, with the presence of pyknotic or necrotic keratinocytes. In macular lesions, epidermal necrosis is infrequent and is always focal. In the classical iris lesion, however, the whole epidermis overlying the oedematous papillary dermis appears completely necrotic, composed of cells with pyknotic nuclei of amorphous acidophilic bodies. The strateum corneum is always normal in erythema multiforme (Fig. 12).

Blister formation in erythema multiforme can be caused by three different mechanisms.

17.1.1 Papillary Oedema

Almost all lesions of erythema multiforme show a variable degree of papillary oedema, appearing as a washed out zone in the subepidermal region. This is most marked in the iris and bullous lesions, where massive subepidermal oedema results in a subepidermal bulla, over which the epidermis shows generalised or focal necrosis. In such bullae, the basal lamina is situated in the roof of the blister (MACVICAR et al. 1963).

17.1.2 Spongiosis

Most lesions of erythema multiforme show spongiosis, but this is most marked in the papular, iris and bullous lesions. Typically, the epidermal cells show a vertical distortion, suggesting transudation of fluid from the dermal vessels. A variable degree of intracellular oedema is also seen in the majority of lesions, appearing as a clear halo around the nuclei of epidermal cells. This is mild or absent in macular lesions, but may be considerable in more advanced lesions.

Intraepidermal vesiculation is seen in only about 25% of cases, usually associated with a variable degree of exocytosis or polymorphs and mononuclear cells into the epidermis with accumulation of these cells within the spongiotic multilocular intraepidermal vesicles.

17.1.3 Liquifractive Degeneration of the Basal Cell Layer

48% of all clinical lesions show focal areas of basal cell necrosis. When marked this can lead to basal cell liquifractive degeneration and the formation of subepidermal blisters. In such blisters, the basal lamina is in the floor of the lesion (Ackerman et al. 1971).

17.2 Immunohistochemistry

In 30–90% of patients, granular deposits of C_3 and/or IgM are found in the small vessels of the papillary dermis (Kazmierowski and Wuepper 1981; Finan and Schroeter 1984). In one study (Wuepper et al. 1980), granular deposits of C_3 could be induced in normal skin following histamine injection, suggestion that circulating immunoreactions are involved.

17.3 Pathogenesis

Erythema multiforme represents an immunological response by the host to a large number of different factors. The actual mechanism by which the immune system initiates the changes seen in the erythema multiforme is as yet unclear. The onset of erythema multiforme is usually 7–14 days after exposure to the precipitating cause, which is compatible with the generation of a specific immune response, and challenge with a known precipitating factor will induce a rapid recurrence of erythema multiforme.

Some patients show positive delayed skin test reactions to suspected precipitating factors at the time of active erythema multiforme, suggesting that a type 4 response may be involved in the pathogenesis of erythema multiforme (Medeiros et al. 1966).

However, direct immunofluorescence findings of C_3 and IgM in dermal blood vessels, and reduced levels of complement components in blister fluid and in the blood suggest a humoral response as mediating erythema multiforme.

In addition, circulating immune complexes are seen in up to 80% patients with erythema multiforme which may also be involved in the pathogenesis of erythema multiforme (WUEPPER et al. 1980).

18. Toxic Epidermal Necrolysis (Scalded Skin Syndrome)

Toxic epidermal necrolysis encompasses two distinct pathological entities, which share the same clinical picture of generalised erythema, tenderness of the skin and widespread exfoliation of the epidermis, giving the skin the appearance of having been scalded with boiling water. These two entities, staphylococcal scalded skin syndrome and adult toxic epidermal necrolysis will be considered separately.

18.1 Staphylococcal Scalded Skin Syndrome

This usually affects children under the age of 5 years, although rare adult cases have been reported. This syndrome represents a spectrum of disease induced by staphylococcus aureus, with impetigo neonatorum at one end and Ritter's disease at the other end.

Impetigo neonatorum presents as slowly enlarging blisters with an erythematous margin, which tend to be localised to one area of the body. The blister fluid is initially clear but does become purulent. Staphylococcus aureus may be isolated from the blister fluid.

Ritter's disease starts as a faint macular eruption with associated generalised tenderness of the skin. After 28–48 h, the skin becomes spontaneously wrinkled and desquamates in sheets. Large flaccid bullae also develop which rupture to leave erythematous erosions. Mucosal surfaces are rarely involved. Blister fluid is invariably sterile.

18.1.1 Histology

Histology shows an intraepidermal blister below the stratum granulosum. The blister cavity frequently contains acantholytic cells and may be confused with pemphigus foliaceus (FEINSTEIN et al. 1971) although immunofluorescence is negative in staphylococcal scalded skin syndrome.

Within the dermis there is a moderately dense perivascular infiltrate of mononuclear cells and neutrophils. There is no evidence of vasculitis.

18.1.2 Pathogenesis

Staphylococcal scalded skin syndrome is due to an infection with a phage group 11 staphylococcus aureus (types 3A, 3B, 3C, 55 or 71) LYELL 1979. A staphylococcal epidermolytic toxin was described by MELISH et al. in 1972 which was able to induce the clinical signs of toxic epidermal necrolysis in a baby mouse model (MELISH and GLASGOW 1970). It seems likely that all forms of the disease are due to local production (impetigo neonatorum) or distant production (Ritter's disease) of the epidermolytic toxin.

18.2 Adult Toxic Epidermal Necrolysis

This is a rare condition usually occurring in adults over 40 years of age, but rarely affects children. It is an acute eruption usually preceded by a mild prodromal illness consisting of malaise, fever, anorexia and skin tenderness. The eruption starts as either a generalised morbilliform rash or a discrete macular erythema on acral sites which rapidly progresses to a generalised erythema. Flaccid bullae develop in the areas of erythema and Nikolski's sign is positive. In fulminant cases, the entire thickness of the epidermis is involved leading to large areas of ulceration, particularly over pressure areas.

Mucosal surfaces are involved, often extensively, including the respiratory and gastrointestinal tracts.

Healing occurs in 2–4 weeks, but there is a high morbidity and a mortality of up to 25–50% (SNYDER and ELIAS 1983). Toxic epidermal necrolysis may be associated with erythema multiforme. In a report from BERGOEND et al. in 1968, the use of long acting sulphonamides in the treatment of an epidemic of meningococcal meningitis, led to an outbreak of toxic epidermal necrolysis. Many of these patients also had typical lesions of erythema multiforme either clinically or histopathologically.

18.2.1 Histology

Early features in the skin are vacuolization and individual necrosis of keratinocytes in the basal and malpighian layers. There is minimal dermal inflammation and no evidence of vasculitis.

In later stages, there is confluent eosinophilic necrosis of the entire epidermis with the formation of a subepidermal blister. Even at this stage, dermal inflammation is only mild.

Ultrastructural studies have shown that the primary attack is an basal and lower malpighian cells leading to vacuolar change and cellular damage.

18.2.2 Pathogenesis

The majority of cases of adult toxic epidermal necrolysis can be trace to a drug. Drugs causing this eruption include the pyrazolones, sulphonamides, barbiturates and anti epileptic drugs (BANDMANN 1970). Although often clinically associated with classical erythema multiforme, and histologically resembling the epidermal form of erythema multiforme, toxic epidermal necrolysis has not been reported in association with herpes simplex viruses.

A number of infections and miscellaneous conditions have been reported in association with toxic epidermal necrolysis (Snyder and Elias 1983) and a small number of idiopathic cases are recognised.

19. Mechano-Bullous Diseases

This group of blistering skin diseases includes the rare genodermatoses epidermolysis bullosa simplex, junctional, dystrophic and acquired form. They are characterised by the development of blisters at sites of trauma which in the normal individual, would not induce blister formation.

In the genetically inherited epidermolysis bullosa, there is a structural abnormality of the skin which renders it more fragile and more susceptible to minor injury.

The different forms of epidermolysis bullosa can be differentiated on clinical and pathological criteria. They can be broadly divided into two groups:

1. Non scarring, in which the blister arises above the basal lamina. These include:

a) Epidermolysis bullosa simplex – autosomal dominant.

b) Weber-Cockayne or localised epidermolysis bullosa simplex – autosomal dominant.

c) Junctional epidermolysis bullosa of the Herlitz or the less severe adult form – autosomal recessive.

2. Scarring in which the blister arises below the basal lamina. These include:

a) Dystrophic epidermolysis bullosa – autosomal dominant.

b) Dystrophic epidermolysis bullosa – autosomal recessive.

19.1 Epidermolysis Bullosa Simplex

Bullae first appear in early childhood, usually as the child starts to crawl. Occasionally the onset of blistering may be delayed until adult life and in such cases the differentiation from epidermolysis bullosa acquista rests on a family history of a blistering disease.

Blisters occur at sites of recurrent minor injury, and tend to be more numerous in the summer months. The blister heal without scarring unless the blisters become secondarily infected. The severity of the disease improves after puberty.

19.2 Localised Epidermolysis Bullosa Simplex – Weber-Cockayne Varient

In this varient of epidermolysis bullosa simplex, blisters are confined to the palms and soles. Frequently, blister do not appear until adolescence or early adult life and tend to be more numerous on the feet (Weber 1926; Cockayne 1947).

19.2.1 Histology

In spontaneous blisters or in friction induced blisters, the first changes observed are of degeneration of basal keratinocytes which become swollen and vacuolated. This leads to cytolysis of the basal keratinocytes with the formation of vesicles or bullae at the dermo epidermal junction. In PAS preparations, the basal lamina is always found in the floor of the blister (PEARSON and SPARGO 1961).

There is little or no inflammatory cell infiltrate in the dermis or epidermis, unless the blister becomes secondarily infected. Elastic tissue is normal.

If the blister does not rupture, regeneration of the basal cells may give the appearance of an intraepidermal cleft. As the lesion ages, the cells in the roof of the blister become pyknotic and essentially become a focal area of parakeratosis.

19.2.2 Electron Microscopy

The first changes seen in blister formation is oedema of the subnuclear cytoplasm of basal keratinocytes. Small vacuoles then develop in the cytoplasm of basal keratinocytes. Small vacuoles then develop in the cytoplasm which enlarge and merge, leading to a cytolytic blister developing between the lower most part of the cell and the cell nucleus (HANEKE and ANTON-LAMPRECHT 1982).

The structures comprising the dermoepidermal junction remain intact and normal throughout the development of the blister.

19.3 Junctional Epidermolysis Bullosa

In this form of epidermolysis bullosa, bullae are present at birth at sites exposed to minor injury and in sites clinically protected from injury.

Blisters rupture to leave denuded areas, which heal slowly but without scarring. Large areas of the skin are involved leading to severe fluid and protein loss and sepsis, which are major causes of death (HERLITZ 1935).

If the child survives beyond the age of 1 year, the disease seems to become less aggressive. It may well be that children that survive early childhood, have a more benign variant of the disease.

19.3.1 Histology

The change seen in junctional epidermolysis bullosa are of a subepidermal bulla. The overlying epidermis is normal except when secondary infection is present. There is little dermal inflammatory infiltrate unless secondary infection is present.

In hair follicles, separation of the epidermis from dermis tends to occur at the level of the sebaceous glands. In PAS preparations, the separation is seen to be above the basal lamina.

19.3.2 Electron Microscopy

In junctional epidermolysis bullosa, the blister forms within the lamina lucida. In unseparated areas, there is hypoplasia of hemidesmosomes and a mild reduction of tonofilaments. A characteristic feature is the absence or an abnormal development of subbasal dense plaques and attachment plaques (Hashimoto et al. 1976).

Focal widening of the lamina lucida is observed as the blister forms, usually in areas deficient in hemidesmosomes. In fully developed blisters the cleavage plane is through the lamina lucida, but at sites of normal hemidesmosomes, the blister may form through the basal keratinocytes with attachment of remnants of the basal keratinocytes to the basement membrane.

In adults with junctional epidermolysis bullosa, normal skin shows large numbers of hemidesmosomes are present with almost normal numbers of subbasal dense plaques. It is possible that these patients represent a milder variant of the disease with only focal structural abnormalities and blisters only occur at these sites.

It is also possible, however, that if patients survive he first year of life, they are able to elaborate more normal hemidesmosomes, which corresponds to the improvement of their clinical disease.

19.4 Dystrophic Epidermolysis Bullosa

19.4.1 Dominant Dystrophic Bullosa

These children present with haemorrhagic blister of the hands, feet, knees and elbows either at birth or in early infancy. Mucosal surfaces are also involved, including mouth, pharynx, genitalia and perianal areas.

Healing of the blisters leads to atrophic or hypertrophic scarring. Epidermal cysts or milia are frequently found within the scars, either singularly or in groups.

Nails may be absent or may become thick and claw-like.

19.4.2 Recessive Dystrophic Epidermolysis Bullosa

Blistering may occur in utero and is present at birth. Blisters lead to scarring and milia formation. Nail dystrophy, dental abnormalities and mucous membrane involvement are invariably present. Frequently the child shows retarded growth and development and occasionally mental retardation.

Scarring of mucous membranes leads to trismus and strictures of the pharynx and oesophagus. Rectal prolapse is a common complication. Leukoplakia and squamous cell carcinoma may develop in scarred mucous membranes. Conjunctival or corneal involvement may occur which can lead to blindness. The more severely affected children often die in childhood as a result of fluid loss from extensive ulceration, infection or from malnutrition resulting from the oesophageal strictures.

19.4.3 Histology

The earliest signs of dystrophic epidermolysis bullosa are of vesiculation in the dermal papillae and fragmentation of collagen bundles in the upper dermis.

The cleavage plane is subepidermal, with the entire epidermis and PAS staining basal lamina forming the roof of the blister. The floor of the blister is composed of fragmented collagen bundles, often with extravasated red blood cells and a cellular infiltrate of histiocytes and lymphocytes.

If the blister remains unruptured, the basal cells regenerate and the separation cleft becomes intraepidermal. The overlying keratinocytes become pyknotic and evolve into a parakeratotic scale.

If secondary infection occurs, there is a marked increase in the inflammatory cell infiltrate within the dermis and epidermis, and focal degeneration or absence of elastic fibres.

Milia develop within adnexal structures, particularly eccrine sweat ducts, which are damaged in the blister formation. With healing, the adnexal structures lose continuity with the surface and keratin filled cysts develop within them.

19.4.4 Electron Microscopy

An early and consistent feature in dystrophic epidermolysis bullosa is the degeneration of collagen fibres and phagocytosis of swollen collagen fibres by histiocytes (Pearson 1962).

In the more aggressive forms of both dominant and recessive dystrophic epidermolysis bullosa, the anchoring fibres of the dermoepidermal junction may be absent or rudimentary. This is not a consistent finding in all patients, and in the less severely affected patients, the anchoring fibrils may be present in normal numbers and may be well formed (Anton-Lamprecht and Schnyder 1973; Anton-Lamprecht and Hashimoto 1976).

19.4.5 Pathogenesis

A consistent finding on light and electron microscopy in both dominant and recessive dystrophic epidermolysis bullosa, is the alteration in the collagen within the upper epidermis. Eisen (1969) has shown that collagenase activity in skin from frictional bullae in recessive dystrophic epidermolysis bullosa is six times higher than in normal skin, and is higher in non blistered skin than in normal skin. This evidence strongly suggests that the primary defect in dystrophic epidermolysis bullosa is an increase in tissue collagenase which further increases with injury to the skin and leads to damage to the dermal collagen and blister formation (Pearson 1971). Lazarus (1972), however, feels that the increased collagenase levels seen in these patients, represents a secondary tissue reaction to chronic injury. The collagenase theory would also not explain the abnormality of anchoring fibrils observed in this disease.

19.5 Epidermolysis Bullosa Acquista

This disease is defined as an acquired abnormal fragility of the skin, with formation of blisters and erosion in response to minor mechanical insult to the skin (WISE and LAUTMAN 1915). It is usually associated with an underlying disease and has been reported with amyloidosis, Crohn's disease, ulcerative colitis, multiple myeloma, carcinoma of the lung, tuberculosis, penicillamine therapy, porphyria cutanea tarda and congenital porphyria. Clinically it resembles epidermolysis bullosa dystrophica with evidence of scarring and milia formation.

19.5.1 Histology

On light microscopy the bulla in epidermolysis bullosa acquista is subepidermal, and frequently shows accompanying dermal changes resulting from the primary disease. In most cases, dermal changes are minimal or absent, but collagen degeneration, elastosis and amyloidosis have been reported.

On electron microscopy, the cleavage plane is below the lamina densa and the overlying epidermis is normal but the lamina densa may show reduplication. A consistent finding is of a fine granular material in close proximity to the anchoring fibrils close to the lamina densa. Anchoring fibrils may be normal or reduced in number (NILSEN et al. 1981).

19.5.2 Immunohistochemistry

On direct immunofluorescence, a continuous granular band of IgG is found along the basement membrane zone. Immunoelectron microscopy shows the deposition to be below the lamina densa and associated with the anchoring fibrils (NILSEN et al. 1981). C_3 has been demonstrated at the basement membrane zone and both IgG and C_3 have been observed in the walls of upper dermal blood vessels (LIVDEN et al. 1978). Indirect immunofluorescence shows the presence of circulating anti basement membrane zone IgG in patients with epidermolysis bullosa acquisita.

19.5.3 Pathogenesis

Epidermolysis bullosa acquisita seems to be an autoimmune disease associated with other systemic diseases. WOODLEY et al. (1984) have isolated the putative epidermolysis bullosa acquisita antigen as a 290,000 dalton (reduced) protein which is not type 1, 4 or 5 collagen, laminin, fibronectin or elastin, but seems to be a matrix protein which is quite distinct from all known skin components. The native protein is a large molecule of over 800,000 daltons and is trypsin sensitive. It is localised in the immediate sub-lamina densa region. It is quite distinct from the bullous pemphigoid antigen which is found in the lamina lucida.

Acknowledgements: Dr. A.C. CHU is a Wellcome Senior Research Fellow. We wish to thank Mr. B. BHOGAL, St John's Hospital for Diseases of the Skin for his help in preparing the photomicrographs.

References

Ackerman AB, Penneys NS, Clark WH (1971) Erythema multiforme exudativum: Distinctive pathological process. Br J Dermatol 84:554–566

Anton-Lamprecht I, Schnyder UW (1973) Epidermolysis bullosa dystrophica dominous – ein defekt der anchoring fibrils? Dermatologica 147:289–298

Anton-Lamprecht I, Hashimoto I (1976) Epidermolysis bullosa dystrophica dominous (Passini) – a primary structural defect of anchoring fibrils. Hum Genet 32:69–76

Bandmann HJ (1970) Medikamente als krandheitlosende Faktoren des Lyell-Syndroms. In: Braun-Falco O, Bandmann HJ (eds) Das Lyell-Syndrom Berne H. Huber Press

Bedi TR, Pinkus H (1976) Histological spectrum of erythema multiforme. Br J Dermatol 95:243–250

Beutner EH, Jordan RE (1964) Demonstration of skin antibodies in sera of pemphigus vulgaris patients by indirect immunofluorescence staining. Proc Soc Exp Biol Med 117:505–510

Beutner EH, Chorzelski TP, Jordan RE (1970) Autosensitisation. In Pemphigus and Bullous Pemphigoid, Charles C Thomas, Springfield, Illinois, p 41

Blackman HJ, Rodrigues MM, Peck GL (1980) Corneal epithelial lesions in keratosis follicularis (Darier's disease). Ophthalmology 87:931–943

Blenkinsopp WK, Haffenden GP, Fry L, Leonard JN (1983) Histology of linear IgA disease, dermatitis herpetiformis and bullous pemphigoid. Am J Dermatopathol 5:547–554

Brunsting LA, Perry HO (1957) Benign pemphigoid? A report of seven cases with chronic scarring herpetiform plaques about the head and neck. Arch Dermatol 75:489–501

Bystryn J-C (1979) Immunofluorescence studies in transient acantholytic dermatosis (Grover's disease). Am J Dermatopathol 1:325–327

Castillo G (1983) Chronic bullous disease of childhood: Linear IgA dermatosis of childhood. Dermatologic Clinics 1:231–234

Caufield JB, Wilgram GF (1963) An electron microscope study of dyskeratosis and acantholysis in Darier's disease. J Invest Dermatol 41:57–65

Center DM, Cruikshhank W (1982) Modulation of lymphocyte migration by human lymphokines. 11. Purification of a lymphotactic factor. J Immunol 128:2569–2573

Center DM, Wintroub BU, Austen KF (1983) Identification of chemoattractant activity for lymphocytes in blister fluid of patients with bullous pemphigoid: evidence for the presence of a lymphokine. J Invest Dermatol 81:204–208

Chalet M, Grover RW, Ackerman AB (1977) Transient acantholytic dermatosis: Reevaluation. Arch Dermatol 113:431–435

Chorzelski T (1962) Experimentally induced acantholysis in Hailey's benign pemphigus. Dermatologica 24:21–30

Chorzelski TP, Jablonska S (1979) IgA linear dermatosis of childhood (chronic bullous disease of childhood). Br J Dermatol 101:535–545

Cockayne EA (1947) Recurrent bullous eruption of the feet. Br J Dermatol 59:109–112

Connors BL, Marks R, Wilson Jones E (1972) Dermatitis herpetiformis: histological discriminants. Trans St Johns Hosp Dermatol Soc 58:191–198

Dabrowski J, Chorzelski T, Jablonska S (1979) Immunoelectronmicroscopic studies in IgA linear dermatosis. Arch Dermatol Res 265:289–298

Diaz-Perez JL, Jordan RE (1976) The complement system in bullous pemphigoid. IV. Chemotactic activity in blister fluid. Clin Immunol Immunopathol 5:360–370

Dvorak AM, Mihm MC, Osage JE, Theodore BA, Kwan H, Austen KF, Wintroub BU (1982) Bullous pemphigoid, an ultrastructural study of the inflammatory response: eosinophil. basophil and mast cell granule changes in multiple biopsies from one patient. J Invest Dermatol 78:91–101

Eisen AZ (1969) Human skin collagenase: relationship to the pathogenesis of epidermolysis bullosa dystrophica. J Invest Dermatol 52:449–453

Emmerson RW, Wilson Jones E (1968) Eosinophilic spongiosis in pemphigus: a report of an unusual histological change in pemphigus. Arch Derm 97:252–257

Feinstein RP, Einbinder J, Shapiro L (1971) Absence of pemphigus-type autoantibodies despite the presence of pemphigus like histopathology. Int J Dermatol 10:115

Finan MC, Schroeter AL (1984) Cutaneous immunofluorescence study of erythema multiforme: Correlation with light microscopic patterns and etiologic agents. J Am Acad Dermatol 10:497–506

Fine J-D, Neises GR, Katz SI (1984) Immunofluorescence and immunoelectron microscopic studies in cicatricial pemphigoid. J Invest Dermatol 82:39–43

Fry L, Seah PP, Riches DJ, Hoffbrand AV (1973) Clearance of skin lesions in dermatitis herpetiformis after gluten withdrawl. Lancet 1:288–290

Fry L, Seah PP (1974) Dermatitis herpetiformis evaluation of diagnostic criteria. Br J Dermatol 90:137–146

Gottlieb SK, Lutzner MA (1970) Hailey Hailey disease: an electronmicroscopic study. J Invest Dermatol 54:368–376

Gottlieb SK, Lutzner MA (1973) Darier's disease: An electron microscopic study. Arch Dermatol 107:225–230

Grover RW (1970) Transient acantholytic dermatosis. Arch Dermatol 101:426–437

Hall RP, Lawley TJ, Katz SI (1981) Dermatitis herpetiformis. Springer Semin Immunopathol 4:33–43

Haneke E, Anton-Lamprecht I (1982) Ultrastructure of blister formation in epidermolysis bullosa hereditaria: V Epidermolysis bullosa simplex localisation type Weber-Cockayne. J Invest Dermatol 78:219–223

Harrington CI, Bleehen SS (1979) Herpes gestationis: immunopathological and ultrastructural studies. Br J Dermatol 100:389–399

Hashimoto I, Gedde-Dahl T, Schnyder UW, Anton-Lamprecht I (1976) Ultrastructural studies in epidermolysis bullosa hereditaria. V. Recessive dystrophic types with junctional blistering. Arch Dermatol Res 257:17–32

Hashimoto K, Lever WF (1967) The intercellular cement in pemphigus vulgaris: An electron microscope study. Dermatologia 135:27–34

Heehan PJ, Quirk CJ (1980) Transient acantholytic dermatosis. Br J Dermatol 102:515–520

Herlitz G (1935) Kongenitaler, nicht syphilitischer Pemphigus: Eine Übersicht nebst Beschreibung einer neuen Krankheitsform (Epidermolysis bullosa hereditaria letalis). Acta Paediat Scand 17:315–371

Hertz KC, Katz SI, Maize J, Ackerman AB (1976) Herpes gestationis: a clinicopathological study. Arch Dermatol 112:1543–1548

Hodge L, Black MM, Ramnarain N, Bhogal B (1978) Indirect complement immunofluorescence in the immunopathological assessment of bullous pemphigoid, cicatricial pemphigoid and herpes gestationis. Clin Exp Dermatol 3:61–67

Hodge L, Marsden RA, Black MM, Bhogal B, Corbett MF (1981) Bullous pemphigoid: the frequency of mucosal involvement and concurrent malignancy related to indirect immunofluorescence findings. Br J Dermatol 105:65–69

Holmes RC, Black MM, Dann J, James DCO, Bhogal B (1982) A comparative study of toxic erythema of pregnancy and herpes gestationis. Br J Dermatol 106:499–501

Hori Y, Tsuru N, Nilmura M (1982) Bullous Darier's disease. Arch Dermatol 118:278–279

Jablonska S, Chorzelski T, Blaszczyk M (1977) Pathogenesis of pemphigus erythematosus. Arch Dermatol Res 258:135–140

Jegasothy BV, Humeniuk JM (1981) Darier's disease: A partially immunodeficient state. J Invest Dermatol 76:129–132

Judd KP, Lever WF (1979) Correlation of antibodies in skin and serum with disease severity in pemphigus. Arch Dermatol 115:428–432

Kazmierowski JA, Wuepper KD (1981) Erythema multiforme: clinical spectrum and immunopathogenesis. Springer Semin Immunopathol 4:45–53

Knight AG, Black MM, Delaney JJ (1976) Eosinophilic spongiosis: Clinical, histological and immunofluorescent correlation. Clin Exp Dermatol 1:141–153

Lawley TJ, Strober W, Yaoita H, Katz SI (1980) Small intestinal biopsies and HLA types in dermatitis herpetiformis patients with granular and linear IgA skin deposits. J Invest Dermatol 74:9–12

Lazarus G (1972) Collaginase and connective tissue metabolism in epidermolysis bullosa. J Invest Dermatol 58:242–249

Lever WF (1965) Pemphigus and pemphigoid. Charles C Thomas, Springfield Ill.

Livden JK, Nilsen R, Thunold S, Schjonsky H (1978) Epidermolysis bullosa acquisita in Crohn's disease. Acta Dermatovener 58:241–244
Lyell A (1979) Toxic epidermal necrolysis (the scalded skin syndrome): A reappraisal. Br J Dermatol 100:69–86
Lyles TW, Knox J, Richardson JB (1958) Atypical features in familial benign chronic pemphigus. Arch Dermatol 78:446–453
MacVicar DN, Graham JH, Burgoon CF (1963) Dermatitis herpetiformis, erythema multiforme and bullous pemphigoid: A comparative histological and histochemical study. J Invest Dermatol 41:289–300
Mann PR, Haye KR (1970) An electron microscope study on acantholytic and dyskeratotic processes in Darier's disease. Br J Dermatol 82:561–566
Marks J, Shuster S, Watson AJ (1966) Small bowel changes in dermatitis herpetiformis. Lancet 11:1280–1282
Marks JG, Thor DE, Lowe RS (1978) Darier's disease: An immunologic study. Arch Dermatol 114:1336–1339
Marsden RA, McKee PH, Bhogal B, Black MM (1980) A study of benign chronic bullous dermatosis of childhood. Clin Exp Dermatol 5:159–172
Medeiros AA, Marty SD, Tosh FE, Chin TD (1966) Erythema nodosum and erythema multiforme as clinical manifestations of histoplasmosis in a community outbreak. N Engl J Med 274:15–21
Melish ME, Glasgow LA (1970) The staphylococcal scalded skin syndrome. Development of an experimental mouse model. N Engl J Med 282:1114–1119
Melish ME, Glasgow LA, Turner MD (1972) Staphylococcal scalded skin syndrome: isolation of partial characterisation of the exfoliative toxin. J Infect Dis 125:129–140
Michel B (1982) Commentary: Hailey and Hailey disease: Familial benign chronic pemphigus. Arch Dermatol 118:781–784
Montes LF, Nankates AJ, Hunt D (1970) Microbial flora in benign chronic pemphigus. Arch Dermatol 101:140–144
Nilsen R, Livden J, Matre R (1981) Ultrastructural and immuno-electron microscopic study in a case of epidermolysis bullosa acquisita. Acta Path Microbiol Scand 89:451–454
Orfanos CE, Schaumburg-Lever G, Lever WF (1974) Dermal and epidermal types of erythema multiforme. Arch Dermatol 109:628–688
Pearson RW (1962) Studies on the pathogenesis of epidermolysis bullosa. J Invest Dermatol 39:551–575
Pearson PW (1971) The mechano bullous diseases. In: Fitzpatrick TB, Eisen AZ, Wolff K, Freedberg IM, Austen KF (eds) Dermatology in General Medicine. McGraw-Hill, New York, p 621–643
Pearson RW, Spargo B (1961) Electron microscopic studies of dermal – epidermal separation in human skin. J Invest Dermatol 36:213–224
Pierard J (1968) Le pemphigus familial benin chronique estil la forme bulleuse de la dyskeratose folliculaire de Darier? Bull Acad R Med Belg 8:693–747
Provost TT, Tomasi TB (1974) Evidence for the activation of complement via the alternate pathway in skin disease. 11. Dermatitis herpetiformis. Clin Immunol Immunopathol 3:178–181
Rand R, Baden HP (1983) Commentary: Darier-White disease. Arch Dermatol 119:81–83
Reitamo S, Reunala T, Konttinen YT, Saksela O, Salo OP (1981) Inflammatory cells, IgA, C_3, fibrin and fibronectin in skin lesions in dermatitis herpetiformis. Br J Dermatol 105:167–177
Riches DJ, Martin BG, Seah PP, Fry L (1973) Ultrastructural observations on uninvolved skin in dermatitis herpetiformis. Br J Dermatol 88:323–330
Russell B, Thorne NA (1957) Herpes gestationis. Br J Dermatol 69:339–357
Sams WM, Gleich GJ (1971) Failure to transfer bullous premphigoid with serum from patients. Proc Soc Exp Biol Med 136:1027–1031
Schaumburg-Lever G, Orfanos CE, Lever WF (1972) Electronmicroscopic study of bullous pemphigoid. Arch Dermatol 106:662–667
Schiltz JR, Michel B (1976) Production of epidermal acantholysis in normal human skin in vitro by the IgG fraction from pemphigus serum. J Invest Dermatol 67:254–260
Schiltz JR, Michel B, Papay R (1978) Pemphigus antibody interaction with human epidermal cells in culture: a proposed mechanism for pemphigus acantholysis. J Clin Invest 62:778
Seah PP, Fry L, Hoffbrand AV, Holborow EJ (1971) Tissue antibodies in dermatitis herpetiformis and adult coeliac disease. Lancet 1:834–836

Simon R, Bloom D, Ackerman AB (1976) Persistent acantholytic dermatosis. A varient of transient acantholytic dermatosis (Grover's disease). Arch Dermatol 112:1429–1431

Singer KH, Hashimoto K, Lazarus GS (1981) Antibody-induced proteinase activation: a proposed mechanism for pemphigus. Springer Semin Immunopathol 4:4–17

Skeete MVH, Black MM (1977) The evaluation of a special liquid fixative for direct immunofluorescence. Clin Exp Dermatol 2:49–56

Stingl G, Honigsmann H, Holubar K, Wolff K (1976) Ultrastructural localisation of immunoglobulins in skin of patients with dermatitis herpetiformis. J Invest Dermatol 67:507–512

Snyder RA, Elias PM (1983) Toxic epidermal necrolysis and staphyloccal scalded skin syndrome. Dermatologic Clinics 1:235–246

Susi FR, Shklar G (1971) Histochemistry and fine structure of oral lesions of mucous membrane pemphigoid. Arch Dermatol 104:244–253

Tolman MM, Moschella SL, Schneiderman RN (1959) Dermatitis herpetiformis: Specific entity or clinical complex? J Invest Dermatol 32:557–561

Van der Meer JB, Remme JJ, Nelkins MJJ (1977) IgA antibasement membrane antibodies in a boy with pemphigoid. Arch Dermatol 113:1462

Waisman M, Stewart JJ, Walker AE (1976) Bullous transient acantholytic dermatosis. Arch Dermatol 112:1440–1441

Weber FP (1926) Recurrent bullous eruption on the feet in a child. Proc Roy Soc Med 19:72

Weinstein WM (1974) Latent coeliac sprue. Gastroenterology 66:489–493

Wintrobe BU, Soter NA, Mihm Mc, Goetzel EJ, Austin KF (1977) Functional and morphological evidence of mast cell involvement in bullous pemphigoid. Clin Res 25:288

Wise F, Lautman MF (1915) Epidermolysis bullosa beginning in adult life: The acquired form of the disease. J Cut Dis 33:441–462

Wojnarowska F, Levene GM, Bhogal B (1982) The distribution of immunoglobulins and C_3 in multiple biopsies from perilesional and clinically uninvolved skin in pemphigus, pemphigoid and its varients. Br J Dermatol 107, Suppl 22:11

Woodley DT, Briggaman RA, O'Keefe EJ, Inman AO, Quenn LL, Gammon WR (1984) Epidermolysis bullosa acquisita autoantibodies bind a unique matrix molecule in human skin basement membrane. J Invest Dermatol 82:396

Wuepper KD, Watson PA, Kazmierowski JA (1980) Immune complexes in erythema multiforme and the Stevens-Johnson syndrome. J Invest Dermatol 74:368–371

Yaoita H, Katz SI (1976) Immunoelectronmicroscopic localisation of IgA in skin of patients with dermatitis herpetiformis. J Invest Dermatol 67:502–506

Yaoita H, Katz SI (1977) Circulating IgA anti-basement membrane zone antibodies in dermatitis herpetiformis. J Invest Dermatol 69:558–560

Yaoita H, Gullino M, Katz SI (1976) Herpes gestationis. Ultrastructure and ultrastructural localisation of in vitro bound complement. J Invest Dermatol 66:386–388

Zone JD, LaSalle BA, Provost TT (1980) Circulating immune complexes of IgA type in dermatitis herpetiformis. J Invest Dermatol 75:152–155

Subject Index

The numbers set in *italics* refer to those pages on which the respective catch-word is discussed in detail

Index of Volumes 69–73 Current Topics in Pathology

Volume 72

Volume 73

www.ingramcontent.com/pod-product-compliance
Lightning Source LLC
Chambersburg PA
CBHW061202240926
51846CB00006B/1091
* 9 7 8 3 6 4 2 6 9 5 7 6 6 *